Clinician's Guide to
SURGICAL CARE

KZ

Notice

Medicine is an ever-changing science. As new research and clinical experience broaden our knowledge, changes in treatment and drug therapy are required. The authors and the publisher of this work have checked with sources believed to be reliable in their efforts to provide information that is complete and generally in accord with the standards accepted at the time of publication. However, in view of the possibility of human error or changes in medical sciences, neither the authors nor the publisher nor any other party who has been involved in the preparation or publication of this work warrants that the information contained herein is in every respect accurate or complete, and they disclaim all responsibility for any errors or omissions or for the results obtained from use of the information contained in this work. Readers are encouraged to confirm the information contained herein with other sources. For example and in particular, readers are advised to check the product information sheet included in the package of each drug they plan to administer to be certain that the information contained in this work is accurate and that changes have not been made in the recommended dose or in the contraindications for administration. This recommendation is of particular importance in connection with new or infrequently used drugs.

Clinician's Guide to
SURGICAL CARE

Editor
John P. Pryor, MD, FACS
Assistant Professor of Surgery
Trauma Program Director
Division of Traumatology and Surgical Critical Care
Department of Surgery
University of Pennsylvania School of Medicine

Associate Editors
Barbara A. Todd, MSN, CRNP, FAANP
Director
Clinical Surgical Specialists & Practitioners
University of Pennsylvania School of Nursing

Michael Dryer, PA-C, DrPH
Director
Physician Assistant Program
Chair
Department of Medical Science and Community Health
Arcadia University

Assistant Editor
Abigail Tripp Berman, AB
University of Pennsylvania School of Medicine

Project Assistant
Lauren Platt, BS
Division of Traumatology and Surgical Critical Care
Department of Surgery
University of Pennsylvania

New York   Chicago   San Francisco Lisbon   London   Madrid   Mexico City   Milan
New Delhi   San Juan   Seoul   Singapore   Sydney   Toronto

The **McGraw·Hill** Companies

Clinician's Guide to Surgical Care

Copyright © 2008 by The McGraw-Hill Companies, Inc. All rights reserved. Printed in the United States of America. Except as permitted under the United States Copyright Act of 1976, no part of this publication may be reproduced or distributed in any form or by any means, or stored in a data base or retrieval system, without the prior written permission of the publisher.

1 2 3 4 5 6 7 8 9 0   DOC DOC   0 9 8

ISBN   978-0-07-147897-7
MHID   0-07-1478973

This book was set in Adobe Garamond by Aptara, Inc.
The editors were Catherine A. Johnson and Karen Edmonson.
The production supervisor was Phil Galea.
Project management was provided by Aptara.
The designer was Mary McKeon.
The cover designer was Mary McKeon.
RR Donnelly was printer and binder.

This book is printed on acid-free paper.

Library of Congress Cataloging-in-Publication Data

Clinician's guide to surgical care / [edited by] John P. Pryor, Barbara A. Todd,
    Michael Dryer.
        p. ; cm.
    Includes index.
    ISBN-13: 978-0-07-147897-7 (pbk.)
    ISBN-10: 0-07-147897-3 (pbk.)
        1. Surgical nursing—Handbooks, manuals, etc.   2. Nurse practitioners—Handbooks, manuals, etc.   3. Physician's assistants—Handbooks, manuals, etc.   I. Pryor, John P. (John Paul), 1966-   II. Todd, Barbara, 1955-   III. Dryer, Michael.
        [DNLM: 1. Perioperative Care.   2. Intraoperative Comlications. WO 178 C641 2008]
    RD99.24.C55 2008
    617'.0231—dc22

                                                                        2008008353

International Edition ISBN: 978-0-07-128724-1
MHID: 0-07-128724-8
Copyright © 2008. Exclusive rights by the McGraw-Hill Companies, Inc., for manufacture and export. The book cannot be re-exported from the country to which it is consigned by McGraw-Hill. The International Edition is not available in North America.

For Carmela, Danielle, Frankie, and John.
I apologize for the "lost" summer of 2007
—J. P.

For all of my surgical colleagues and mentors
during my career
—B. T.

To my family, friends, and faculty, who, make my work meaningful and fun
—M. D.

Contents

Contributing Authors

John N. Awad, MD
Orthopaedic Specialty Group, PC
Fairfield, Connecticut
Orthopaedic Surgery
Bridgeport Hospital, Yale New Haven
Health System
Bridgeport, Connecticut

Susan Baker-Sample, RN, MSN, CRNP
Director of Nursing
Department of Nursing
Lancaster General Hospital
Lancaster, Pennsylvania

Benjamin Braslow, MD
Assistant Professor of Surgery
Division of Traumatology and Surgical
Critical Care
Department of Surgery
University of Pennsylvania School
of Medicine
Philadelphia, Pennsylvania

Jessica Brown, RN, MSN, ACNP-BC, CLNC
Acute Care Nurse Practitioner
Division of Trauma & Surgical
Critical Care
Pitt County Memorial Hospital
Greenville, North Carolina

Jeffrey Cope, MD
Cardiothoracic Surgeon
Department of Surgery
Lancaster General Hospital
Lancaster, Pennsylvania

Bryan A. Cotton, MD
Assistant Professor of Surgery
Department of Surgery/Trauma and Emergency
Surgery
Vanderbilt University Medical Center
Director of Surgical Critical Care
Middle Tennessee Valley VA Medical Center
Nashville, Tennessee

Michael Daly, MSN, MBA, ACNP/APRN-BC
Manager Surgical ICU/Trauma Nurse
Practitioner
Vanderbilt University Medical Center
Nashville, Tennessee

Robert V. Dawe, MD
Clinical Instructor in Orthopedics and
Rehabilitation
Yale University School of Medicine
New Haven, Connecticut
Chief of Orthopaedic Surgery
Bridgeport Hospital, Yale New Haven Health
Bridgeport, Connecticut

Donovan D. Dixon, MD
Generalist
Department of Obstetrics and Gynecology
Womack Army Medical Center
Fort Bragg, North Carolina

Jeffrey A. Drebin, MD, PhD
Professor of Surgery
Chief, Division of Gastrointestinal Surgery
Vice-Chairman, Department of Surgery
University of Pennsylvania School of Medicine
Attending Surgeon
Division of Gastrointestinal Surgery
Hospital of the University of Pennsylvania
Philadelphia, Pennsylvania

Joanna C. Ellis, MSN, CRNP-BC
Adult Acute Care Nurse Practitioner
Division of Traumatology and Surgical
 Critical Care
Department of Surgery
University of Pennsylvania School of Medicine
Trauma Nurse Practitioner
Division of Traumatology and Surgical
 Critical Care
Department of Surgery
Hospital of the University of Pennsylvania
Philadelphia, Pennsylvania

Michael David Fejka III, PA-C
Physician Assistant
Division of Colon and Rectal Surgery
Department of Surgery
Hospital of the University of Pennsylvania
Philadelphia, Pennsylvania

Virgen Milagros Figueroa, RPA-C
Physician Assistant
Division of Obstetrics and Gynecology
New York Methodist Hospital
Brooklyn, New York

Mary Kate FitzPatrick, RN, MSN, CRNP
Clinical Director, Nursing Operations
Department of Nursing
Hospital of the University of Pennsylvania
Philadelphia, Pennsylvania

Adam D. Fox, DPM, DO
Clinical Instructor in Surgery
Division of Traumatology and Surgical
 Critical Care
Department of Surgery
University of Pennsylvania School of Medicine
Philadelphia, Pennsylvania

Jenna Gates, PA-C, MHS
Physician Assistant
Division of Gastrointestinal Surgery
Department of Surgery
University of Pennsylvania School of Medicine
Philadelphia, Pennsylvania

Claudia E. Goettler, MD, FACS
Assistant Professor of Surgery
Division of Trauma & Surgical Critical Care
The Brody School of Medicine
East Carolina University
Staff Surgeon
Division of Trauma and Surgical Critical Care
Pitt County Memorial Hospital
Greenville, North Carolina

Michael D. Grossman, MD, FACS
Assistant Professor of Surgery
University of Pennsylvania School
 of Medicine
Philadelphia, Pennsylvania
Chief
Division of Traumatology and Surgical
 Critical Care
St. Luke's Hospital
Bethlehem, Pennsylvania

Oscar Guillamondegui, MD
Assistant Professor of Surgery
Division Trauma, Surgical Critical Care and
 Emergency Surgery
Vanderbilt University Medical Center
Nashville, Tennessee

Mary E. Haskell, APN, TNS
Acute Care Nurse Practitioner, Ventilator
 Management Team
OSF St Francis Medical Center
Peoria, Illinois

Elliott R. Haut, MD, FACS
Assistant Professor of Surgery and
 Anesthesiology Critical Care Medicine
Division of General and Gastrointestinal
 Surgery, Section of Trauma and
 Critical Care
Department of Surgery
The Johns Hopkins University School
 of Medicine
Baltimore, Maryland

Martha M. Kennedy, PhD, RN, ACNP
Nurse Practitioner
Weinberg Intensive Care Unit
Education Coordinator
ICU Advanced Practice and PA Post-Graduate
 Residency Program
Director, ICU Advanced Practice Residency
 Program
Instructor, Anesthesia and Critical Care
 Medicine
The Johns Hopkins Hospital
Baltimore, Maryland

**Ruth M. Kleinpell, PhD, RN, FAAN,
 FCCM**
Professor
Rush University College of Nursing
Nurse Practitioner
Our Lady of the Resurrection Medical Center
Chicago, Illinois

James S. Krinsley, MD, FCCM, FCCP
Associate Clinical Professor of Medicine
Columbia University College of Physicians and
     Surgeons
New York, New York
Director of Critical Care
Stamford Hospital
Stamford, Connecticut

Teresa Krosnick, PA-C
Physician Assistant
Division of Critical Care Medicine
Department of Perioperative Evaluation
Johns Hopkins Outpatient
Baltimore, Maryland

Joshua M. Levine, MD
Assistant Professor
Department of Neurosurgery
Co-Director Neurocritical Care Program
Department of Neurology, Neurosurgery,
     Anesthesiology and Critical Care
University of Pennsylvania School of Medicine
Philadelphia, Pennsylvania

Najjia N. Mahmoud, MD
Assistant Professor of Surgery
Division of Colon and Rectal Surgery
Department of Surgery
University of Pennsylvania School of Medicine
Philadelphia, Pennsylvania

J. Stephen Marshall MD, FACS
Associate Professor of Clinical Surgery
Department of General Surgery
University of Illinois Chicago College of
     Medicine at Peoria
Medical Director of Bariatric Program
Department of General Surgery
OSF St Francis Medical Center
Peoria, Illinois

Terri R. Martin, MD, FACS
Attending Physician
Division of Trauma and General Surgery
Department of General Surgery
Advocate Lutheran General Hospital
Park Ridge, Illinois

Susan R. McGinley, MSN, CRNP-BC
Trauma Nurse Practitioner
Division of Traumatology & Surgical
     Critical Care
Department of Surgery
Hospital of the University of Pennsylvania
Philadelphia, Pennsylvania

Courtney C. Morton, MPA, PA-C
Physician Assistant
Division of Health Professions
Master of Physician Assistant Program
Eastern Virginia Medical School
Norfolk, Virginia

Heidi B. Nebelkopf Elgart, RN, MSN, CRNP
Trauma Nurse Practitioner
Division of Traumatology and Surgical
     Critical Care
Department of Surgery
Hospital of the University of Pennsylvania
Philadelphia, Pennsylvania

Judy Nunes, PA-C
Adjunct Assistant Professor
Physician Assistant Program
Quinnipiac University
Hamden, Connecticut
Lecturer
Division of Physician Associate Program
Department of Internal Medicine
Yale University School of Medicine
New Haven, Connecticut
Chief Physician Assistant
Department of Neurosurgery
Yale-New Haven Hospital
New Haven, Connecticut

Rita Rienzo, MMSc, PA-C
Manager, Surgery Physician Assistants
Department of Surgery
Yale-New Haven Hospital
New Haven, Connecticut

Michael F. Rotondo, MD, FACS
Professor and Chairman
Chief, Trauma and Surgical Critical Care
Department of Surgery
The Brody School of Medicine
East Carolina University
Chief of Surgery
Director, Center of Excellence for Trauma and
     Surgical Critical Care
Pitt County Memorial Hospital
University Health Systems of Eastern Carolina
Greenville, North Carolina

Babak Sarani, MD
Assistant Professor of Surgery
Division of Traumatology and Surgical
     Critical Care
Department of Surgery
University of Pennsylvania School of Medicine
Philadelphia, Pennsylvania

David W. Scaff, DO
Clinical Assistant Professor of Surgery
Department of Surgery
Penn State University
Hershey Pennsylvania
Trauma Surgeon
Division of Trauma Surgery and Surgical
  Critical Care
Department of Surgery
Lehigh Valley Hospital
Allentown, Pennsylvania

C. William Schwab II, MD
Assistant Professor or Urology
Department of Surgery
Division of Urology
University of Pennsylvania School of Medicine
Pittsburgh, Pennsylvania

Corinna P. Sicoutris, CRNP
Lead Nurse Practitioner
Surgery Critical Care Service
Division of Traumatology and Surgical
  Critical Care
Department of Nursing
Hospital of the University of Pennsylvania
Clinical Associate Professor
Adult Care Nurse Practitioner Program
Department of Nursing
University of Pennsylvania School of Medicine
Philadelphia, Pennsylvania

Ruby A. Skinner, MD, FACS, FCCP
St. Fraucts Medical Center
Division of Trauma and Surgical and
  Critical Care
Los Angeles, California

Laurie L. Strockoz-Scaff, PA-C
Adjunct Faculty
King's College
Wilkes-Barre, Pennsylvania
Physician Assistant
Division of Cardiothoracic Surgery
Department of Surgery
St. Luke's Hospital
Bethlehem, Pennsylvania

**Shannon Sweeney, RN, MSN, ACNP/
APRN-BC**
Nurse Practitioner
Division of Trauma
Department of Surgery
Vanderbilt University Medical Center
Nashville, Tennessee

Kenneth Vives, MD
Associate Professor
Division of Stereotactic and Functional
  Neurosurgery
Department of Neurosurgery
Yale-School of Medicine
Chief of Stereotactic and Functional
  Neurosurgery
Yale-New Haven Hospital
New Haven, Connecticut

**Eileen Maloney-Wilensky, MSN,
  ACNP-BC**
Director, Clinical Research Division and
  Mid Level Provider Program
Department of Neurosurgery
Hospital of the University of
  Pennsylvania
Philadelphia, Pennsylvania

G. Melville Williams, MD
Professor of Surgery
Division of Vascular Surgery
Department of Surgery
John Hopkins University School
  of Medicine
Former Surgeon-in-Charge
Division of Vascular Surgery
Department of Surgery
John Hopkins Hospital
Baltimore, Maryland

**Mary A. Williams, RN, MSN,
  CRNP**
Cardiac Transplant Nurse Practitioner
Division of Cardiovascular Medicine
Department of Surgery
Hospital of the University of
  Pennsylvania
Philadelphia, Pennsylvania

**Denise M. Zappile, RN, MSN,
  CRNP-BC**
Surgical Critical Care Nurse Practitioner
Division of Traumatology and Surgical
  Critical Care
Departments of Surgery and Nursing
Hospital of the University of
  Pennsylvania
Philadelphia, Pennsylvania

Preface

In many ways, *The Clinician's Guide to Surgical Care* represents a new approach to surgical education. First and foremost, it is the first textbook in surgery specifically developed for nonphysician clinicians, both nurse practitioners and physician assistants. Each chapter has been written as a collaborative effort by clinicians and surgeons, guided by an editorial staff of a surgeon, nurse practitioner, and physician assistant. Our goal is to fill the educational gap that exists between the materials available for surgical trainees and surgical nursing, none of which fits the unique educational needs of nonphysician clinicians.

Recognizing that clinicians are on the front line of preoperative, perioperative, and postoperative care, we felt that the guide should provide clear, up-to-date, and useful information on how to solve clinical problems seen in patients with surgical disease. Therefore, throughout the book we emphasize critical thinking and clinical decision making, instead of simply providing information on each disease.

The first section gives an overview of surgical care and logistics of caring for patients before and after surgery. In the second section, the chapters are arranged in a problem-based approach, similar to what is encountered in real life on the wards each day. For each surgical problem, the guide provides information on what to look for in the medical history and physical exam, which laboratory and radiographic studies to consider, and advice on how to develop a diagnostic plan. The final section of each chapter is a discussion of the most common surgical conditions that can cause the problem, along with treatment options. The format mirrors the decision-making process that occurs in the minds of surgeons and clinicians faced with a surgical problem.

To augment the discussion of each chapter, we have provided summaries of over 55 different surgical procedures, supplemented with figures, including 60 original drawings. The goal is to give the clinician a better understanding of the anatomic changes that occur during major operations, along with the physiologic consequences.

The guide is meant to be used to improve critical thinking in surgical disease. It is not meant to be a comprehensive textbook of all general surgery. After the guide is used to make a final diagnosis, the reader is encouraged to refer to a surgical text with a full discussion of the pathophysiology, epidemiology, and detailed management of specific diseases. Although the guide was not specifically written as such, the editors recommend using the very successful *Current Surgical Diagnosis and Treatment* text by McGraw-Hill as a companion reference.

The editorial staff and contributing authors look forward to your comments about the guide in hopes of continuing to improve the contents in subsequent editions. Please feel free to contact us with your comments and suggestions at pryorj@uphs.upenn.edu.

John P. Pryor

Barbara Todd

Michael Dryer

GENERAL SURGICAL CARE

A Team Approach to Surgical Care

Michael Dryer, PA-C, DrPH ■ *Barbara Todd, MSN, CRNP, FAANP* ■ *John P. Pryor, MD, FACS*

Key Points

- Although from different origins and educational backgrounds, the nurse practitioner and physician assistant fields are developing similar practices.

- The increased complexity of surgical care, coupled with the decreased resident work-hour rules and increased pressure for surgeons to be in the operating room have created a surgical workforce vacuum that clinicians are now filling.

- Nurse practitioners and physician assistants have evolved from the role of "assistant" to integral members of the surgical team.

- The team model of surgeons and clinicians provides a framework for the collaborative schemes that the field of medicine will adopt in the next decade.

■ THE SURGICAL CARE TEAM

Surgical care encompasses the initial appreciation of a surgical problem, making a clinical diagnosis, providing operative and perioperative treatment, and caring for long-term complications. Most surgical problems are first identified by a nonsurgeon, such as primary care physicians, nurse practitioners (NPs), or physician assistants (PAs). The surgical consult often involves clinicians, residents, and subspecialists such as radiologists and gastroenterologists. Operative procedures are performed by surgeons in coordination with anesthesiologists, surgical assistants, operating room nurses, and technologists. Finally, perioperative care is provided by clinicians who may include NPs, PAs, intensivists, hospitalists, and surgeons. Thus, it is clear that surgical care is not provided solely by the surgeon, but by a large and varied surgical team.

The delivery of surgical care in the United States is currently undergoing major changes. Although these changes are not unique to surgery, they are amplified in surgical care because it is more often hospital based and has a higher acuity than many other fields of medicine. The increasing complexity of surgical operations, the economic pressures to perform more procedures, and the evolving limitation on resident work hours, have merged to create a need for nonsurgeons, and nonphysician clinicians to take on many of the perioperative care roles once delegated only to surgeons or surgeons in training.

In the role of "gatekeepers," primary care and emergency medicine providers are charged with the responsibility to initially see patients with surgical problems. Likewise, patients who have had a surgical procedure are often quickly released back to the primary care provider for follow-up care. Thus, understanding the process of moving from a surgical problem to a clinical diagnosis is extremely important. Likewise, having a basic understanding of what happens during major procedures will improve the care patients receive in the postoperative period.

The concurrent growth and success of the NP and PA professions has started to positively impact the care of surgical patients in many settings, but most notably in the inpatient, high-acuity environment of academic medical centers. For example, at the hospital of the University of Pennsylvania, the number of nonphysician clinicians that provide care to inpatient surgical patients grew from 12 employees in 1990 to more than 50 in 2007. In many cases, nonphysician clinicians provide all direct patient perioperative care, including admitting, making clinical decisions, performing procedures, first assisting, providing patient and family education, case management, and facilitating discharges—tasks traditionally only carried out by surgeons or house staff.

With this tremendous growth, it is important to delineate resident role, surgeon role, and the non-physician clinician role. The addition of these new clinicians to the surgical team helps to optimize patient outcomes, patient and staff satisfaction, while allowing compliance with the resident work-hour reform.

■ CLINICIANS

NPs and PAs have become a major force in the U.S. health care system. This is particularly true in primary care where together they represent one fourth of the primary care workforce. While the roots of the PA and NP professions are quite different, their development over the past 40 years has followed a

TABLE 1-1.
A Comparison of Clinician Types

Requirement	Nurse Practitioner	Physician Assistant
Philosophy	Nursing and medical model	Medical model
Education	Master's degree	Master's degree
Licensure	Nursing board	Medical board
Certification	National certification is voluntary. Several agencies provide certification. Acute care certification is only provided by the American Nurse's Credentialing Center. Master's degree is required to sit for the examination	National certification required. Certifying agency is National Commission on Certification of Physician Assistants (NCCPA)
Recertification	Every 5 yr with clinical practice and continuing education. Recertification may also be obtained by reexamination, but is not mandatory	Reexamination every 6 yr, and 100 h of continuing education every 2 yr
Scope of practice	Varies with each state, physician collaboration and/or supervision required. In some states, scope of practice is authorized by both the nursing and medical boards	Works under supervision of the physician and board of medicine
Reimbursement	Medicare and Medicaid. Reimbursement from other third-party payers variable	Medicare and Medicaid. Reimbursement from other third-party payers variable

near parallel course (Table 1-1). The one major distinction has been the PA commitment to the medical model and dependent practice which contrasts with NPs who continue to strive for independent practice through the advanced practice of nursing.

The Physician Assistant

The origins of the PA profession date back to 1650, when Peter the Great introduced feldshers into the Russian army. After their military service, many feldshers went on to provide primary care in rural areas across Russia. Physicians often supervised their practice, although many practiced independently as well. Currently, there are more than a million feldshers still practicing in Russia. It is estimated that as many as 30% of the physicians in the former Soviet Union started out as feldshers.

The Chinese barefoot doctors originated in 1965 as a product of Mao's Cultural Revolution. Like the feldshers, they were expected to provide many of the medical services that had previously been the exclusive domain of physicians. Today, the barefoot doctors support China's primary care infrastructure and serve as the point of first contact for Chinese patients seeking medical care.

The concept of an assistant to the physician had developed at Duke University in the late 1950s and early 1960s. The first program was initiated by a nurse Thelma Ingles, who, in conjunction with Dr. Eugene Stead, then Chairman of Medicine at Duke University, developed "an advanced medical education program for nurses." The program trained registered nurses to perform general medical duties that had been in the exclusive domain of physicians. This 1-year program could have been the precursor to the NP movement if not for the opposition of organized nursing. On each of three successive attempts, the National League of Nursing refused to accredit the program, claiming that it was "inappropriate and perhaps dangerous for nurses to assume medical tasks." Dr. Stead abandoned the program for nurses and turned his focus to the training of medical corpsmen who were returning from Vietnam. The first PA class was composed of four Navy corpsmen and was funded in large part by the National Heart Institute. The program began in 1965 and graduated its first class in 1967.

The 1960s was a time of political turmoil and expanded social consciousness. The importance of health and health care was gaining acceptance, as evidenced by the enactment of Medicaid and Medicare. This, combined with an unequal distribution and shortage of physicians, created a fertile environment for the introduction of the PA.

The Nurse Practitioner

The first NPs were formally educated at the University of Colorado in 1965 as pediatric NPs, under the leadership of Dr. Ford and Silver. The premise of the early role was to expand nursing knowledge of the public health nurse in the care of well babies in underserved rural areas. The role of the NP has evolved over the past 40 years in direct response to society's need for primary and specialty care. The graduates of NP programs may function in primary care as well as acute care. The scope of practice for NPs varies from state to state.

NPs are registered nurses who are prepared, through advanced education and clinical training, to provide a wide range of preventive and acute health care services to individuals of all ages. NPs complete graduate-level education preparation that leads to a master's degree. NPs take health histories and provide complete physical examinations; diagnose and treat many common, acute, and chronic problems; interpret laboratory results and X-rays; prescribe and manage medications and other therapies; provide health teaching and supportive counseling with an emphasis on prevention of illness and health maintenance; and refer patients to other health care professionals as needed.

NPs are authorized to practice across the nation and have prescriptive privileges, of varying degrees, in 49 states. The most recent Health Resources and Services Administration Sample Survey report (2004) shows 141,209 NPs in the United States, an increase of more than 27% in comparison to 2000 data. The actual number of NPs in 2007 is estimated to be at least 145,000.

■ REIMBURSEMENT ISSUES

Reimbursement for surgical services provided by a PA or NP is complex and variable. Patient care services provided outside of the operating room are often bundled into the fees paid to the hospital or the primary surgeon. The Medicare formula for reimbursement of PAs and NPs who first assist during surgery is set at 85% of the physician fee schedule. Medicare currently reimburses a physician who first assists at the rate of 16% of the primary surgeon's fee. Therefore, PAs and NPs who first assist are covered at 85% of 16%, or 13.6% of the fee paid to the primary surgeon. It should be noted that Medicare must deem that a first assistant is necessary in order to justify reimbursement. There are approximately 1900 surgically related CPT codes for which Medicare will not pay for a first assistant. While some third-party payers will follow the Medicare formula for reimbursement, others will follow their own methodology.

In general, PAs and NPs are cost-efficient providers of surgical care. This was highlighted in a recent survey by the Medical Group Management Association, which found that in surgical practices, the employer only paid their PA 31 cents for every dollar of charges they generated.

The paradigm of clinicians and surgeons provide a framework for safe, efficient surgical care to be provided. We will need to continue to evaluate this model of care in regards to patient outcomes, patient safety, cost benefits, and patient/staff satisfaction.

2

The Surgical Consultation

Laurie L. Strockoz-Scaff, PA-C ■ *David W. Scaff, DO*

Key Points

- Clinicians will be involved in both performing consults and requesting consults from other surgical services.

- Surgical consultations are appropriate for patients with an identified surgical disease or when expert advice of a surgical specialty is needed to provide ongoing medical care.

- When requesting a consult, a concise reason and a level of urgency are indicated.

- When requested to perform a consult, a prompt response assures that urgent surgical problems will be identified and cared for quickly.

- A full surgical consult includes a thorough review of the medical record and radiographic findings, a patient interview, directed examination, and discussion with the nursing and clinician staff caring for the patient.

- Full communication with the requesting service, patient, and patient's family is paramount.

■ THE SURGICAL CONSULT

The idea of obtaining or completing a surgical consultation can be anxiety-provoking for the service requesting the consult, the clinician providing the consult, and for the patients receiving the consult. In reality, a surgical consult can bring a new perspective to the care for the patient and provide insight into any surgical interventions that may be necessary. Medical physicians, emergency medicine physicians, and nonphysician clinicians request surgical consults as part of their daily practice. Surgical teams receive essentially all of their patient practice from surgical consultation either in the outpatient office, emergency department or hospital. Clinicians that work on a surgical service are in the unique position of having the responsibility to perform consults and request consults from subspecialty services.

■ REQUESTING A SURGICAL CONSULT

For nonsurgical clinicians and physicians, requesting a surgical consult is considered a collaborative process rather than a failure of medical therapy. Patients are informed by the primary service that a surgical consultation is going to be requested. This allows a discussion to occur between the patient and primary service concerning the need for a surgical opinion. During this discussion, patients may voice concern over having to undergo invasive surgery. Their fears should be addressed by explaining that a surgical consult does not always mean "surgery" is necessary and more often than not a surgical consult does not result in a surgical intervention. The consult should be viewed as an educational tool for both the patient and the primary service. The surgical service can discuss invasive and noninvasive treatments, educating patients on all of the options available. This educational experience will allow patients to participate in their own care and empower them to be in control of the situation. This autonomy will help improve the patient's mental well-being. If a patient has had prior operative intervention, and the patient is agreeable, attempt to consult the same surgeon or surgical group to allow for continuity of care.

Surgical consultations are appropriate for patients with an identified surgical disease that cannot be treated by medical intervention alone, such as appendicitis or colon cancer. In these situations, patients may be appropriately transferred to the surgical service if other preexisting conditions are not a factor in the current situation. However, some patients with a complex case benefit from having medical physicians manage nonsurgical issues in collaboration with the surgical team. This is most common in elderly patients with numerous comorbidities.

In other cases, having a surgeon "on board" during a situation that may progress to a surgical intervention may be useful, such as a patient with a bowel obstruction or Crohn's disease. The surgeon will follow the patient's clinical course and offer recommendations on further workup or continued treatment. With daily patient contact, the surgical team will be able to assess a failure of nonoperative treatment and optimize the timing of surgical procedures.

Patients who have a chronic disease may benefit from an early surgical evaluation regarding the risks and benefits of medical versus surgical treatment. For example, advanced coronary artery disease can be treated with stents, angioplasty, or coronary artery bypass grafting (CABG). Certainly, CABG is the most invasive and carries the highest risks. However, electing the less invasive procedure of stenting may preclude operative intervention in the future. Therefore, obtaining a surgical consultation early allows the patient to be properly informed of the possible treatment options.

Patients who have a nonoperative disease, such as metastatic cancer or renal failure, may benefit from a surgical clinicians involvement to assist with minor surgical interventions. This is often in the form of minimally invasive procedures that allow the medical treatment to continue, such as a chemotherapy port placement or a thoracentesis. The surgical team will perform interventions and follow the patient for a period of time after the procedure. If no complications from the procedure occurred and no further intervention is warranted, surgery teams will often "sign off" and be available on an as-needed basis. This practice allows medical therapies to proceed in a focused manner under a single physician. It is the responsibility of the surgeon to inform the medical team that they will not be following the patient on a daily basis in the future.

In requesting a surgical consultation, a clear, concise reason should be stated, such as "management of bowel obstruction" or "evaluation for cancer resection." Also, a sense of the urgency of the consult is necessary to assure that the proper resources are deployed to have the patient seen. If the request is of a routine surgical nature, a consultation may be placed in the usual manner available, such as a computer order entry, or through unit clerks or office staff. If the request is of an urgent nature or the patient's clinical course is complex, having a conversation with the consulted surgical clinician is ideal for all parties. This will allow specific issues to be addressed more efficiently and improve the patient's care.

■ PERFORMING A SURGICAL CONSULT

In performing a surgical consultation, be as complete as possible in every patient encounter. Each encounter should yield knowledge of the patient's past medical history and current clinical course, using data from the medical record, completed diagnostic tests, and interviews with the managing team and patient. The comprehensive surgical consultation may be divided into three phases: data review, patient interview and examination, and recommendations.

Data Review

Review the patient's medical record as the most important source of patient data. This provides an overview of the patient's original presentation and course of events. Since surgical consultations are sometimes obtained after patients have been treated medically for a period of time, it may be necessary to review a large amount of information. This step is important, because often the need for a surgical consultation is the result of complications from other therapies. For example, a patient who suffers an acute myocardial infarction and undergoes CABG, may develop abdominal pain suspicious for ischemic bowel. Thus, understanding the chain of events will influence the subsequent surgical decision making. The chart review will also reveal other consultants participating in the patient's care. These consultants may have important insight to surgical issues and the disease process. Lastly, review all past and current medication regimes.

Take time to review all laboratory data looking for abnormalities suggestive of disease processes. All potential surgical patients should have a workup including a recent complete blood count, complete metabolic panel, protime, and prothrombin time. Often patients will have many previous laboratory studies, and attention is then made to the trends of values, such as the lactate, creatinine or hemoglobin. In some cases, additional studies are suggested by the consulting clinician.

Similarly, take time to review all radiographic studies done up to the point of consultation. Reviewing the actual images, not just the report, will allow the clinician to see subtle changes that correlate to physical findings that may not have been reported by the radiologist. If new studies are warranted, discuss the recommendation with the primary service that will order and coordinate the tests.

Patient Interview and Examination

Patient Interview

Once the data review is complete, the next phase of the surgical consultation commences with the patient interview. Begin with defining the patient's chief complaint (CC) and the history of present illness. The CC is a simple statement in the patient's own words of what brought them to the hospital, or what event initiated a surgical consult. Use the history of present illness to further delineate the CC in regards to onset, duration, location, radiation, exacerbation, and relief of symptoms. Other helpful information, such as recent travel and contact with people who may be sick, is sought.

The patient's past medical history is reviewed directly with the patient when possible. This history may offer some key information about the current problem. Ask specific questions about the medical history to highlight areas of current concern. These areas include cardiovascular, hematologic, endocrine, infectious disease, neurologic, gastrointestinal, renal, and musculoskeletal histories. Open-ended questions, such as "were you ever admitted to the hospital," will help uncover a patient's remote history that they had previously forgotten.

Knowing a patient's past surgical history may help formulate a differential diagnosis for the current problem. Recurrent hernias, intra-abdominal adhesions, and cancer recurrences often result in surgical consultations. Also, if the patient's current medical condition warrants surgery, it is important from a planning standpoint to know in detail what procedures have already been performed. Prior abdominal procedures can cause intra-abdominal adhesions making additional surgery more difficult. Implantable devices pose infectious and electrocautery risks. Knowing of prior difficulties with anesthesia is vital to care concerning upcoming procedures.

Obtaining an allergy history of environmental allergens, foods, and medications is important given the need for perioperative antibiotic therapy and postoperative care. Especially pertinent is any allergy to latex and adhesive tape. Patients with latex allergies require operating room notification well in advance of the surgery time.

All current and recent medications used by the patient are reviewed. This will include all prescribed medicine as well as over-the-counter therapies. Recent steroid therapy may result in delayed wound healing or adrenal insufficiency. Antiplatelet and anticoagulant agents may increase bleeding risks, and chemotherapy regimens can alter the patient's immune system resulting in overwhelming infections. Over-the-counter medications, including vitamins and herbal supplements, can also have varied, deleterious side effects. Patients will often subconsciously exclude them from a medication list because they are not prescribed and thought to be safe.

A patient's social history is reviewed with special attention to support systems, work history, and recent history of drug, alcohol, or tobacco use. Patients with a significant tobacco history are more at risk for pulmonary complications. Patients with chronic alcohol usage may have increased sedative requirements and necessitate withdrawal prophylaxis. Those suffering from drug addiction may have difficulty with anesthesia, future drug dependency and drug-seeking behavior, as well as poor IV access resulting from vascular deterioration.

The patient's family history is reviewed to identify a possible genetic disease process. Having a strong family history of cardiac disease, diabetes, or cancer may impact the preoperative workup, hospital course, or postoperative follow-up. Identifying any possible issues before surgical intervention will result in the best possible outcome for the patient.

Physical Examination

Having successfully reviewed the patient's history, perform a directed physical examination. Although the examination will focus on the condition referred for consultation, a more general examination may be needed if the diagnosis is not clear or if the patient has a systemic disease that can affect several body systems. Begin with a review of the patient's vital signs along with trends and a general observation of the patient. Determine if the patient is comfortable or in pain by observing body position and facial expression. Note the skin color and temperature. Patients who have pale, ashen, and diaphoretic skin are in acute shock and resuscitation is begun as diagnostic maneuvers are started.

Examination of the head and neck should focus on the identification of masses, jaundice, or bruits. Identification of lymphadenopathy in cervical, groin, or axilla regions may signify an infectious or neoplastic disease process. The chest examination includes evaluation of the cardiorespiratory system to include heart, lungs, and peripheral vasculature. The abdomen should be examined for tenderness, distension, and palpable masses. Old surgical scars should be noted and palpated for fascial integrity and clues about previous surgeries. Examine the integumentary system looking for open wounds or lesions resulting from chronic disease processes or poor wound healing. The neurologic system should be evaluated for abnormalities in motor or sensory function that can result from central or peripheral pathology. A rectal examination is always performed to evaluate for masses, sphincter tone, and presence of occult blood. A gynecologic examination is indicated in women with abdominal pain or with abnormal vaginal bleeding.

Recommendations

The final phase of a surgical consult is making recommendations regarding further testing or interventions. For the consultant, using terms such as, "must proceed with" or "the patient needs" are not appropriate for the chart. This language forces the primary service into following this action plan or having to explain in the chart why it is not appropriate at this time. Consider using terms such as "recommend" and "consider." This allows the primary service the ability to consider and plan the appropriate timing based on the patients overall condition.

Recommendations may include further studies required to accurately diagnose a disease process. These may include laboratory work, radiographic studies, or minimally invasive testing, such as percutaneous biopsies. Other nonoperative recommendations can include a period of observation (serial examinations) or additional consultations with other subspecialist.

If the recommendation is a surgery, the patient is prepared for the operation. A surgical consent is obtained after explaining to the patient and their loved ones the reason for intervention, the procedure to be performed, the risks and benefits of the procedure, and potential complications of the procedure (see Chapter 4). Realistic expectations in the postoperative phase are clearly stated so that false hopes are not created. Allow time for the patient and family to raise questions and concerns. In cases where the patient is incapacitated and cannot make an informed consent, the patient's surrogate decision maker or power of attorney is contacted and fully informed.

In preparing a patient for an operative procedure, complete all medical testing for clearance and proceed with the planned intervention. Continue perioperative medications such as beta blockers or therapies such as hemodialysis, in cooperation with the primary team. Order appropriate antibiotic coverage as well as preoperative therapies including special skin cleansers or bowel preparations. In general, patients are kept NPO (nothing by mouth) for 6 hours prior to operative procedures, if the situation allows.

In rare cases, although surgery would be indicated, the clinical situation is such that continued care may be futile or overly heroic. The surgical team may recommend no intervention for a process that ordinarily would require surgery. This is often a difficult, but acceptable management decision in patients who are not expected to survive even with surgery. These decisions are made in conjunction with the patients' loved ones, and primary team. Rarely, the conversation can include the patient.

3

General Care of the Surgical Patient

Barbara Todd, RN, MSN, CRNP ■ *Mary A. Williams, RN, MSN, CRNP*

Key Points

■ A meticulous preoperative preparation is critical to the care of the surgical patient.

■ A preoperative checklist includes orders, medication adjustments, a medical record notation, and notification of the operating room and anesthesiologist.

■ Preoperative anesthetic risk assessment is discussed with the surgeon and anesthesiology team before surgery.

■ The surgical consent must be complete, informed, and executed by a clinician or physician on the surgical team.

■ Postoperative pain is addressed with a combination of narcotics, nonsteroidal medication, and regional analgesia. The patient care analgesia is a very effective way to deliver postoperative analgesia.

■ Prophylaxis for deep vein thrombosis includes early ambulation, mechanical compression devices, and low-dose anticoagulants.

■ Perioperative antibiotics are given 2 hours before skin incision and are administered for 24 hours after surgery.

■ PREOPERATIVE CARE

Preoperative Evaluation

Perform a comprehensive **preoperative evaluation** of patients preparing for surgery. The role of the preoperative evaluation is to document the patient's health history, medical condition, and medical stability to undergo the procedure. It is important to identify factors that may contribute to an increased mortality or morbidity risk for the patient. It also allows for the opportunity to optimize or improve a patient's medical status or stability prior to the procedure.

A preoperative evaluation includes a detailed history and physical examination of the patient. When taking the history, include all past and present medical illness along with the dates of any hospitalization and reasons for the hospitalization. Include a **surgical history** with all types of surgeries, dates, and any history of difficulty with anesthesia, intubation, or extubation. A current list of **medications** is compiled, including herbals or supplements used by the patient. Some herbals and supplements are associated with increased risk of perioperative bleeding.

Assess for aspirin or non-steroidal anti-inflammatory drug (NSAID) use, which may potentiate bleeding. **Aspirin**, which inhibits platelet aggregation, should be stopped 5–7 days prior to surgery. **Warfarin** should be stopped 4 days before surgery to allow for normalization of the international normalized ratio. Patients who are taking warfarin for atrial fibrillation, previous mechanical valve replacement, cardiac abnormality, previous stroke, or other high-risk patients should be considered for admission prior to the date of surgery for conversion to intravenous heparin.

Patients who are actively using or have taken **corticosteroids** for more than 2 weeks during the previous year will require postoperative coverage with parenteral steroids sufficient to cover the stress of surgery. Document all allergies and assess for history of **latex sensitivity**. It is very important to get a **social history** that includes all current or prior alcohol, tobacco, and drug use.

A history of heavy alcohol use identifies potential problems with perioperative bleeding and postoperative delirium tremens. Identify any **religious preference**, which may impact surgery such as the refusal of blood products. Identify if the patient has a **living will** or durable power of attorney for an alternate medical decision maker. If so, obtain a copy and place in the patient's chart. In the **social history**, include the patient's current home living situation that may impact postoperative care or discharge planning. Assess for a **family history** of medical disease, particularly cardiovascular disease, and anesthetic allergies or reactions. A complete **systems review** should be used to identify any new or undiagnosed problems that may impact surgical risk or require interventions and/or treatment prior to surgery.

A head-to-toe **physical examination**, along with a mental status examination and cranial nerve testing should be performed to serve as a baseline in the advent that a postoperative change occurs. It also allows comparisons to be made. Examine the neck and oropharynx to note if the patient may present difficulty

with endotracheal intubation. If so, have a member of the anesthesi-
uate the patient prior to arrival in the operating room.

Order laboratory and diagnostic testing based on the history and physical
examination findings and any procedural-specific protocols. **Routine testing** generally includes a complete blood count with differential, comprehensive chemistry including liver function testing, coagulation studies, chest X-ray, urinalysis,
and urine **pregnancy testing** for females of childbearing age. **Electrocardiograms**
are generally ordered for patients older than 40 years, or for a patient undergoing any type of cardiothoracic procedure. **Pulmonary function tests** are not
routinely ordered unless a patient is undergoing thoracic surgery, has a history
of pulmonary disease, or a history of smoking more than 10 pack years.

A **preoperative plan** for each patient will include any consults or further diagnostic testing needed as identified from the history, review of systems, physical
examination, or previous diagnostic results. If the patient is unstable for surgery
or their medical condition is not optimal, notify the surgeon and a member of
the anesthesia team and consider postponement of an elective procedure.

The Preoperative Checklist

If the patient is medically stable and the plan is to proceed with surgical intervention, complete a **preoperative checklist** ("preop"). A preop includes patient
care orders, notification of the operating room, and a notation in the medical
record. In general, patients are made nothing by mouth ("**NPO**") and given intravenous **fluids** the night before surgery. Consider holding continuous and bolus
total **enteral nutrition** given in the stomach or small bowel, as per hospital policy.
Consider procedure-specific orders such as bowel preparation or preprocedure
skin preparation. Determine the potential **blood product** need and order a type
and cross for blood products as indicated.

Review the active **medication list** and make decisions on which medicines to
continue and which to hold. In general cardiac medications, such as beta blockers
are continued through the perioperative period, whereas anticoagulants such as
aspirin or Plavix may be withheld. Insulin doses may be adjusted during the NPO
period. If the patient is on a heparin drip, it is often stopped 4–6 hours before
surgery. The ultimate decision on what medications to withhold are made jointly
by the surgical and anesthesiology teams. Medications that may be ordered before
surgery include anxiolytics and sleeping aids.

A **preoperative notation** is made to demonstrate that all of the details of
the checklist have been completed. The note includes the proposed procedure,
surgical team involved, and results of pertinent studies and biopsies. The consent
is placed in the chart along with copies of any relevant study results.

Risk Assessment

A major component of the preoperative preparation and evaluation is an
assessment of the patient's perioperative risk. **Surgical risk** is the possibility of
morbidity or mortality associated with the surgical procedure, anesthesia, or the
postoperative recovery. **Risk stratification** is the ability to predict outcomes of

...the patient's severity of illness. A number of risk ...een developed, but risk stratification is based on four ...sk: (1) demographic data of the patient, which includes ...uch as age, gender, and body surface area; (2) urgency of ...ergent and urgent procedures carry more risk than elective ...presence of comorbidities that are unrelated to the surgical ... ...have a significant impact on the patient's ability to recover succe... ...m the procedure; and (4) the presence of cardiac disease.

In det... ...ning anesthesia and surgical risk, the American Society of Anesthesiologists has adopted a physical **classification system** to assist with the prediction of anesthetic morbidity and mortality (Table 3-1). In 2002, The American

---

TABLE 3-1.
American Society of Anesthesiology (ASA) Classification System for Preoperative Risk

ASA Class 1
  No organic, physiologic, biochemical, or psychiatric disturbance
  The pathologic process for which the operation is to be performed is localized
    and does not entail a systemic disturbance
ASA Class 2
  Mild to moderate systemic disease disturbance caused either by the condition to
    be treated surgically or by other pathologic processes
  Well-controlled hypertension
  Status post-CABG without symptoms
  History of asthma
  Anemia
  Cigarette use
  Well-controlled diabetes mellitus
  Mild obesity
  Age <1 yr or >70 yr
  Pregnancy
ASA Class 3
  Severe systemic disturbance or disease from whatever cause, even though it
    may not be possible to define the degree of disability with finality
  Angina
  Poorly controlled hypertension
  Symptomatic respiratory disease (e.g., asthma, COPD)
ASA Class 4
  Indicative of the patient with severe systemic disorders that are already
    life-threatening
  Not always correctable by operation
  Unstable angina
  Congestive heart failure
  Debilitating respiratory disease
  Hepatorenal failure
ASA Class 5
  The morbid patient who has little chance of survival but is submitted to operation
    in desperation
Modifier: Emergency operation (E)

TABLE 3-2.
Clinical Predictors of Increased Perioperative Risk from Myocardial Infarction, Heart Failure, and Death

Major Risk

Unstable coronary syndromes

- Acute or recent myocardial infarction with evidence of ischemic risk by clinical symptoms or noninvasive study
- Unstable or severe angina (Canadian Class III or IV)

Decompensated heart failure

Significant arrhythmias

- High-grade atrioventricular block
- Symptomatic ventricular arrhythmias in the presence of underlying heart disease
- Supraventricular arrhythmias with uncontrolled ventricular rate

Severe valvular disease

Intermediate Risk

Mild angina pectoris (Canadian Class I or II)

Previous myocardial infarction by history of pathologic Q waves

Compensated or prior heart failure

Diabetes mellitus (particularly insulin-dependent)

Renal insufficiency

Minor Risk

Advanced age

Abnormal ECG (left ventricular hypertrophy, left bundle branch block, ST abnormalities)

Rhythm other than sinus (e.g., atrial fibrillation)

Low functional capacity (e.g., inability to climb one flight of stairs with a bag of groceries)

History of stroke

Uncontrolled systemic hypertension

College of Cardiology (ACC) and the American Heart Association (AHA) published updated guidelines for the perioperative cardiovascular evaluation for noncardiac surgery (Table 3-2). These guidelines provide a framework for considering cardiac risk of patient's undergoing noncardiac surgery. The ACC/AHA guidelines outline a format for combining major clinical predictors of cardiovascular risk, surgery-specific risk, and the patient's functional capacity in metabolic equivalent or MET levels (Table 3-3). The guidelines outline in algorithmic form which patients are candidates for cardiac testing prior to their noncardiac surgery. Patients who are unable to meet a 4-MET demand during most of their normal daily activities have increased perioperative cardiac and long-term risks. The last component of the ACC/AHA guidelines is the surgery-specific risk of cardiac surgery that includes two components: the type of surgery and the degree of hemodynamic stress associated with the procedure (Table 3-4).

The ACC/AHA guidelines also incorporate an algorithm of a stepwise approach to preoperative cardiac assessment. The algorithm includes the major clinical predictors, functional capacity, and cardiac risk stratification. It assists the clinician with estimation of risk for the individual patient. The algorithm

TABLE 3-3.
Estimated Energy Requirements for Various Activities

1 MET	Can you take care of yourself?
	Eat, dress, or use the toilet?
	Walk indoors around the house?
	Walk a block or two on level ground at 2–3 mph or 3.2–4.8 kmph?
	Do light work around the house like dusting or washing dishes?
4 METs	Climb a flight of stairs or walk up a hill?
	Walk on level ground at 4 mph or 6.4 kmph?
	Run a short distance?
	Do heavy work around the house like scrubbing floors or lifting or moving furniture?
	Participate in moderate recreational activites like golf, bowling, dancing, tennis, or throwing a baseball or football?
>10 METs	Participate in strenuous sports like swimming, singles tennis, football, basketball, or skiing?

also assists the clinician in determining which patients require further cardiac testing and a cardiology consult prior to proceeding with the surgical procedure.

If patients are considered for elective surgery and have increased risk as outlined by these assessment tools, obtain a **cardiology consult**. Consider functional and anatomic testing that may lead to cardiac stabilization prior to surgery. **Echocardiography** gives information about the structure and gross function of the cardiac chambers and valves. Use echo to determine the ejection fraction and the presence of significant wall motion abnormalities. Consider traditional **cardiac stress** and **thallium stress** tests to determine myocardium as risk for eventual infarct. If indicated, consider performing **coronary angioplasty** to determine if

TABLE 3-4.
Cardiac Risk for Noncardiac Surgical Procedures

High	**(Reported cardiac risk often >5%)**
	Emergent major operations, particularly in the elderly
	Aortic and other major vascular
	Peripheral vascular
	Anticipated prolonged surgical procedures associated with large fluid shifts and/or blood loss
Intermediate	**(Reported cardiac risk generally <5%)**
	Carotid endarterectomy
	Head and neck
	Intraperitoneal and intrathoracic
	Orthopedic
	Prostate
Low	**(Reported cardiac risk generally <1%)**
	Endoscopic procedures
	Superficial procedures
	Cataract
	Breast

angioplasty with stenting or **coronary bypass** is warranted to improve or stabilize coronary perfusion (see Chapter 12).

The Surgical Consent

Before any surgical procedure, a surgical consent must be obtained which fully informs the patient about their illness and the proposed treatment. If a valid consent is not obtained by the health care practitioner responsible for performing the treatment, the team is open to liability and even worse, it could be considered a crime (battery). When obtaining consent, assure that consent is being given by a legally competent person, is given voluntarily, and that it is informed.

The American Medical Association and the American College of Surgeons note that the **informed consent** conducted by the health care practitioner will include the following: the patient's diagnosis, the nature of the proposed operation including estimated risks of mortality and morbidity, the common complications of the procedure as well as the benefits of the proposed treatment, the alternative forms of treatment both operative and nonoperative, and the risks and benefits of not receiving or undergoing the proposed treatment.

The conversation regarding consent is obtained in a private setting and before the patient has received any sedation. The patient is given the opportunity to ask questions and fully understand the proposed procedure so he or she can make an informed choice. If the patient expresses concerns or has unanswered questions, the consent is not signed until all concerns have been addressed. Finally, only licensed professionals, such as clinicians, nurses, or physicians, should obtain and witness the patient's signature.

■ POSTOPERATIVE CARE

Pain Control

Pain is universal after a surgical procedure and it is imperative to provide adequate pain control in the postoperative period. Inadequate pain control is not only distressing for the patient, but can also lead to serious complications, such as pneumonia and depression. Evaluate each patient after surgery and rate his or her pain on a scale of 1 to 10. Trending the subjective pain scale will allow the clinician to judge how well pain relief treatment is working.

For all major surgeries, order a **narcotic** pain medicine to control postoperative pain. Narcotics are most effective when given by the intravenous route, although this can be associated with side effects such as respiratory depression and mental status changes. The **patient-controlled anesthesia** has been shown to be an effective way for patients to deliver medication when needed, leading to better pain control with smaller doses of narcotic. It should be considered standard of care for postoperative patients unless there is a contraindication or if the patient cannot operate the device independently. **Nonsteroidal anti-inflammatory** medications are considered as adjuncts to narcotics, and work best in patients

TABLE 3-5.
Types of Postoperative Analgesia

Analgesic Type	Respiratory Depression	Steady Level	Hypotension	Anti-inflammatory
NSAID	0	+	0	++
Intermittent dose narcotic	++	+	+	0
Patient-controlled analgesia (PCA)	+	++	+	0
Spinal analgesia	0	0	+	0
Epidural analgesia	+	++	++	0

with musculoskeletal injury or involvement in the surgical site. NSAIDs are associated with bleeding complications, and thus, use these agents with care and after consultation with the operating surgeon (Table 3-5).

Most advanced anesthesia techniques such as **spinal anesthesia** and **epidural infusions** are very effective in decreasing pain while sparing many of the side effects seen with parenteral administration of narcotics (Figure 3-1). Continuous epidural infusion often contain a mixture of local anesthetic and a narcotic, but can function with one or the other used alone. **Complications** of epidural catheters include venous dilation with hypotension and cerebrospinal fluid leaks at the site of puncture.

In the later postoperative period, patients are often transitioned to oral pain medication. Although rare, patients can develop a **dependency** to prescription pain medications and clinicians must evaluate ongoing need for narcotic medications carefully in the outpatient setting.

Deep Vein Thrombosis Prophylaxis

On account of the immobility during surgery, associated disease processes such as cancer and the hypercoaguable state induced by tissue injury, surgical patients are at high risk for deep vein thrombosis (DVT). The **risk** of DVT is also increased with obesity, oral contraceptive use, history of thrombosis, congestive heart failure, age greater than 40 years, major hip or knee surgery, fractures, or the patient's undergoing major abdominal, urologic, or gynecologic surgery.

DVT prophylaxis is therefore addressed in all surgical patients. Attention is made to the promotion of early ambulation. If the patient will be on bedrest or unable to ambulate for a period of time postoperatively, order either mechanical or anticoagulant prophylaxis. **Mechanical devices** include thromboembolitic stockings, intermittent pneumatic leg compression, or pneumatic boots. In patients at moderate risk for DVT, consider subcutaneous **heparin** or **enoxaparin** therapy. In high-risk patients, such as patients who undergo hip or knee surgery or superobese patients, consider stronger anticoagulants such as **warfarin** or prophylactic **vena cava filter** placement.

EPIDURAL AND SPINAL ANALGESIA

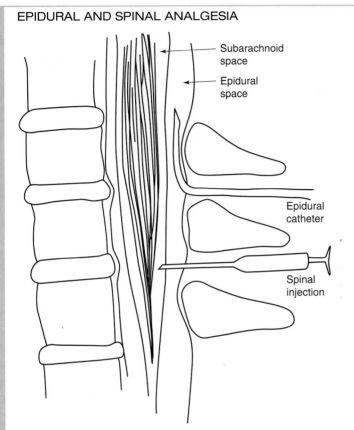

Subarachnoid space

Epidural space

Epidural catheter

Spinal injection

FIGURE 3-1

Placement of Analgesia by Way of an Epidural Catheter and Spinal Injection

Both spinal and epidural analgesia provide a regional analgesic to the peripheral nerves of the spinal cord. Because the analgesic is given locally in the cord, systemic effects of the medications are reduced, although not completely removed. **Spinal analgesia** is often used for short procedures of the pelvis or lower extremities. With the patient in the sitting position, and after skin preparation and local infiltration with lidocaine in the skin, a catheter is introduced through the spinous process of the lumbar vertebrae into the subarachnoid space. The confirmation is made by aspirating cerebrospinal fluid into the syringe. A bolus injection of anesthetic is then injected into the space causing immediate numbness below the level of injection. The catheter is then removed, and the analgesic lasts for several hours.

An **epidural analgesia** catheter is placed when a longer period of analgesia is desired. The patient preparation is similar, but the technique differs in that the catheter is introduced into the space outside the dural sheath, thus the term epidural. A test dose of analgesic is given to make sure that the catheter is in the right location, and then a continuous infusion of analgesic is given. The epidural catheter has the advantage that it can provide pain relief during, and for several days after a major operation. Complications include hypotension from vasodilatation and leakage of cerebrospinous fluid from the site of puncture.

Stress Ulcer Prophylaxis

Stress ulceration is a serious and potentially fatal complication in critically ill postoperative patients. The development of stress ulceration is thought to be multifactorial, including ischemic injury of the gastric mucosa as a result of hypoperfusion, loss of cytoprotectants, and increased gastric acid. Patients who are considered to be at high risk for increased incidence of stress ulceration are those with respiratory failure, prolonged intubation, or those with a coagulopathy, head injury, or burn. Other major risk factors for increased stress ulceration include sepsis, liver failure, hypotension, renal failure, preexisting ulcer disease, and multisystem trauma.

In patients at-risk who can take medications into the stomach, consider **sucralfate** given in divided doses throughout the day. For higher-risk patients, or those with a history of bleeding, consider an intravenous **histamine type 2 blocker** or proton pump inhibitor. Continuous infusion of **proton pump inhibitor** is reserved for patient with active bleeding.

Perioperative Antibiotics

Postoperative wound infections are a major cause of infectious morbidity and mortality in the surgical patient. The goal of prophylactic antibiotics is to reduce the incidence of postoperative wound infections and has become the standard of care in virtually all surgical procedures. Antibiotics should be selected on the basis of the organism most likely to be surgically encountered, avoiding broad-spectrum therapy that may lead to the development of antimicrobial resistance. First- or second-generation **cephalosporins** are generally used as first line agents in most surgical procedures because of their effectiveness against gram-positive cocci. **Vancomycin** is typically reserved for the patient who is penicillin allergic or has a documented history of MRSA.

Some common **guidelines** regarding antibiotic prophylaxis are generally well accepted. The selected antibiotic should be selected based on the most likely contaminating organism, most often skin flora. The initial dose of the antibiotic is administered within 2 hours *prior* to the surgical incision to allow adequate blood levels when the skin incision is made. For prolonged procedures, antibiotics are readministered every 3 hours with the exception of vancomycin and aminoglycosides, which have longer half-lives. Antibiotic coverage should provide an adequate dose based on the patient's body weight or body mass index. Finally, in most procedures, prophylactic antibiotic therapy is not to exceed 24 hours. There is no evidence that continuing antibiotics until all drains or catheters are removed will lower infection rates.

Selected Readings

Hutchison RW. Challenges in acute post-operative pain management. [Review]. *Am J Health Sys Pharm.* 2007;64(6 Suppl 4):S2-S5.

Reynolds TM. National Institute for Health and Clinical Excellence. Clinical Science Reviews Committee of the Association for Clinical Biochemistry. National Institute for Health and Clinical Excellence guidelines on preoperative tests: the use of routine preoperative tests for elective surgery. [Review]. *Ann Clin Biochem.* 2006;43(Pt 1):13-16.

Segal JB, Streiff MB, Hoffman LV, Thornton K, Bass EB. Management of venous thromboembolism: a systematic review for a practice guideline. [Review]. *Ann Int Med.* 2007;146(3):211-222.

Sesler JM. Stress-related mucosal disease in the intensive care unit: an update on prophylaxis. [Review]. *AACN Adv Crit Care.* 2007;18(2):119-126; quiz 127-128.

Snow V, Qaseem A, Barry P, et al. Management of venous thromboembolism: a clinical practice guideline from the American College of Physicians and the American Academy of Family Physicians. *Ann Int Med.* 2007;146(3):204-210.

Terry PB. Informed consent in clinical medicine. [Review]. *Chest.* 2007;131(2): 563-568.

4

Tubes, Drains, and Ostomies

Shannon Sweeney, RN, MSN, ACNP-BC ■ *Bryan A. Cotton, MD*

Key Points

■ Surgical drains are used to drain fluid from a body cavity. Common complications include infection and erosion into surrounding tissues or organs.

■ Drains may be open or closed. Open systems are associated with higher rates of infection.

■ The type of drain or tube placed depends largely on the viscosity of fluid to be drained, length of time the drain should remain in place, and body cavity to be drained.

■ Having a full understanding of the purpose, date of insertion, and internal location of drains will help assure appropriate postoperative management.

■ The clinician should address with the surgeon the time frame for removal of the drains, as well as indications for removal.

■ In order to appropriately manage patients with colostomies and ileostomies, the clinician should understand both the type of colostomy or ileostomy present, the reason for its creation, complications associated with the particular type of diversion, and any plans for revision.

■ AIRWAY

Endotracheal Tube

An endotracheal tube (ETT) is inserted into the trachea to establish a secure airway or to protect the airway in patients at risk for compromise. Endotracheal intubation is indicated in patients who are unable to protect the airway because of altered mental status, drugs, or other pathology, or those with severe chest wall injury or other condition resulting in inadequate ventilation. Intubation is also indicated in patients with inadequate oxygenation not corrected with nasal cannula or face mask, or in patients suffering injury to the face or neck or other mechanical airway obstruction.

Endotracheal tubes include both orotracheal and nasotracheal tubes. In most patients, **orotracheal intubation** is the safest and most effective means of intubation, as well as the preferred route for establishing an airway. Key components to successful intubation include preoxygenation, adequate suctioning, and knowledge of available equipment (see Figure 5-2). Confirmation of placement with **end tidal CO_2** assessment and auscultation must follow every intubation (see Figure 5-3). **Complications** include esophageal intubation, right mainstem intubation, bronchospasm or laryngospasm, laryngeal nerve injury, pneumonia, aspiration, tracheal stenosis, and tracheomalacia. In addition, oral ETT tubes impede oral hygiene and may cause erosion of oral mucosa.

In certain populations, **nasotracheal intubation** (NT) is necessary in patients with contraindications to laryngoscopy such as cervical spine injury, maxillofacial fractures, or oropharyngeal injury or deformity. Since they are passed through the nasopharynx, nasotracheal tubes have smaller lumens. Nasotracheal intubation is a **blind technique**, inserted without direct visualization of the vocal cords. Thus, misplacement into the esophagus is possible. **Epistaxis** is a real and frequent complication of this approach, and thus, coagulopathy should be corrected if possible before attempting NT intubation. Other complications specific to NT tubes include sinus infection, kinks in the tubing, tracheal erosion, and trauma to nasal polyps.

Laryngeal Mask Airways

The laryngeal mask airway (LMA) is a supraglottic device used as a method of airway protection for routine anesthetic procedures and occasionally as a rescue device when endotracheal intubation has failed. It can be placed easily by providers with minimal training. It is a nondefinitive airway, since it sits in the pharynx to obstruct the esophagus and allows air to passively enter trachea (Figure 4-1, H). Since the tube is not passed through the vocal cords, there is less trauma to the tracheal structures. Contraindications include patients who have eaten prior to intubation (risk of aspiration), morbidly obese patients, pregnant patients of more than 14-week gestation, patients with abdominal or other injury that could slow GI motility, patients with high peak airway pressures, and patients with compromised pulmonary compliance.

TUBES USED IN SURGERY

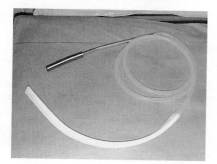

A. Jackson-Pratt (JP) Drain

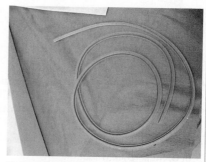

B. Blake Drain

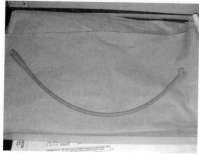

C. Malecot Tube

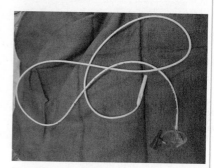

D. Dobhoff Feeding Tube

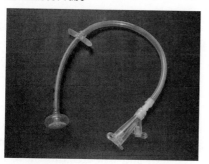

E. PEG Tube

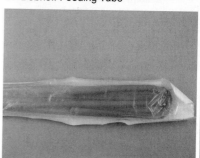

F. 'T' Tube

FIGURE 4-1
Tubes Used in Surgical Care

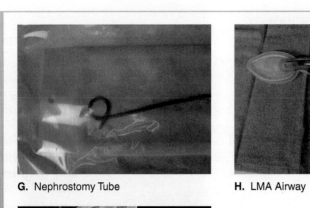

G. Nephrostomy Tube

H. LMA Airway

I. Bivona (top) and Shiley
(bottom) Airways

FIGURE 4-1
(Continued)

Tracheotomy

A tracheotomy is a surgical opening created in the trachea for the purpose of establishing a secure airway. Tubes are characterized by the **lumen size** (4–8 mm), whether they have a balloon at the tip (cuffed) and whether they have holes in the side of the lumen (fenestrated). **Cuffed tubes** are used mostly for patients on a ventilator since it prevents air leaking from around the tracheostomy (Figure 4-1, I). **Fenestrated** tubes allow air to escape around the tube, and pass through the vocal cords allowing limited speech.

Tracheotomy is **indicated** in patients where need for endotracheal tube is anticipated for more than 14 days and in severe maxillofacial or upper airway trauma. When compared with ETT, tracheotomy allows many patients to communicate more easily, is associated with increased patient comfort, decreased work of breathing and airway resistance provides oral hygiene more easily, and allows patients the ability to ambulate and mobilize while maintaining a secure airway. **Contraindications** include bleeding diathesis, deformity of the neck structures that makes tube insertion impossible, tracheomalacia, and known infection in the neck structures. Special care must be given to patients with cervical spine injury as extension is not possible.

Complications of tracheotomy include infection, tracheoesophageal fistula, tube obstruction, tracheoarterial fistula with massive hemorrhage, tracheal stenosis, and prolific granulation tissue leading to hemorrhage or tracheal obstruction. Fenestrated tracheotomy tubes, placed often during weaning, provide a surface favorable to formation of granulation tissue and can lead to significant obstruction and bleeding.

Care of tracheotomy tubes should be meticulous to decrease the risk of infection. **Suctioning** should be performed on an as-needed basis to assist with removal of secretions. Sterile technique must be maintained during deep tracheal suctioning. **Humidification** of air is required as physiologic humidification is lost as a result of bypassing the sinuses. The site should be inspected at least daily for signs of maceration or soft tissue infection. **Cleansing** should be accomplished with sterile saline or 50% strength hydrogen peroxide and sterile saline. A small 2 × 2 drain sponge may be placed against the skin to protect it from maceration and ulceration.

Downsizing of the tracheotomy may be undertaken approximately 7 days after the surgical procedure. Intermittent capping of the tracheotomy with or without a Passy–Muir valve should be undertaken prior to downsizing or decannulation. The **Passy–Muir** device is a one-way valve that allows speech to be possible with the tube in place. Prior to decannulation, patients should be able to demonstrate the ability to clear secretions, and to breathe easily through the upper airway. Upon decannulation, most tracheotomy sites close within a few days.

■ THORACIC

Thoracic cavity drains include both pleural and mediastinal tubes. They play critical roles in the management of thoracic and cardiac surgery patients. These tubes are also utilized in the management of a wide variety of clinical scenarios such as traumatic hemo-pneumothorax, malignant effusions, and empyema.

■ THORACOSTOMY

Thoracostomy (chest) tubes are inserted into the **pleural space** to evacuate fluid or air from the space. The drains are 28–42 French tubes with radiopaque markers and multiple holes at the distal end. Indications include symptomatic pneumothorax (tension, spontaneous, iatrogenic), large pneumothorax over 15%–20%, hemothorax, recurrent effusion, malignant effusion, chylothorax, parapneumonic effusion or empyema, penetrating chest trauma, bronchopleural fistula (Figure 4-2). The most important relative contraindication to thoracostomy tube insertion is known coagulopathy, which should be corrected, where possible, prior to insertion.

THORACOSTOMY

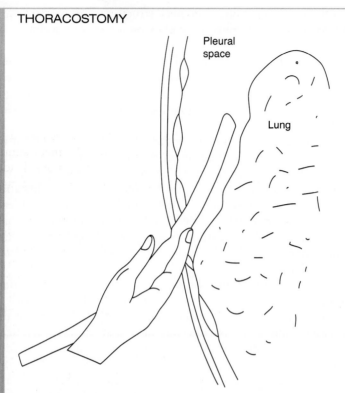

Pleural space

Lung

FIGURE 4-2
Proper Placement of a Thoracostomy Tube into the Pleural Space

A sterile environment must be maintained at all times. Insertion is at the third to fifth intercostal space, midaxillary line. A large-bore tube is used for trauma (36 French or greater) since smaller tubes may not efficiently drain blood or viscous fluid. Prep with antiseptic solution and draping in sterile fashion, the incision site is identified and 1% lidocaine with epinephrine is injected. A skin incision is made large enough to admit the provider's finger and tube together. Sharp dissection is continued to the chest wall. The intracostal area is perforated with a heavy clamp and the muscle is spread to enlarge a hole between the ribs. Before insertion of the tube, the pleura is explored digitally. The tube should be directed toward the apex and posteriorly so that the last hole is approximately 3 cm into the pleural cavity. The tube is then connected to the appropriate drainage system. Large braided suture is used to secure the tube. Petrolatum gauze is sometimes placed around the tube at the insertion site for purpose of occlusion and the tube secured with silk/adhesive tape.

Recent guidelines suggest preprocedure antibiotic administration is associated with decreased risk of empyema. To maximize the benefit of antibiotics, the first dose is administered prior to insertion whenever possible. In instances where the antibiotic cannot be administered prior to insertion, administration is initiated as soon as possible. Although some authors suggest continuation of antibiotics for a 24-hour period, there is no benefit of extending their duration beyond this.

Perform a Postinsertion chest radiograph to assess tube placement. Daily chest radiographs are not indicated but reserved for any respiratory or cardiac decompensation that may be related to tube function.

Complications include local insertion-site infection, empyema, pulmonary artery laceration, and tube dislodgement. Misplacement of the tube into the abdominal cavity can cause diaphragmatic injury and laceration of the intra-abdominal organs. Rarely, a cardiac injury can also occur.

Mediastinal

Mediastinal tubes include both large bore and smaller bore tubes placed after cardiac or thoracic surgery to drain blood and fluid from the mediastinum and pericardium. In most cases after **cardiac surgery**, the pleura are divided so that the mediastinum communicates with one or both of the pleural spaces.

Understanding the three-chamber **collection system** is important for troubleshooting problems with both thoracostomy and mediastinal tubes. The first chamber collects fluid, but allows air to escape along the top of the chamber to chamber two. The second chamber is the water seal. Here air must flow through a water column, essentially making it impossible for air from outside to reflux back into the pleural space. The third chamber is another column of water that determines how much suction is applied to the system. The amount of suction transmitted to the plural space is related to the height of the water column, typically 20 cm.

The drainage system should be inspected frequently to assess for any air leaks, quality and consistency of output, amount of drainage, and assessment of criteria for discontinuation of the tube. New air leak should prompt detailed inspection of the tube and drainage system. If no mechanical reason for the leak can be found, chest X-ray may be warranted to assess tube position and any new anatomic abnormality. In general tubes are **pulled** when there is resolution of the pathology prompting the tube, no evidence of air leak, and less than 100 cc of drainage for a 24-hour period (Figure 4-3).

■ GASTROINTESTINAL

Nasogastric

Nasogastric (NG) and orogastric tubes (OG) are inserted through the nose or mouth, respectively, and guided into the stomach (see Figure 13-1). Gastric decompression is often indicated after gastrointestinal surgery or in patients with a physiologic or anatomic obstruction of the bowel. Also, these tubes are often used as a conduit to provide enteral nutrition. Thus, the **indications** include need for gastric lavage, decompression, obstruction or partial obstruction, ileus, and administration of enteral nutrition.

The **NG** route is preferred since it is the most comfortable for the awake and alert patient. It is contraindicated in known cranio-facial fractures or nasal or pharyngeal obstruction. **OG** tubes are poorly tolerated in those who are not

THORACOSTOMY TUBE REMOVAL

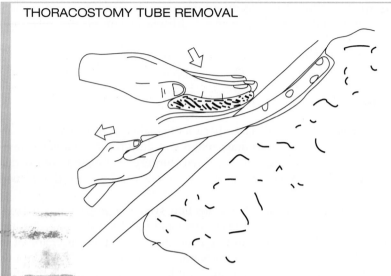

FIGURE 4-3
Proper Hand Positioning During Removal of a Thoracostomy Tube

Obtain a chest X-ray when placing the patient on water seal from suction. The tube should remain on water seal for 6–8 hours prior to removal to allow for detection of any occult pneumothorax. Administer analgesics and/or anxiolytics before removal. After sedation is given and the sutures are removed, the chest tube is removed quickly with the patient at maximal deep inspiration and Valsalva. Remove the tube with one hand as the other hand covers the hole with an occlusive dressing. Dress the site with 4″ × 4″ gauze (with or without Vaseline gauze) and silk/adhesive tape. A complete pulmonary examination including auscultation of all lung fields (anterior and posterior), percussion and phonation, and assessing the work of breathing is performed. After removal, routine upright chest radiograph is mandatory.

adequately sedated and/or intubated secondary to protective gag reflexes. Oral tubes have less risk of local tissue trauma than NG tubes.

Complications of both approaches include gastric or esophageal perforation, reflux secondary to compromise of the lower esophageal sphincter, pressure ulcers of oral or nasal skin, aspiration of gastric contents, dislodgement, and erosion of the esophagus. With NG tubes, sinusitis, epistasis, and trauma to nasal polyps may also occur.

Management of both types of tubes includes flushing every 4–6 hours with at least 30 mL water, and after feeding or medication administration, to maintain patency. Tubes should be placed on **intermittent low-wall suction** to avoid trauma to gastric mucosa. These tubes should be **securely fastened**, as dislodgement is frequent. In both tubes, **tube position** should be changed every 2 hours to avoid pressure ulcer formation.

Nasojejunal

Nasoenteric tubes, also known as Dobhoff tubes, are specially designed to be inserted past the stomach into the proximal small bowel (Figure 4-4). They are primarily placed for the purpose of enteral nutrition; however, small bowel decompression may also be accomplished with nasojejunal (NJ) tubes (Figure 4-1, D). Postpyloric tubes are associated with less risk of aspiration and lower gastric residual volumes than NG/OG tubes. Often, these tubes are of smaller bore and can be more susceptible to obstruction.

Maintenance of NJ tubes includes flushing the tube with 30 mL water after medication, and every 4–6 hours as with NG/OG tubes. Complications are similar to those associated with NG/OG tubes. Since the stomach is bypassed, feeding must be accomplished through continuous method rather than by boluses, as with gastric feeding. Feeding intolerance and diarrhea are common with nasoenteric tubes.

Gastrostomy

The stomach may be accessed directly by surgically placed catheters that exit the abdominal wall usually in the left upper quadrant. They are **indicated** for the long-term administration both of medications and enteral nutrition, and occasionally for gastric decompression. They are utilized in patients with various conditions causing dysphagia, anorexia, persistent weight loss with cancer or other pathology, altered mental status and vegetative state necessitating medication, and nutrition administration for more than 4 weeks. **Contraindications** include coagulopathy, which should be corrected prior to surgery.

The most common serious complication of these tubes is **dislodgement**, which requires immediate attention. Other **complications** include ulceration of the gastric mucosa, peritonitis, necrotizing fasciitis, colocutaneous fistula, local infection, and hemorrhage.

Gastrostomy tubes can be placed endoscopically or by open method. Endoscopic placement is associated with decreased cost and decreased recovery time. **Percutaneous endoscopic gastrostomy** (PEG) involves utilization of endoscopy to visualize a needle punctured through the abdominal wall by an assistant (Figure 4-1, E). A wire mechanism is then used to pull a catheter through the patient's mouth, into the stomach and than out the abdominal wall. Because the peritoneal cavity is never visualized, the complications include damage to organs such as the colon or liver. The procedure can be done at the bedside.

Open techniques include the **Stamm gastrostomy**, the most common type of open gastrostomy. The Stamm procedure may be accomplished with a small left upper quadrant or upper midline incision. A tube is placed into a gastrostomy and brought out through a separate incision in the anterior abdominal wall. Various types of tubes can be used, such as a Foley catheter, Malecot (Figure 4-1, C), or red rubber catheter.

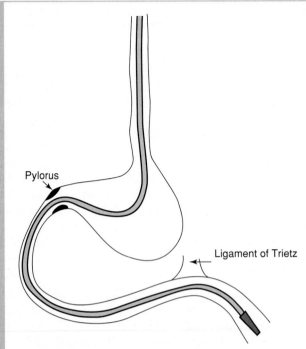

FIGURE 4-4
Proper Placement of a Nasoenteric Tube

Assure the head of the bed is elevated prior to insertion and the patient positioned with neck in flexion. As with NG insertion, encouraging the patient to swallow will assist with guiding the NJ tube through the esophagus. To stimulate gastrointestinal motility, administer metoclopramide 10 minutes prior to the procedure. The NG aspirate may be obtained prior to the procedure, if desired, and the pH measured prior to NJ tube insertion. The stylet hub is then inserted into the NJ tube port (medication port should be capped). Flush the device with at least 10 mL of water to inspect for any break or lack of patency. Some tubes have hydrophilic coatings activated by this action. Pass the tube through the nostril into the nasopharynx and then the esophagus. Flexion of the patient's neck and having the patient swallow will facilitate passage of the tube into the esophagus.

At approximately 60 cm, attempt aspiration, and if fluid is obtained, check the pH to ensure gastric placement (gastric fluid may appear bilious and have a pH of 1–7 depending on any antacid therapy). The tube is advanced gently toward the pylorus at around 70 cm. Slow injection of 60 mL air as the tube advances will assist with pylorus opening. At 100 cm, attempt to aspirate contents again, looking for a pH >7 indicating entry into the duodenum. If the tube is felt to be in place, the stylet is removed, and the tube is then fastened carefully. A KUB should be obtained postprocedure to verify placement prior to medication administration, or initiation of enteral feeding.

Verify output, drain location, patient, surgeon plan for drain removal, and type of drain. In closed drains, suction must be released prior to discontinuation. Remember to remove any anchoring device or sutures present. Grasp the tube as close to the skin as possible, and with the other hand, place two fingers on either side of the tube with firm pressure. Gently and continuously pull on the drain to remove. If resistance is encountered, stop, anchor the drain, and contact the surgeon. Place a dry dressing over the insertion site.

Removal or replacement of a gastrostomy tube can usually be accomplished at the bedside or in the outpatient setting. Care must be taken to assure that the tube is not removed prior to establishment of a mature tract, which typically can be assured after 4–6 weeks. PEG tubes and most rubber tubes can be simply pulled out, with variable amounts of resistance. If a Foley balloon catheter is in place, the balloon must first be deflated. Gastrostomy sites typically heal in 1–7 days, and usually do not require surgical closure. Tubes that are pulled inadvertently before 4 weeks should prompt involvement of the surgeon immediately. Options include attempting replacement, imaging with computed tomography, or operative intervention.

Gastrostomy–jejunostomy

A gastrostomy–jejunostomy (G–J) tube is a small lumen catheter placed through an existing gastrostomy tube (usually a PEG) into the proximal jejunum. Similar to Dobhoff tubes placed, they offer benefits in patients who cannot tolerate enteral feeding in the stomach. The G–J tube has two lumens, one allowing for jejunal feeding and a second for gastric decompression. Placement of a jejunostomy tube through a gastrostomy has been shown to be associated with fewer enteral leaks than jejunostomy tube alone. It is important to confirm the ports with the operative team so that the correct ports are used for each purpose.

Biliary

T-tubes are named for the "T" shaped end of the tubes that are specifically designed to be placed into a lumen for decompression and access (Figure 4-1, F). T-tubes are usually placed into the **common bile duct** beside or though the cystic duct after biliary surgery, hepatic surgery, or liver transplant to facilitate gravity drainage of bile into a collection bag. T-tubes may also be used to facilitate interventional procedures and for cholangiography. Typical drainage may be 300–500 mL output during the initial 24 hours. This may decrease to 200 mL/24 h within 4 days.

Skin surrounding the tube should be kept clean and dry to prevent maceration and infection. Patient education regarding this risk should be provided as patients often care for the tubes at home.

Nasobiliary

These are uncommonly used tubes in patients who require relatively noninvasive way to decompress the biliary tree. These tubes are inserted endoscopically, and offer an alternative to biliary stenting. Benefits include the fact that they usually can be removed easily and allow interval tube cholangiogram. Gentle traction applied to the tube can enable removal in most patients.

Cholecystostomy

Cholecystostomy tubes are inserted to decompress the gallbladder, most often because of an obstructed cystic duct. The tube can be placed during open surgery or as a percutaneous technique. **Percutaneous cholecystostomy** is a reasonable choice for management of acute cholecystitis in patients who could not tolerate cholecystectomy (see Chapter 10). Interval cholecystectomy may be undertaken after acute inflammation has resolved. Approximately 40% of cultured fluid from cholecystostomy tubes is positive for bacteria (usually gram negative). Cholecystostomy tubes should not be removed prior to establishment of a mature tract. This occurs in most patients after a 10-day period has elapsed.

Rectal Tubes

Management of rectal effluent is possible using soft, large bore tubes placed in the rectum, often by the patient's bedside nurse. They may be indicated in patients with open perineal or sacral wounds, severe diarrhea, or where contamination and maceration is deemed to be placing the patient at high risk for infection or other morbidity.

Although used frequently, the clinician should assure that such a tube is truly necessary, since there are significant potential complications to long-term use. Many rectal tubes have a balloon or Malecot tip, which can lead to pressure erosion of the rectum because of lack of repositioning and constant pressure on the tissues. Therefore, these tubes should be for the shortest period of time possible to prevent necrosis and subsequent infection.

■ CLOSED SUCTION DRAINS

Closed suction drains are drains that communicate with the area being drained, but remain closed to other cavities or the external environment. They are used to drain pus, blood, or other fluid within a body cavity. As with all drains, it is imperative to define the location and purpose for each surgical drain after surgery. Daily, drains should be assessed for air leaks and/or obstructions. The amount and character is recorded as an ancillary vital sign. Some drains are flushed on a routine basis, and others are not; therefore, it is important to clarify the plan on each tube. Drains are pulled when drainage is minimal and there is no need to sample fluid.

Jackson-Pratt

These are silicone drains with a flat smooth functional end fitted with many holes, connected to a long round tubing that ends in a suction bulb (Figure 4-1, A). These are one of the most popular postoperative drains, used for a wide variety of indications. They have a **radiopaque marker** that makes them visible on radiographs, which can help in determining location of placement.

Blake

Blake drains are fluted drains with multiple channels to facilitate drainage from a body cavity (Figure 4-1, B). The channels provide increased surface area for evacuation of fluid, and allow injection and irrigation of fluid in one port while draining a second port. Blake drains are also more comfortable for the patient and may also be used in the mediastinum and pleural spaces.

HemoVac

Often used in orthopedic procedures, HemoVac drains offer covalently bonded hydrogel that allows blood and debris to be evacuated with less incidence of tube obstruction. They are composed of a soft, round tubing that is collapse-resistant attached to a saucer type collection chamber. These drains can be used in a wide variety of settings including neurosurgery, orthopedics, urology, gynecology, and general surgery settings.

Percutaneous

Interventional radiologist (IR) can insert a variety of drainage catheters into various body cavities guided by computed tomography, fluoroscopy, or ultrasound. An "IR" catheter is usually connected to a closed suction container. The procedure is relatively safe except in the setting of a coagulopathy. The most common complication of abscess drainage catheters is catheter dislodgement. It is thus important to assure the catheter is secured to the skin and adequate patient and nursing education is provided.

Radiographs may be helpful in determining **catheter location**. Many of these catheters are relatively small bore and, depending on location, may need to be flushed with 5–10 mL sterile saline daily to maintain patency. With clinical improvement, repeat CT scan may be performed prior to removal. In some instances, contrast injection may be indicated to look for any fistulae.

Negative Pressure Devices

The use of negative pressure therapy is a newer technology that allows both wound coverage and drainage in one device. These devices create negative pressure that maintains a moist wound environment while draining fluid and exudates from the wound bed. In addition, it provides debridement with sponge changes and encourages wound approximation by contraction.

In uninfected wounds, **dressing changes** may be done every 48 hours. Indications include surgical wounds, acute and chronic wounds, traumatic wounds, partial thickness burns, dehisced wounds, diabetic wounds, pressure ulcers, flaps, and grafts. **Contraindications** include wound malignancy, untreated osteomyelitis, unexplored fistula, wound with necrotic tissue and eschar, and placement over exposed blood vessels or organs.

■ OPEN DRAINS

Penrose

These traditional drains are made of soft latex rubber that is open at both ends. They work by passive drainage and are enhanced both by gravity drainage and by capillary action, "wicking" fluid from a given cavity. Penrose drains are indicated to drain purulent fluid, blood, serum, and other fluids. They function best when positioned dependently. The risk of infection with an open drain is higher than that with a closed drain, and thus they are only used for infected collections. The drain is secured on the skin, and collection bag or gauze is placed over the external opening to avoid skin irritation. Open drains are usually removed incrementally with clinical improvement ("cracking").

■ OSTOMIES

Enterostomy

An enterostomy is a surgical opening of a portion of the bowel to the skin surface. Enterostomies may be temporary or permanent. **Permanent ostomies** are typically created in the setting of cancer or severe inflammatory bowel disease whereas **temporary enterostomies** are often created emergently in the setting of obstruction, trauma, infection, or perforation. Enterostomies can be an **end ostomy** where the bowel is divided and the distal end brought out, or a **loop ostomy** where the bowel continues on past the site where it is brought through the wall. Complications include ischemia, retraction of the stoma, stenosis, prolapse, and peristomal hernia. New enterostomies should be inspected for ischemia and/or retraction in the first few postoperative days.

Esophagostomy

In rare cases it is necessary to bring the proximal esophagus to the skin surface to divert saliva away from the thoracic esophagus (**spit fistula**). In cases of emergent esophageal resection, such as esophageal perforation or cancer, the diversion may be permanent. In other cases, a temporary spit fistula may be created to divert saliva from a tenuous esophageal repair or anastomosis. The ostomy is usually placed along the anterior border of the left sternocleidomastoid muscle in the neck.

Colostomy

END COLOSTOMY is constructed after resection of a segment of colon that can not be reanastomosed for some reason. Leading causes for this are gross peritoneal contamination after a perforation, such as diverticulitis (see Chapter 10) or as part of a cancer resection (see Chapter 14). The distal part of the colon can be left in place, stapled off (Hartman's procedure; Figure 14-1) or exteriorized as a **mucous fistula**. The location of the ostomy depends on the segment of colon that was removed.

LOOP COLOSTOMY is a temporary colostomy created to divert the fecal stream from reaching the distal bowel. The loop allows communication of both the proximal and distal bowel with the skin surface, decompressing both proximally and distally. It also allows both for diversion of fecal material and for instrumentation and preparation of the distal colon. The most common reason to create a loop colostomy is to divert the fecal stream from a distal obstruction that can not be resected (unresectable cancer) or from an injury that needs to heal (rectal gunshot wound).

Ileostomy

An ileostomy involves a segment of small bowel that is brought through the abdominal wall. The location along the bowel is variable, and proximal ileostomies will have different physiologic consequences than distal ones. An ileostomy is indicated in primary diseases, such as inflammatory bowel disease after colectomy, or as a diversion to protect a distal anastomosis. Since the average daily output from ileostomies is approximately 500–800 mL, the most significant morbidity of an ileostomy is **dehydration**. Patients often need additional intravenous hydration and electrolyte repletion. Additionally, attention must be provided to peristomal skin to ensure proper care. Continent ileostomies are created at times with an internal reservoir, but the procedure is associated with higher complications and obstruction.

■ URINARY DIVERSION

Ileal Conduit

An ileal conduit is a means of urinary diversion through transplantation of the ureters into an isolated segment of the ileum that is closed on one end. The other end is connected to an opening in the abdominal wall. Thus, the external appearance is exactly the same as an ileostomy.

Urine is collected in an ostomy bag, making it convenient for patients because of ease of stoma care. Ileal conduit is contraindicated in patients with short bowel syndrome and inflammatory bowel syndrome. Complications include infection, bowel obstruction, stoma stenosis, and extravasation of urine. Bacteruria is present in 75% of specimens, and typically does not require treatment, but patients should be thus appropriately educated regarding signs and symptoms of infection.

Nephrostomy

Another form of urinary diversion is the nephrostomy tube, which is indicated for temporary urinary diversion after obstruction, most often a result of renal calculi. These are percutaneous tubes often placed by CT guidance, into the renal pelvis to drain urine (Figure 4-1, G). Nephrostomy tubes also offer access for instillation of antimicrobial agents, chemotherapy in malignancy, and for agents to dissolve calculi in cases of obstruction. Complications include hemorrhage, pain, intra-abdominal organ damage, extravasation of urine, inability to retrieve the tube, sepsis, and catheter dislodgement.

Catheters should be firmly anchored to prevent dislodgement. If dislodgement occurs, the fistula often will rapidly close, and thus patient and nursing education must be thorough regarding need for two point anchors. As the renal pelvis only has a capacity of 5–8 mL, it is imperative that any obstruction of the nephrostomy tube be addressed immediately. Again, appropriate patent and nursing education is a priority.

Patients should be instructed to maintain hydration of 2–3 L/d to prevent infection, and should be educated regarding signs and symptoms of pyelonephritis.

Selected Readings

Adrales G, Huynh T, Broering B, et al. A thoracostomy tube guideline improves management efficiency in trauma patients. *J Trauma.* 2002;52(2):210–214.

Blackbourne, L. *Advanced Surgical Recall*, 3rd ed. Baltimore, MD: Lippincott Williams & Wilkins, 2007.

Cline D, Ma J, Tintinalli J, Kelen G, Stapczynski S (eds). *Emergency Medicine.* 5th ed. New York: McGraw-Hill, 2000.

Klingensmith ME, Amos K, Green D, Halpin V, Hunt S, Eberlein T (eds). *The Washington Manual of Surgery.* 4th ed. Philadelphia: Lippincott Williams & Wilkins, 2005.

Laws D, Neville E, Duffy J. Pleural Disease Group, Standards of Care Committee, British Thoracic Society. BTS guidelines for the insertion of a chest drain. *Thorax* 2003;58(Suppl 2): ii53–ii59.

Luchette FA, Barie PS, Oswanski MF, et al. Practice management guidelines for prophylactic antibiotic use in tube thoracostomy for traumatic hemo-pneumothorax: EAST Practice Management Guidelines Work Group. http://www.east.org/tpg/chesttube.pdf. Accessed February 6, 2008.

Reynolds SF, Heffner J. Airway management of the critically ill patient: rapid sequence intubation. *Chest* 2005;127:1397–1412.

5

Respiratory Compromise

Martha M. Kennedy, PhD, RN, CCRN, ACNP ■ *Elliott R. Haut, MD, FACS*

Key Points

- Assess each patient with respiratory compromise with attention to the priorities of airway, breathing, and circulation.
- Urgent treatment must often be instituted, even before the definitive diagnosis is made.
- Oxygen therapy is the first-line treatment in all cases of respiratory deterioration. Endotracheal intubation can stabilize almost any respiratory emergency.
- Pulse oximetry is a simple, rapid, portable, bedside test that should be performed early in the evaluation of respiratory distress. However, pulse oxymetry does not reveal any information about adequacy of ventilation or acid base balance.
- Atelectasis is the most common cause of respiratory compromise in surgical patients, most often caused by poor pain control and recumbent positioning.
- The diagnosis of pneumothorax, hemothorax, and symptomatic pleural effusions can be made by physical examination and chest x-ray (CXR). Both will respond to intervention with tube thoracostomy.
- Pulmonary embolism is considered in the differential diagnosis of every surgical patient in respiratory distress. In patients with a high suspicion and in whom diagnosis is delayed, presumptive anticoagulation is started immediately.

■ HISTORY

Investigate the history of the **recent events** that may be related to the presentation of respiratory compromise. Determine the type of recent surgery, recent trauma, or infectious exposure, especially in immunocompromised patients.

Review the **medical record** for changes in medication therapy, especially with cardiac or pulmonary medications as well as any changes in activity level that could be accompanied by changes in thromboembolism risk.

Interrogate the **rapidity of symptoms** as the first clue to the source of respiratory compromise. Sudden onset of symptoms may indicate acute obstruction of air or blood to the lungs, such as acute bronchoconstriction, pulmonary embolism, or acute pneumothorax. Symptoms that develop slowly are seen in chronic airway inflammation processes such as chronic bronchitis or heart failure. Long-term malnutrition, muscle wasting, or muscular disorders such as muscular dystrophy may progress from chronic compromise to acute respiratory failure. In addition, the causative agent in cases of pneumonia may be differentiated by time to onset. Bacterial pneumonia often has a more abrupt onset with fever and chills. Viral pneumonia may come on more slowly and have a prodrome including upper respiratory symptoms, malaise, headache, and cough.

It is important to identify pertinent past or current surgical and **medical conditions** and recognize their role in pulmonary function. Consider both the disease itself and the effect of treatments when working up the differential diagnosis. Cancer patients may have respiratory compromise related to chemotherapy or radiation therapy such as cardiomyopathy, pulmonary fibrosis, pleural effusion, or capillary leak. Long-term asthma patients may have tracheal stenosis from multiple intubations.

Determine if the patient has had similar **pulmonary problems** in the past, and assess the cause. Patients with asthma, chronic obstructive pulmonary disease (COPD), cancer and/or heart failure may have baseline symptoms under control but exacerbations of the disease may lead to acute shortness of breath and respiratory failure. Consider that the patient may have a delayed complication from an earlier procedure or trauma, such as airway edema after intubation. Always consider anaphylaxis in patients receiving new medications or contrast dye.

Obtain names of physicians and/or medical institutions that have provided care to this patient, especially pulmonologists and cardiologists. Obtain names of medications used routinely and/or emergently for relief of shortness of breath.

Elicit a **family history** of cardiac or lung disease that may give clues as to why the patient is now acutely compromised.

■ PHYSICAL EXAMINATION

The examination begins with assessment of the airway, breathing, and circulation. Rapidly assess **airway patency** by asking the patient to speak a full sentence; those who can most likely have a secure airway. Inspect the mouth and neck for obstructions or swellings. If the airway patency is in doubt, have a low threshold to secure the airway with endotracheal intubation. Patients who are already intubated must have the endotracheal or tracheotomy tube checked for patency and proper position.

Breathing is assessed by inspecting, auscultating, and percussing the chest. A visual **inspection** will determine if the chest wall is rising adequately, whether accessory muscles are being used, and whether there are any external signs of chest injury that can cause respiratory compromise. Observe chest wall movement: Unequal expansion can result from a mucous plug or airway compression from tumor, flail chest, intercostal injury from trauma limiting musculoskeletal activity, as well as pneumothorax, hemothorax, or pleural effusion impinging on lung expansion.

Auscultate the chest to reveal the location and severity of airway pathology. Stridor is a high-pitched sound found on inspiration that indicates high airway obstruction such as in the trachea or pharynx. Gurgling indicates blockage of the posterior pharynx with saliva, blood, or the base of the tongue. Wheezing is evidence for small airway edema such as in asthma or early fluid overload. Crackles indicate fluid in the small airways in conditions such as pulmonary edema and pneumonias.

Percussion may give added clues to the cause of the problem. Dullness to percussion is found with consolidation, atelectasis, or pleural effusion. Hyperresonance may indicate pneumothorax or emphysema. In addition, evaluate the **work of breathing**. A patient who uses accessory muscles for inspiration or any muscles for expiration is likely to fatigue. **Paradoxical breathing**, where the chest rises but the abdomen sinks during inspiration, is indicative of diaphragmatic fatigue and/or weakness. While **tachypnea** is often recognized as a sign of respiratory distress; a patient who was tachypneic and is now slowing their rate may not always be getting better. Evaluate for increasing failure and carbon dioxide retention leading to bradypnea and impending respiratory arrest.

Evaluate the quantity and nature of **sputum** produced for indications of source and extent of disease. Bacterial infections may be yellow, green, rust, clear, or transparent, and sometimes purulent and/or blood-streaked. If chronic in nature, the patient may report that sputum production is more abundant in the morning. Tuberculosis and pulmonary infarction may present with large amounts of bleeding and/or clotting blood. Pulmonary edema may result in pink, frothy sputum.

Extrapulmonary signs may give clues as to the source or extent of respiratory problems. **Cyanosis** can result from disturbance in either cardiac (circulatory failure) or pulmonary (oxygenation failure) function. Cyanosis of the sclera and mucous membranes is associated with inadequate oxygen absorption by the lungs, and is more evenly distributed. Cyanosis of the digits and protrusions (fingers, toes, nose, and lips) is associated with overreduction of hemoglobin related to sluggish circulation or flow obstruction. **Clubbed fingers** may provide clues to a history of long-standing low-oxygen levels. Tachycardia may be due to an underlying stressor such as pain, anxiety, or sepsis, but may also be due to hypoxemia and the stress state associated with it. Evaluate the patient for other causes of decreased respiratory excursion such as tense ascites or distended hollow viscera, such as the stomach, small bowel, or colon.

Although many different problems can lead to a change in level of **consciousness**, hypoxemia, and hypercarbia should always be considered a potential source of a patient's deteriorating mental status (see Chapter 8). When mental status changes with oxygen therapy or wakefulness improves with increased ventilation, respiratory insufficiency should be addressed.

■ LABORATORY STUDIES

Pulse oximetry is a simple, rapid, portable, bedside test that is performed early in the evaluation of respiratory distress. The pulse oximeter determines the degree to which each hemoglobin molecule is saturated with oxygen. A low reading, or a "desaturation," is indicative of a primary oxygenation disorder. Recall that the oxygen-carrying content is influenced by the hemoglobin level as well as the saturation. Thus, a pulse oximetry reading of 100% is possible even if the hemoglobin level is dramatically low, resulting in inadequate oxygen delivery to the tissues. In addition, pulse oximetry is not reliable during two distinct physiologic conditions: in patients with methemoglobinemia and those with carbon monoxide (CO) intoxication. Both of these conditions involve hemoglobin molecules that are binding substances other than oxygen but are read erroneously by the oximeter as carrying oxygen.

Consider drawing an **arterial blood gas** (ABG) as the best way to determine the patient's oxygenation, ventilation, and acid–base status (see Table 5-1). Oxygenation requires sufficient contact of blood with the alveolar membrane allowing diffusion of oxygen into the deoxygenated pulmonary blood flow to bind with hemoglobin and be carried into the systemic circulation. Thus, the value assesses the alveolar–capillary complex. Ventilation is defined as the body's removal of CO_2. Inadequate ventilation will result in primary respiratory acidosis, whereas hyperventilation will lead to primary respiratory alkalosis. Acidosis from metabolic sources is evidenced by a compensation of hyperventilation and/or an increase in the serum bicarbonate level on the ABG.

Order a **complete blood count** to ensure that anemia is not contributing to the respiratory compromise. A low-hemoglobin level can cause respiratory insufficiency because the majority of oxygen carried in the blood is bound to hemoglobin. An elevated **white blood count** may indicate infection as the underlying cause. Obtain a basic **electrolyte panel** to gain information regarding volume status, chronic respiratory problems (i.e., increased CO_2 with COPD patients), chronic metabolic disturbances, and renal function. All of these abnormalities may influence the respiratory system as well. Consider drawing **cardiac markers** to determine if the patient's respiratory distress is due to a primary cardiac disturbance (Chapter 12). **Cardiac enzymes** (CPK, CPK-MB, cardiac troponin) may be warranted. A serum **brain natriuretic peptide** will be elevated in cases of heart failure causing hypoxia and is sent to the laboratory, if this is a concern. **Phosphate** levels are checked in cases of chronic respiratory

TABLE 5-1.
Interpretation of the Arterial Blood Gas

Arterial Blood Gas	CO_2	HCO_3
Respiratory acidosis, uncompensated	⇑	Within normal limits
Respiratory acidosis, compensated	⇑	⇑
Respiratory alkalosis, uncompensated	⇓	Within normal limits
Respiratory alkalosis, compensated	⇓	⇓
Metabolic acidosis, uncocompensated	Within normal limits	⇓
Metabolic acidosis, compensated	⇓	⇓
Metabolic alkalosis uncocompensated	Within normal limits	⇑
Metabolic alkalosis compensated	⇑	⇑

Arterial blood gas (ABG) testing is the best way to determine the patient's oxygenation and ventilation status. Any process that diminishes alveolar ventilation (small and/or infrequent breaths, increased anatomic dead space), diffusion across the alveolar-capillary membrane (poor perfusion, loss of surface area, change in gas concentrations, and diffusion gradients), or transport of gases throughout the body (decreased cardiac output, decreased hemoglobin) will potentially alter oxygenation, ventilation, and acid-base balance.

Ventilation is defined as the body's removal of CO_2. Appropriate ventilation requires the coordination of the respiratory musculature allow movement of air into and out of the lungs. CO_2 diffuses into the alveolar space from the returning systemic blood for removal during exhalation. Inadequate ventilation will result in primary respiratory acidosis, whereas hyperventilation will lead to primary respiratory alkalosis.

Four main acid-base disturbances can be seen on ABG testing.

***Respiratory acidosis** results from inadequate clearance of CO_2, such as in decreased mental status or splinting from postoperative pain. **Metabolic acidosis** is caused by the accumulation of organic acids, most often from inadequate tissue perfusion during shock. **Respiratory alkalosis** results from hyperventilation that can be related to anxiety, or hypoxemia that causes the patient to be tachypneic during "air hunger." Finally, **metabolic alkalosis** is caused by excess serum bicarbonate, most likely iatrogenic.*

***Interpretation** starts by noting whether the pH is acidotic (<7.4) or alkalotic (>7.4). Next, the CO_2 is used to determine whether the disorder is respiratory or metabolic in nature. Thus, an ABG with a pH of 7.2 with a high CO_2 is an evidence for a respiratory acidosis, whereas a result of pH 7.5 with a low CO_2 reflects a metabolic alkalosis. Lastly, the partial pressure of oxygen is interpreted in the context of the fraction of inspired oxygen (FiO_2) the patient is receiving. A PaO_2 of 110 is normal if the patient is breathing room air, but abnormal if the patient is on 100% non-rebreather mask (where the PaO_2 should be around 300). The difference between the oxygen supplied and the oxygen noted in the saturated blood is the **a-A difference**, and reflects the degree of hypoxia.*

failure since patients with low levels may have profound muscle weakness (including the diaphragm) leading to severe hypoventilation.

In patients with acute respiratory failure, a normal **D-dimer** level definitively rules out pulmonary embolism as the cause of hypoxia. However, in postoperative surgical patients, the use of D-dimer assays to determine the presence or absence of pulmonary embolism (PE) is limited because it is often elevated as a result of the surgical procedure. These assays are only helpful when the level is low.

■ RADIOGRAPHIC STUDIES

In all cases of respiratory compromise order a **chest X-ray** (CXR) as the first radiographic examination. Review the CXR in a systematic fashion to ensure no findings are missed (Figure 5-1). Consider a **Chest CT** as the definitive test for almost any pathology within the chest. It gives anatomic information about the lungs, pleura, pleural spaces, mediastinum, vasculature, and soft tissues. It has replaced conventional angiogram for diagnosis of pulmonary embolism at many medical centers. The two distinct **disadvantages** of the chest CT are the requirement to transport the patient to the scanner, and the need for IV contrast administration. Risks of the intravenous contrast include both iodine dye allergy and the risk of acute renal failure for patients with renal insufficiency. Renal dysfunction can be attenuated by pretreating with intravenous hydration, sodium bicarbonate, or n-acetylcesteine (Mucomyst).

Ventilation–perfusion (V/Q) scan remains a sensitive and specific test for the diagnosis of pulmonary embolism. Although it has basically been replaced by computed tomography, V/Q scan may still be used in cases of patients who cannot receive IV dye due to an allergy or impending renal failure. Conventional **pulmonary angiogram** is not commonly performed because of its invasive nature. However, it still may have a limited role to diagnose and potentially treat pulmonary embolism by directed thrombolysis or catheter embolectomy. **Pulmonary function tests** have no role in patients with acute respiratory compromise. After stabilization, pulmonary function tests can be used to determine the character of the underlying pulmonary function as obstructive, restrictive, or diffusion related.

■ DIAGNOSTIC PLAN

Acute respiratory compromise can be immediately life-threatening. Lack of oxygen to the brain for as little as 2–4 minutes can cause permanent neurologic defects (see Chapter 17). Thus, quickly assess for life-threatening respiratory failure that requires immediate intervention. If airway obstruction is suspected, determine if it is fixed or removable. Use **suction** liberally in cases of acute aspiration or retained secretions. **Position** the airway open using basic life-support techniques, and consider sitting the patient upright if possible. Administer **oxygen** by high flow non-rebreather mask, and establish **venous access** if not already present. If respirations are shallow and inadequate, consider assisting ventilations with a **bagged valve mask** (BVM) ventilator. If there are severe derangements in the airway, breathing, or circulation, consider early **endotracheal intubation** using the rapid sequence intubation (RSI) technique by a trained clinician (Figure 5-2). *Securing the airway with intubation, and providing positive pressure ventilation will stabilize almost every type of respiratory failure.*

INTERPRETATION OF THE CHEST RADIOGRAPH

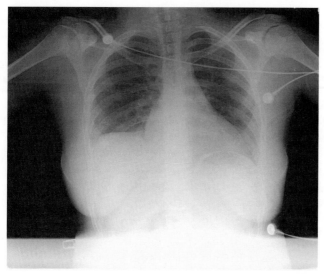

A

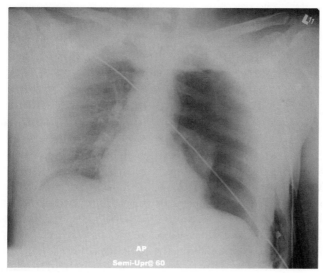

B

FIGURE 5-1
A) Normal CXR, and B) Large Left pneumothorax

It is imperative that the clinician develops one systematic way of looking at each chest radiograph so that subtleties are not missed. One helpful way is to scan the radiograph using the "airway, breathing, circulation, disability, and everything else" format (A).

Airway: If the patient is intubated, confirm that the tube is in the trachea and in the correct position. It should end approximately 2 cm above the carina.

The trachea should be midline. It may be deviated toward the side of lung collapse or away from the side of a tension pneumothorax. Look for pneumomediastinum. This air outside the trachea and lungs could signify esophageal rupture or pneumothorax.

(Continued)

Breathing: Examine the lung fields for a pneumothorax (air in the pleural space). This will be confirmed by noting the absence of lung markings all the way out to the parietal pleura (B). There will also be a thin lung edge line (visceral pleura). A pneumothorax in a patient with respiratory compromise mandates immediate tube thoracostomy (chest tube).

Complete opacification of one lung ("white-out") has a large differential diagnosis, although it is most commonly atelectasis or fluid. In atelectasis (lung collapse), the mediastinum and trachea are deviated toward the side of whiteout. In the acute setting, this is often caused by mucus plugging. In massive pleural effusion (fluid), the mediastinum and trachea are deviated away from the side of white-out. The fluid may be blood (hemothorax), serum (hydrothorax), lipid (chylothorax), or pus (empyema). Other possible causes include pneumonia (consolidation, tumor, or absence of a lung after surgical pneumonectomy. Examine the lungs for signs of consolidation (lobar atelectasis), infiltrates (often pneumonia), interstitial lung disease (most often pulmonary edema), lung masses (lung cancer), or diffuse patchy infiltrates (acute respiratory distress syndrome [ARDS]).

Circulation: Review the cardiac silhouette. An enlarged heart (>50% of the width of the chest) suggests cardiac enlargement or a pericardial effusion. A widened mediastinum may suggest aortic dissection (nontraumatic), aortic transaction (trauma setting), adenopathy, or mediastinal mass, which may cause acute shortness of breath.

Disability: Examine all bones on the film for fractures (especially after trauma). This includes the spine, ribs, clavicles, and humerus.

Everything else: The film should be examined in detail in order to avoid missing another alternative cause for respiratory compromise. Abdominal pathology is a common cause of respiratory distress. Examine the area beneath the diaphragm for other clues about the cause of respiratory distress. Intra-abdominal free air signifies bowel perforation that may cause respiratory distress and is always a surgical emergency. Acute gastric dilatation can cause shortness of breath because the patient cannot take a deep breath. This can also cause chest pain that can mimic a myocardial infarction. Foreign bodies in the tracheobronchial tree can cause respiratory distress from airway obstruction. These are most commonly ingested coins or toys in the case of children. In adults, aspirated teeth may cause similar symptoms.

If no immediate, life-threatening issues are identified on the primary survey, then further diagnostic workup is indicated. Perform a complete pulmonary and general **physical examination**, looking for clues to the etiology of the failure. The **CXR** will often lead to a definitive diagnosis and guide appropriate therapy. However, a normal CXR does not rule out certain etiologies such as pulmonary embolism or early heart failure. Use the **pulse oximetry** as an easy bedside procedure to give immediate information about the patient's ability to oxygenate. Oxygen therapy should be instituted (by face mask or nasal cannula) to alleviate symptoms of hypoxia. Even if supplemental oxygen relieves the patient's symptoms, further workup is indicated to determine the cause and to plan the most appropriate therapy.

Since pulse oximetry does not give any information about elimination of CO_2, consider drawing an ABG to assess ventilation. Common causes for poor ventilation in surgical patients include poor pain relief with splinting and atelectasis. Assess current and past **pain levels** and ability of the patient to cough and perform on the incentive spirometer. Other patients at risk for ventilation failure are obese patients, especially after bariatric surgery. Determine if **continuous**

ENDOTRACHEAL INTUBATION

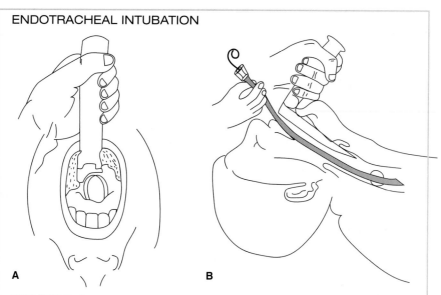

A   B

FIGURE 5-2
A) Placement of the Endotracheal Tube, and B) View into the Larynx During Intubation

Rapid sequence intubation (RSI) and all endotracheal intubations are performed by clinicians specifically trained and credentialed to perform the procedure. RSI allows for the sedation and paralysis of patients to allow smooth airway control where spontaneous breathing and a full gag reflex would not allow unaided intubation.

The procedure starts by preoxygenating the patient with high-flow non-rebreather mask or blow by tent. Active manual ventilation is avoided if possible to decrease forced insufflation of the stomach. An assistant performs the Sellick maneuver, manual pressure on the cricoid cartilage to push the larynx into a better position for view, and compress the esophagus. Sedation and paralytic medications are given; the types and doses may vary among clinicians and hospitals.

After paralysis is confirmed, the procedure begins by grasping the intubation blade in the left hand and opening the mouth with the right hand (A). The blade sweeps the tongue from right to left and lifts it anteriorly to allow a view of the vocal cords. This must be performed by lifting straight up, not by twisting the wrist which can injure the teeth. Once the vocal cords are visualized, an endotracheal tube can be passed between them and the balloon inflated (B).

More than one test is mandatory to confirm appropriate endotracheal tube placement. Auscultation is performed over both lung fields and the epigastrium. Proper tube placement will reveal breath sounds in both lungs and absence of sound over the epigastrium. Breath sounds only on one side may indicate a mainstem intubation. Second confirmation of tracheal placement is accomplished with an end-tidal CO_2 detector. Lack of end-tidal CO_2 is an evidence of incorrect placement, and intubation is reattempted.

positive airway pressure therapy has been used before and consider beginning new treatments.

In surgical patients, pulmonary embolism must be considered high in the differential diagnosis of any patient with acute respiratory compromise. If suspicion is very high and there are no absolute contraindications, start heparin therapy immediately while further diagnostic tests are performed. Consider a **chest CT** or **ventilation–perfusion scan** as the noninvasive test of choice to make the diagnosis.

■ DIFFERENTIAL DIAGNOSIS AND TREATMENT

Atelectasis

Generalized collapse of the alveolar respiratory units is common after surgery of both the abdomen and chest can have significant impact on respiratory function. Both postoperative abdominal and chest wall pain can lead to "splinting," ineffective cough, atelectasis, hypoxemia, and eventually pneumonia. Adequate postoperative **pain control** is essential in the prevention and treatment of atelectasis (see Chapter 3). Supportive care includes adequate analgesic therapy to allow for improved pulmonary toilet. Intravenous narcotics given as a **patient-controlled analgesia** may help control pain effectively; however, continuous **thoracic epidural** pain management may be most effective for patients with multiple rib fractures or in the elderly. Non-steroidal antiinflammatory drugs (NSAIDs) may have some additive benefit.

A consequence of atelectasis is the formation of **mucous plugs** that can cause acute airway obstruction and respiratory failure. Often patients will have a recent history of poor cough, poor pain tolerance, and inactivity, then present with sudden shortness of breath. In the ventilated ICU patient, plugs are heralded by sudden or rapidly progressing desaturation, increased airway pressures, and loss of inspiratory volume. Major mucous plugs will cause large areas of full atelectasis on CXR. First-line treatment includes oxygen therapy, pulmonary toilet, pain relief, and inhaled **beta agonist** or **Mucomyst**. If these treatments fail, **bronchoscopy** with suctioning of the plug is indicated (see Figure 12-4). Bronchoscopy performed in non-intubated patient (awake bronchoscopy) is a difficult skill, and endotracheal intubation may be necessary to facilitate the procedure.

Pulmonary Edema

Hypervolemia commonly causes respiratory distress in hospitalized patients with underlying cardiac disease. Left-sided **ventricular failure** may lead to increased venous pressures that overwhelm the pulmonary vasculature and lead to decreased lung function (see Chapter 12). Alternatively, fluid overload can be an iatrogenic consequence of administering too much fluid in the perioperative period or a result of mobilization of fluids received during surgery (see Chapter 7).

The diagnosis is made by physical examination findings of **crackles** combined with a CXR with increased heart size, increased pulmonary vascular congestion, and pulmonary edema. An attempt at **diuresis** is often indicated but further cardiac evaluation is important as well. Order an EKG and cardiac enzymes to determine if the patient is having an acute myocardial infarction or ischemia. Consider additional testing with echocardiogram, central venous monitoring; or pulmonary artery catheter placement will help determine the cause of cardiac failure and the need for additional diuresis, if volume overloaded. In addition, consider **inotropic support** for better ventricular function, or more sophisticated technologies such as intra-aortic balloon pump or ventricular assist devices for improvement of cardiac function.

Pleural Effusion

The pleural space can fill with blood (hemothorax), serum (hydrothorax), lipid (chylothorax), or pus (empyema). Make the diagnosis of pleural effusion on **upright CXR** where a fluid level with meniscus is appreciated in the pleural space. Approximately 500 mL is needed in the pleural space to cause blunting of the costophrenic angle on CXR. Consider a CT scan or ultrasound evaluation to better define the amount, location, and possible loculation of the fluid.

A **hemothorax** is most often caused by blunt or penetrating trauma, or iatrogenically after central-line or chest tube placement. The major symptoms caused by hemothorax are related to blood loss and resultant shock rather than problems with oxygenation or ventilation. Tube thoracostomy (see Figure 4-2) is usually adequate for evacuation of a traumatic hemothorax in the majority of cases, although patients with ongoing bleeding or bleeding associated with the need for transfusion or hemodynamic instability may require operative intervention.

Simple effusions (hydrothorax) can occur as a transudate or an exudate. **Transudative** pleural effusions are caused by systemic factors which alter the balance of the formation and reabsorption of pleural fluid. Examples include left ventricular failure, pulmonary embolism, cirrhosis, malnutrition, and nephrotic syndrome. **Exudates** are effusions caused by alterations in local factors affecting the formation and reabsorption of pleural fluid. They often occur when inflammation leads to increased capillary permeability. Exudates are caused by bacterial pneumonia, cancer, viral infection, and pulmonary embolism. Simple effusions that become symptomatic are drained by **thoracentesis** (Figure 5-3) or by tube **thoracostomy** (see Figure 4-1).

Chylothorax is the accumulation of chyle within the chest cavity. This is often caused by malignancy or by any type of thoracic surgery in which the thoracic duct is injured. **Empyema**, the collection of pus around the lung, is a significant infectious problem. This requires thoracostomy drainage as well as systemic antibiotics. Empyema can result after pleural or other thoracic procedures, as a secondary infection of other fluid in the chest, or associated with an underlying pneumonia. Both chylothorax and empyemas tend to require long-term pleural drainage, and thus, are not amendable to simple thoracentesis.

Pneumothorax

Although most commonly the result of direct injury to the lung, bronchus or chest wall injury, iatrogenic causes can occur during surgery, central-line placement, or ventilation with high airway pressures in intubated patients. Make the diagnosis by the physical findings of decreased breath sounds, cough, and hyperresonance on the effected side. Although often seen on **CXR**, some small

NEEDLE THORACOSTOMY AND THORACENTESIS

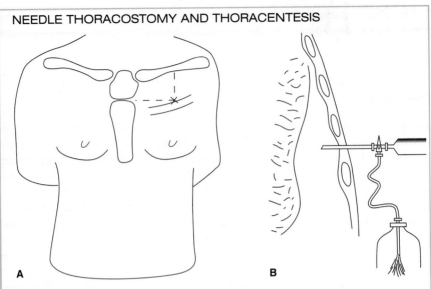

A   B

FIGURE 5-3
A) Location of a Needle Decompression, and B) Thoracentesis

Needle thoracostomy of a tension pneumothorax is performed using a large (14 or 16 gauge) intravenous catheter placed into the pleural space. The area of the second intercostal space at the mid-clavicular line is rapidly prepped with betadine (A). The catheter is placed just over the rib, to avoid injury to the intercostal vessels that run under the rib margin. When the catheter is appropriately positioned, there will be a characteristic rush of air with the decompression of the chest. The angiocath is slid over the needle and the metal needle removed. If the diagnosis is correct, the patient should improve rapidly. Needle thoracostomy must be followed by a formal tube thoracostomy, when available.

Thoracentesis involves the simple drainage of pleural fluid without leaving a permanent tube behind. The patient can be positioned sitting or lying in the lateral decubitus position on the side of the effusion. Whether commercial kits or basic supplies are used, the concept is that a closed system is needed to drain fluid without letting air enter the chest causing a pneumothorax (B). If a simple catheter is used, it is attached to a three-way stopcock that is connected to a collection chamber at one hub, and a syringe on the other. The needle is introduced over the rib into the pleural space, and the three-way stopcock is turned to allow fluid to enter the collection chamber. After fluid is completely drained, the needle and assembly are removed. A CXR is performed to rule out pneumothorax.

pneumothoraces may only become apparent on chest CT. **Simple pneumothorax** is defined by a collection of air around the lung. Depending upon the extent of the injury, find decreased breath sounds, decreased expansion, and increased percussion notes in the affected area. The patient may be symptomatic; however, they will have no hemodynamic compromise.

Tension pneumothorax results from air escaping into the pleural space, with no means of returning into the bronchial tree for exhalation. As a result, with each breath, the pneumothorax grows and compresses the lung pushing the mediastinal structures toward the unaffected side. This causes diminished venous return to the heart and **cardiovascular collapse**. Classic signs include deviation of the trachea away from the injured side, a hyperexpanded chest, and less chest expansion with respiration.

Tension pneumothorax can develop quickly and should be ruled out in any ventilated patient with sudden onset of increased airway pressures, tachycardia, and hypotension even in the absence of the "classic signs." Treatment of tension pneumothorax requires rapid decompression, either with **needle thoracostomy** (Figure 5-3) or chest tube placement. Simple pneumothorax often requires evacuation with either a traditional chest tube or smaller bore catheter, although small ones may be amenable to watchful waiting. In this case, the use of 100% oxygen by face mask will facilitate resolution; then, the nitrogen in the pneumothorax will flow into the lung and be exhaled. This approach is less likely to be followed if the patient requires positive pressure ventilation.

Pulmonary Embolism

Suspect PE in every surgical patient with new onset respiratory symptoms. The **classic symptoms** include tachypnea, dyspnea, tachycardia, and hypoxia. Massive emboli, sometimes called "saddle emboli," occluding the proximal pulmonary artery, may result in profound hypotension, syncope, acute elevations of right ventricular pressure, shock, and severe hypoxemia. However, many patients never have a catastrophic presentation of dyspnea or hypoxia, but instead have progressively worsening oxygenation with only transient tachycardia or tachypnea. Symptoms may develop from a single large PE or a shower of smaller emboli occluding multiple pulmonary arterial segments.

The physical examination is unreliable in making the diagnosis of PE, thus have a **high suspicion** in patients with major risk factors for deep venous thrombosis (see Chapter 3). Obtain a **12-lead EKG** to look for right-sided findings of P pulmonale, right axis deviation, S1-Q3-T3 pattern and right bundle branch block, although the most common findings are simple sinus tacycardia with or without non-specific S-T changes. The **CXR** is often unrevealing, but may show infiltrates, pleural effusion, elevated hemidiaphragm, atelectasis, wedge-shaped infiltrate (with infarction), or cardiomegaly. A normal CXR clearly does not rule out the diagnosis. Consider **echocardiography** at the bedside to show RV dilation, tricuspid regurgitation, pulmonary hypertension, and pulmonary artery dilation. A low-D-**dimer** level in the context of a low pretest clinical suspicion, essentially rules out the disease. **ABG** analysis may show hypoxemia and hypoventilation, but similar to the CXR, it cannot be used to rule out or rule in the diagnosis.

Order a spiral **chest CT** as the definitive study to make the diagnosis of pulmonary embolism. Alternatively, if CT is not available, have a ventilation–perfusion scan or a pulmonary angiogram performed. If the patient is considered high risk and the previous studies are equivocal or unavailable, start **empiric treatment** with heparin. Start **oxygen** therapy immediately and consider the need for full ventilatory support. Consider **inotropic** support of the right ventricle in patients with hemodynamic instability.

Once the diagnosis is made, start anticoagulation therapy with a **heparin** infusion, titrated to an aPTT goal of 2.0 times control. This is often followed by **warfarin** therapy with a goal of INR > 2.0. Alternatively, subcutaneous dosing of **low molecular weight heparin** may also be used to achieve anticoagulation. Monitor closely for signs and symptoms of bleeding as well as thrombocytopenia related to heparin therapy. Therapy with systemic **thrombolytics** is reserved for patients with hemodynamically significant massive PE or life-threatening hypoxemia. The use of thrombolytics requires assessment of the relative and absolute contraindications to therapy including, but not limited to, a history of hemorrhagic stroke (absolute), active bleeding (absolute), recent femoral or large arterial puncture (absolute), surgery within past 10 days (relative, unless intracranial), severe hypertension, or pregnancy (relative).

Embolectomy can be performed by either a surgical or interventional radiological procedure. Removal of a clot from the pulmonary vasculature is a high-risk procedure reserved for those who are near cardiac or respiratory arrest despite aggressive life-saving therapy.

Determine the need for an **inferior vena cava filter** placement may play a significant role in the treatment of patients with PE. Traditional indications for placement have been prevention of further PE in the patient who has a contraindication to anticoagulation, development of a PE and/or DVT despite adequate anticoagulation therapy, hemodynamically unstable patients who will not receive thrombolytic therapy as an adjunct to embolectomy, or the presence of large mobile iliofemoral DVT. With the advent of newer technology and the use of retrievable (or temporary) IVC filters, the indications are changing and expanding rapidly.

Adult Respiratory Distress Syndrome

Characterized by the sudden onset of respiratory distress, adult respiratory distress syndrome (ARDS) is associated with severe hypoxemia and acute diffuse parenchyma infiltration in the absence of cardiac failure. As a result of the injury to the alveolar–capillary membrane from either intrinsic or extrinsic factors, there is leaking of protein-containing fluid into the interstitial and alveolar spaces, effectively decreasing pulmonary compliance and lung aeration as the air sacs fill with fluid. This decreases the ability of the lung to diffuse gases across the alveolar capillary membrane, producing significant hypoxemia. **Primary ARDS** is caused by a local pulmonary process (pneumonia, aspiration, chemical inhalation). **Secondary ARDS** is triggered by systemic factors external to the lung (sepsis, trauma, burns, head injury, shock, and pancreatitis). ARDS has specific defining features. Make the diagnosis by demonstrating **bilateral fluffy infiltrates** on CXR, hypoxia (PaO_2/FiO_2 ratio of <200), and a **low pulmonary capillary wedge** pressure (<18 mm Hg) (see Figure 6-4).

Treatment for ARDS is aimed primarily at the underlying case for the syndrome. Provide mechanical **ventilatory support** as necessary to allow time for the lungs to heal. Long-term care of patients with ARDS is complex, but the primary tenet of treatment is to prevent ongoing secondary damage to the lung.

Use **low tidal volume**, low airway pressure ventilation with **high PEEP** (positive end-expiratory pressure) to improve survival in patients with ARDS. The role of **steroid therapy** in ARDS is controversial and should be guided by local practices.

COPD and Asthma

Reactive airway disease is characterized by airway inflammation, edema, and bronchospasm, which cause intermittent airflow obstruction. Asthma episodes may be triggered by a variety of allergens, irritants, gastroesophageal reflux, stress states, exercise, cold temperature, endotracheal intubation, or suctioning. In a patient with respiratory failure from an asthma attack, treatment is immediate administration of oxygen, **inhaled bronchodilators**, large-dose **corticosteroids** given early in the episode, and intubation if required. Other less commonly used therapies such as **magnesium** and **theophylline** are infrequently needed to control severe bronchospasm.

Heliox therapy, a mixture of helium and oxygen, which reduces turbulent airflow in the larger airways, may increase delivery of bronchodilators to distal airways. Inhaled general anesthetics are another powerful therapy for difficult-to-treat acute asthmatic attack.

Mechanical ventilation may be required for the patient unable to continue to meet the work of breathing or the one who shows signs of failure such as mental status decline or blood gas deterioration despite aggressive therapy.

Ventilator therapy includes use of **low tidal volume** (6–7 mL/kg) strategies with tolerance of acidosis and "permissive hypercapnia," adjustment of flow rates to allow sufficient inspiratory flow and expiratory time, keeping plateau pressures less than 30 cmH20, and use of sedation and paralytics as required until the initial crisis has passed.

Anaphylaxis

Acute allergic reactions can lead to bronchospasm or airway obstruction from laryngeal edema. This is most often seen in surgical patients as a response to a previously unknown intravenous contrast dye or drug allergy. Treatment includes removal of the offending agent as well as immediate delivery of **bronchodilators**, nebulized **racemic epinephrine**, H2 blockers, and steroids to attenuate the allergic response. Consider intramuscular or subcutaneous dosing of epinephrine for prolonged cases. If oral or laryngeal edema is significant, bag-valve-mask ventilation may initially be more productive than endotracheal intubation through an edematous airway, allowing time for medications to take effect. Be prepared to perform **cricothyrotomy** if intubation is not possible secondary to gross edema.

Selected Readings

Airway and Ventilatory Management. In: *Advanced Trauma Life Support (ATLS) Student Course Manual*. 7th ed. Chicago, IL: American College of Surgeons Committee on Trauma; 2004.

Chen H, Sonnenday CJ, Lillemoe KD, eds. *Manual of Common Bedside Surgical Procedures*. 2nd ed. Philadelphia: Lippincott Williams & Wilkins; 2000.

James CR. *Chest Radiology*. 5th ed. Philadelphia: Mosby; 2003.

Marcucci L, Martinez E, Haut ER, Slonim A, Suarez J, eds. *Avoiding Common ICU Errors*. Philadelphia: Lippincott Williams & Wilkins; 2007.

6

Hemodynamic Failure

Denise M. Zappile, RN, MSN, CRNP-BC ■ *Susan R. McGinley, MSN, CRNP-BC* ■ *Babak Sarani, MD*

Key Points

- Shock, regardless of type or cause, represents a state of inadequate tissue and organ oxygenation and perfusion.

- Types of shock include hypovolemia, distributive with inappropriate vasodilation, cardiogenic after pump failure, or obstructive if there is a blockage of normal blood flow.

- Defining the severity of shock may be difficult, since overt symptoms may not be present until the late stages. Symptoms may include systemic hypotension, tachycardia, oliguria, or altered mental status.

- The biochemical hallmark of shock is a lactic acidosis. This can be measured directly with lactate levels or indirectly with bicarbonate or anion gap measurements.

- All types of shock require initial volume resuscitation except left-sided cardiogenic shock, which may require inotropic, vasopressor, and afterload reducing support initially.

- After volume resuscitation, invasive monitoring may be necessary to judge adequacy of fluid status and the need for inotropic and vasopressor support.

■ HISTORY

Begin by assessing for the events leading up to the shock. The **history of the present illness** is especially important in helping to stratify the possible causes of shock. If the patient was involved in a motor vehicle accident, hypovolemic or neurogenic shock is suspected. If an elderly woman is brought from home after a recent illness, sepsis would be high on the differential diagnosis list.

Determine if there has been a **fluid loss** leading to hypovolemia. In addition to obvious blood loss, look for occult sources of volume loss such as severe emesis or diarrhea, high fistula output, inappropriate diuresis (diabetic ketoacidosis, diabetes insipidus, and diuretic abuse), or burns. "**Third spacing**" is the concept of fluid leaving the vascular space and accumulating in the interstitium, associated with severe inflammation such as pancreatitis or ischemic bowel (see Chapter 7).

Determine if there is a possibility of **sepsis** causing distributive shock. Sepsis is common in elderly patients, those with urinary retention or prostatism (urinary sepsis), those with immunosuppression, or those taking steroids. Other patients at risk are those with open wounds or a recent abdominal catastrophe (see Chapter 9).

Consider **neurogenic shock** in patients with a history of spinal cord trauma or in patients who have received a neuroaxial block, such as epidural or spinal anesthesia.

Determine if the patient has any **allergies**, especially any history of severe reactions that can suggest anaphylactic shock.

Determine if there has been a sudden cessation of chronic steroids leading to **adrenal insufficiency**, a rare but potential consideration in shock. Secondary adrenal insufficiency may also present in other types of shock state, such as sepsis and hypovolemia.

Assess risk factors for **obstructive shock** including a predisposition for a pulmonary embolism (PE) such as a hypercoagulable state, recent trauma, recent prolonged bed rest or immobility, and a history of DVT/swollen extremity (see Chapter 5). Cardiac tamponade in the nontrauma setting is often related to uremia, cancer, or pericarditis (see Chapter 12). A rare, but treatable, cause of obstructive shock is a tension pneumothorax, often seen as a spontaneous problem in young, thin males who have a pleural bleb rupture (see Chapter 5).

Look for evidence of **previous heart disease** as a possible indicator of cardiogenic shock. Especially note any recent **chest pain** or **dyspnea**, understanding that both may be absent in patients with diabetes mellitus. Obtain a full cardiac history, including previous myocardial infarctions, hypertension, angina, and previous procedures, such as angioplasty and coronary artery bypass grafting.

■ PHYSICAL EXAMINATION

Start with a constitutional examination looking for **altered mental status** (agitation or stupor) that can be seen in late-stage shock. As in all emergency situations, assess patency of the **airway** and the patient's ability to maintain this airway.

Assess the cardiac system by the rate and character of the pulse. **Tachycardia** and hypotension can be seen in most types of shock. **Bradycardia** and hypotension are associated with neurogenic shock because the sympathetic fibers to the heart have been severed, resulting in an inability to mount a reflex tachycardia. Irregular rhythms can cause hypotension by impairing cardiac filling or ejection.

Assess heart sounds for muffling or new onset murmur. It is helpful to know the patient's baseline blood pressure, since a "normal" pressure may represent relative hypotension in patients with poorly controlled hypertension.

Assess for **jugular venous distention** as a measure of fluid status and determination of right heart failure. Flat veins are consistent with hypovolemia or euvolemia. Distended neck veins suggest impaired right ventricular (RV) output as seen in RV failure, pulmonary embolism, cardiac tamponade, pulmonary hypertension, or late-stage left ventricular failure.

Perform a **pulmonary examination** by listening to lung sounds. Evaluate for left ventricular failure by noting crackles associated with pulmonary edema. Acute respiratory distress, absent or diminished breath sounds, and tracheal shift are clinical findings consistent with potential tension pneumothorax.

Examine the **abdomen**, noting tenderness and masses. A tender abdomen with signs of sepsis can suggest an intra-abdominal source of infection. Hypovolemia with abdominal pain is consistent with peritoneal or retroperitoneal bleeding. Perform a **rectal examination** to determine if there is frank or occult blood loss from a gastrointestinal bleed as the source of hypovolemia. Occasionally a perirectal abscess or a perineal infection (fournier's gangrene) can be a source of undiagnosed sepsis.

Warm **extremities** in a hypotensive patient suggest distributive shock. Examine the nail bed for cyanosis, indicating hypoxemia or severely depressed cardiac output. A diffuse **rash** and skin **wheels** are associated with anaphylactic reactions.

■ LABORATORY STUDIES

Order a **CBC** to determine the **hemoglobin** level in patients suspected of hemorrhage. Recall that the hemoglobin and hematocrit may take time to drop as fluid re-equilibrates from the extracellular space, and thus, levels may be normal in acute blood loss. A **white blood cell** count greater than 12,000 or less than 4000 is consistent with sepsis. Thrombocytopenia can exacerbate volume loss from hemorrhage, and it can be a nonspecific marker of sepsis.

In patients who have active hemorrhage, assure that the patient has a current **type and cross-match**. Order a **prothrombin** and **partial thromboplastin time** to rule out coagulopathy. Order a **chemistry panel** to assess acidosis and renal function. A low bicarbonate level suggests acidosis, and further workup with determination of the anion gap and **arterial blood gas** may be helpful to evaluate degree or cause of acidosis. An elevated **lactate** level is seen with poor tissue perfusion, and it can be present in various forms of shock. A lactate level that fails to normalize over time indicates ongoing shock and inadequate resuscitation.

Consider an **EKG** to assess cardiac rhythm and ischemia associated with cardiogenic shock. A greater-than-2-mm ST **depression** represents cardiac ischemia or strain, whereas a greater-than-1-mm ST **elevation** represents cardiac infarction. Also, consider **cardiac enzymes** every 8 hours to evaluate nonelevated ST segment MI or cardiac strain. An elevation of the **brain naturetic peptide (BNP)** is associated with active congestive heart failure (CHF) and may support a diagnosis of cardiogenic shock.

When evaluating for septic shock, obtain **cultures** of the blood, urine, and sputum. Also, consider cultures of other body fluids or tissue that are suspected of being a source of infection.

■ RADIOGRAPHIC AND INVASIVE STUDIES

Order a **chest X-ray** (CXR) to assess cardiac silhouette and lung fields. Look for pulmonary edema as a sign of cardiac failure or areas of opacity suggesting pneumonia as the cause of sepsis. Other rare causes of shock, such as a spontaneous pneumothorax or chronic pericardial tamponade, can also be ruled out with a CXR.

Consider an **echocardiography** for patients in refractory shock to assess cardiac function, determine intravascular fluid status, and rule out pericardial tamponade. Echocardiography is also useful in distinguishing right from left ventricular dysfunction.

Consider invasive monitoring in patients with ongoing shock. Place an **arterial pressure catheter** to continuously monitor blood pressure. To determine intravascular fluid volume, place a **central venous catheter (CVC)** to monitor right atrial pressure and central venous oxygen saturation (Figure 6-1). Consider a **Swan–Ganz catheter (SGC)** to measure cardiac output, mixed-venous oxygen saturation, cardiac filling pressures, and pulmonary pressure (see Figure 6-2 and 6-3).

Consider following one or more **end points of resuscitation**. Markers of tissue perfusion include mixed venous oxygen saturation, tissue oxygenation, serum lactate levels, and organ function such as urine output. Consider using a continuous mixed venous output catheter or tissue oximeter to guide therapy (see Figure 9-1).

■ DIAGNOSTIC PLAN

Before starting an in-depth diagnostic plan, start active **resuscitation**. Assure that the airway is patent and consider **endotracheal intubation** for patients with a depressed mental status. Place large-bore **intravenous catheters** and begin crystalloid infusion as a first line of treatment for all types of shock. Consider early placement of **invasive monitors** such as a CVC or an SGC. In patients with obvious blood loss, consider **transfusion** of blood and blood products early in the resuscitation. Initiate **warming** techniques to avoid hypothermia. If septic shock is suspected, start **empiric antibiotics** directed at the potential sources dictated by the history and physical examination. If the hemodynamic failure continues despite fluid resuscitation, consider the use of **vasopressor** agents for blood pressure support.

CENTRAL VENOUS ACCESS

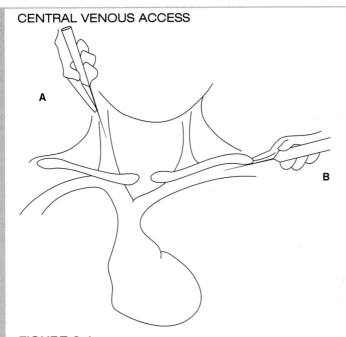

FIGURE 6-1
The Internal Jugular (A), Subclavian (B) and Femoral (C) Approaches to Venous Access

The procedure is performed under sterile conditions. Anatomical landmarks are identified, a wide skin field is sterilized and draped, and the skin is infiltrated with local anesthetic. If the internal jugular or the subclavian veins are to be cannulated, the patient should be placed in the head down (Trendelenberg) position to avoid air embolism and to distend the veins. The central venous catheter (CVC) is placed using the **Seldinger technique**. In this procedure, a needle is introduced into the vein. A J-tipped guidewire is then passed through the needle into the vessel. A dilator is then introduced over the wire and removed until skin dilation has been achieved. The dilator is then removed, and the catheter is placed over the guidewire into the vessel. The lumens are flushed with saline to assure patency and the device by suturing in place and covering with a sterile dressing. A postprocedure chest radiograph is ordered to confirm placement and to rule out a pneumothorax or effusion associated with the procedure.

Cannulation is attempted in one of three different routes. The **internal jugular** approach has the advantages of easy access to the lateral neck, a straight conduit into the right atrium, and ability to tamponade an incidental hematoma (A). The **subclavian** approach has the advantage of comfort for the patient and the ability to easily care for the site on the anterior chest wall (B). The **femoral vein** approach avoids potential damage to the lungs but has a higher eventual infection and DVT rate. Injury to the femoral artery and nerve is also possible on account of the proximity of these structures to the vein (C).

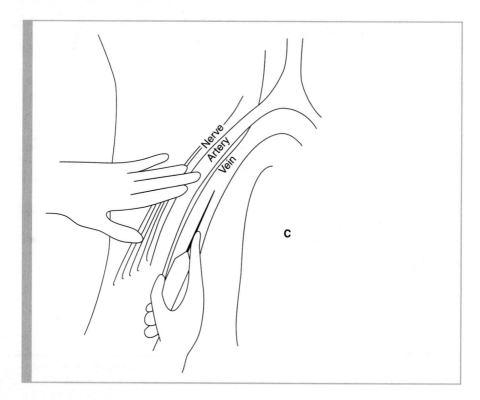

Use the history of the present illness, physical examination, and laboratory findings to determine the most likely category of the shock state. Most cases of hypovolemic and neurogenic shock are easily diagnosed from the history. Septic and anaphylactic shock are often more difficult to identify, since there may be little to no clues from the history. Cardiogenic shock can have many causes, traumatic and nontraumatic, and should be considered in each differential diagnosis.

Consider the early use of **echocardiography** and invasive monitors to help determine the category and the etiology of the hemodynamic failure.

■ DIFFERENTIAL DIAGNOSIS AND TREATMENT

Hypovolemic Shock

Manage first and foremost by volume resuscitation and control of the fluid loss. Attempt to infuse the type of fluid that has been lost. Thus, if there is an acute hemorrhage, transfuse blood and blood products. If there are losses from ileostomy output, replace with crystalloids rich in electrolytes.

In cases of blood loss, resuscitation must occur concurrently with attempts to **control hemorrhage**. This may include surgical procedures or endoscopic maneuvers in cases of gastrointestinal bleeding (see Chapter 13). In acute hemorrhage, balance the infusion of packed red cells with **fresh frozen plasma** and **platelet**

PULMONARY ARTERY CATHETERIZATION

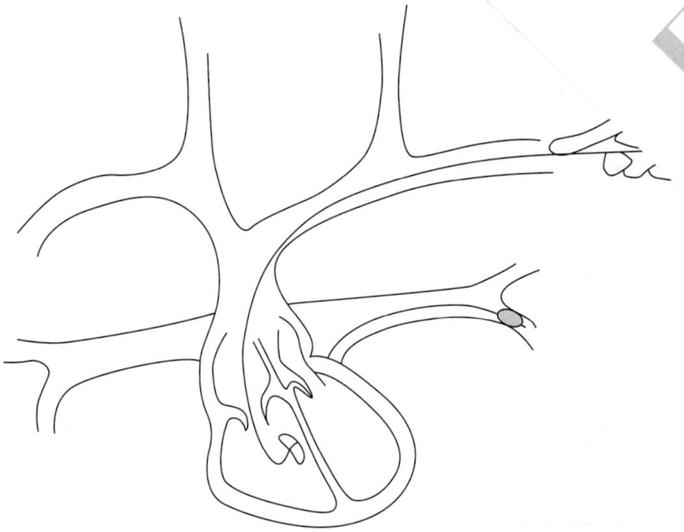

FIGURE 6-2
Proper Placement of the Pulmonary Artery Catheter

Pulmonary artery catheterization (PAC) is performed in the same sterile fashion as CVC insertion with the same full protective barrier (Figure 6-1). The catheter is inserted through an 8.5-French introducer sheath, which is already in place. Start by preparing the PAC by connecting and flushing all tubing. Transduce and zero all tubing prior to insertion. Test balloon by inflating and allow passive deflation.

Pass the catheter through the introducer sheath into the vein. The markings around the catheter indicate 10 cm increments from the tip. Once the catheter has entered venous circulation, approximately 15–20 cm, inflate the balloon with 1.5 cc of air. The balloon should stay inflated as you advance the catheter forward to encourage flow through the right ventricular outflow tract. Any time the catheter is pulled back, deflate the balloon to prevent damage to the valvular structures.

The catheter will advance through the right atrium, across the tricuspid valve, through the right ventricle, across the pulmonic valve, and into the pulmonary artery (PA) where it will wedge into the vascular bed of a branch of the pulmonary artery. Catheter position is determined by interpretation of the waveforms and pressure readings, as it moves through the heart and into the pulmonary circulation (Figure 6-3). Advancement past the PA position will result in a wedge tracing. Once a wedge trace is obtained, deflate the balloon. A PA waveform should return. Otherwise, the catheter has been advanced too far and can result in pulmonary arteriole occlusion and pulmonary infarct. Pull back the catheter slowly until a PA trace appears. Note the position of the catheter and secure. A chest radiograph should be obtained to confirm catheter position. The tip of the catheter should be no further than 3–5 cm from the midline. A daily chest radiograph should be obtained to detect catheter migration.

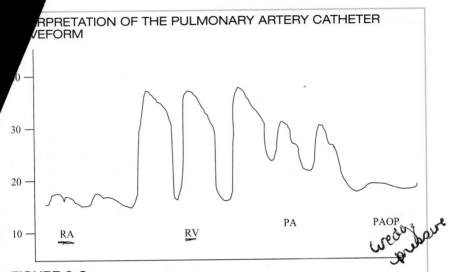

FIGURE 6-3
A Pulmonary Artery Catheter Waveform Tracing

As the tip of the PAC is introduced into the superior vena cava, a relatively flat wave is noted, which corresponds to the central venous pressure. As the catheter is advanced to approximately 30 cm, the waveform will change to reflect the **right atrial** (RA) pressure. The RA waveform is complex, with several ascending (a, v, c) and descending (x, y) waves. Once past the atrium, a dramatic **right ventricular** (RV) waveform is noted. The normal values of the RV pressure are 15–30 mm Hg systolic and 3–12 mm Hg diastolic. With continued advancement, the tip will follow the ventricular outflow into the PA. The PA waveform appears similar to the systemic arterial waveform with much lower pressures. Normal value of the pressures is systolic 15–30 and diastolic 6–16 mm Hg.

Once in the PA, the catheter is gently advanced into a point where forward flow of blood is temporarily obstructed, creating a static fluid column between the PAC tip and the left side of the heart. Here the **pulmonary artery occlusion pressure** (PAOP) or "wedge" pressure is measured. The waveform looks similar to the RA waveform, as it is reflecting atrial contractions from the left atrium. Once the PAOP is measured, the balloon is quickly released so as not to cause damage to the pulmonary artery with prolonged pressure. With release of the balloon, the PA waveform should return.

transfusion, as clinically indicated. For continued bleeding, consider infusion of recombinant **factor VIIa** as an adjunct to traditional resuscitation.

Cardiogenic Shock

Shock from heart failure most often occurs in the setting of an **acute myocardial infarction** (AMI) or an exacerbation of **CHF**. Standard advanced cardiac life support algorithms are recommended for treatment of dysrhythmias. Treatment is directed at re-establishing coronary flow and supporting the cardiac function.

For patients with AMI, consider **anticoagulation** and **antiplatelet** therapy with heparin and aspirin if there are no contraindications. Consider starting a **β-blocker** and **nitroglycerin** unless contraindicated because of hypotension or bradycardia. **Morphine** is recommended in small aliquots if the blood pressure will tolerate. It is utilized to decrease anxiety and to reduce the afterload of the left ventricle.

For unresponsive cardiogenic shock, consider **norepinephrine** for isolated blood pressure support. Dopamine is considered if the patient both requires blood pressure support and is bradycardic. Avoid isoproterenol because it increases myocardial oxygen demand. Consider a cardiology consult regarding an **intra-aortic balloon** pump for patients in refractory shock despite the above measures. All patients with AMI are considered for immediate **cardiac catheterization**. Also, a **cardiac surgery** consult for possible immediate coronary artery bypass grafting should be obtained. **Thrombolytic therapy** is an option if no other contraindications exist and cardiac catheterization and/or surgery are not immediately available.

Septic Shock

Suspect distributive shock in patients with hemodynamic failure and a confirmed or suspected infection. As in all types of shock, early treatment is fluid administration and resuscitation. ① infection

Use a **goal-directed therapy** by trending the central venous oxygen saturation and keeping the value >70%. Keep the mean arterial pressure >65 by using **norepinephrine** as the preferred vasopressor agent (see Chapter 9). Use the serum **lactate level** as a measure of the effectiveness of resuscitation. Use crystalloid infusions, vasopressors, and red blood cell transfusion (in that order) to keep lactate levels in the normal range. Consider **vasopressin** if the blood pressure is not responsive to escalating doses of norepinephrine. Draw **cultures** of the fluids and tissue most likely the cause of the sepsis. Start broad-spectrum **antibiotics** pending the results of the cultures. In patients with hypotension, who are unresponsive to both fluid resuscitation and vasopressor support, consider relative **adrenal insufficiency** and treatment with hydrocortisone.

NE → DA   crystalloids → vasopressor → RBC

Neurogenic and Anaphylactic

These are similar in that they both cause inappropriate vasodilation. The most common cause of neurogenic shock in the hospital setting is the effect of **epidural catheter** infusions. Neurogenic shock is also seen with acute **spinal cord injury** after trauma. Anaphylaxis can be seen in both the hospital and the emergency settings.

Anaphylactic shock is an antigen immunoglobulin E interaction, which causes the release of histamine, serotonin, and proteolytic enzymes resulting in hypotension and possible severe bronchospasm. The usual triggers include bees, insect bite, medications, and certain foods.

First, remove the **offending agent**. This could be stopping the epidural infusion or decontaminating the agent causing an allergic reaction. On account of **vasodilation**, these patients are relatively hypovolemic and thus receive **fluid resuscitation** as the initial therapy. Typically, vasodilation will cause a reflex tachycardia. In those with spinal cord injury, damage to the sympathetic system may cause a paradoxical bradycardia. For shock unresponsive to removing the offending agent or fluids, consider **vasopressor** support with one of the following: epinephrine, norepinephrine, or phenylephrine. Titrate the resuscitation to an acceptable urine output, blood pressure, and mental status. Consider **antihistamines** and **epinephrine** in patients with anaphylaxis (see Chapter 5).

Pulmonary Embolus

This is an uncommon cause of obstructive shock that must be considered in all patients with acute hemodynamic failure. The diagnosis is often made by a **CT angiogram** (CTA) of the chest but can also be seen on echocardiography or ventilation/perfusion scan. If there are no contraindications, start a bolus heparin drip infusion (see Chapter 5). Thrombolytics are considered in very unstable patients with no contraindications. Surgical pulmonary embolectomy can be used in very unstable patients with contraindications to thrombolytic therapy.

Pericardial Tamponade

Diagnosed by **echocardiogram**, this is often a complication of renal or metastatic disease or a result of trauma to the chest. An operative **pericardial window** is the definitive treatment; however, **pericardiocentesis** can be used as a temporizing measure in nonacutely injured patients. If neither of the above procedures is available, fluid administration can temporarily alleviate the hypotension by filling the right side of the heart.

Tension Pneumothorax

A tension pneumothorax is defined by hemodynamic failure associated with a lung collapse. Immediate treatment is indicated. Perform **needle thoracostomy** by placing a large-bore intravenous catheter in the second intercostal space at the mid-clavicular line (see Figure 5-3). The needle is removed, and the plastic angiocatheter is kept in the chest while a chest tube is placed. Definitive treatment for the pneumothorax is placement of a tube **thoracostomy** on the side of the collapse (see Figure 4-2).

Selected Readings

Cinel I, Dellinger RP. Advances in pathogenesis and management of sepsis [review]. *Curr Opin Infect Dis.* 2007;20(4):345–352.

Cohn SM. Potential benefit of vasopressin in resuscitation of hemorrhagic shock [review]. *J Trauma Injury Infect Crit Care.* 2007;62(6 Suppl):S56–S567.

Kelley DM. Hypovolemic shock: An overview [review]. *Crit Care Nurs Q.* 2005;28(1):2–19; quiz 20-1.

Otero RM, Nguyen HB, Huang DT, et al. Early goal-directed therapy in severe sepsis and septic shock revisited: Concepts, controversies, and contemporary findings [review]. *Chest. 2006;130(5):1579–1595.*

Shafi S, Kauder DR. Fluid resuscitation and blood replacement in patients with polytrauma [review]. *Clin Orthop Relat Res. 2004;(422):37–42.*

7

Fluid Imbalance

Heidi B. Nebelkopf Elgart, RN, MSN, CRNP ■ *Michael D. Grossman, MD, FACS*

Key Points

■ Preoperative evaluation of fluid balance is essential in preventing hypovolemia or hypoperfusion during induction of anesthesia and during the perioperative period.

■ The anesthetic record and nursing flow sheets provide valuable information regarding measurable and immeasurable losses to guide fluid resuscitation and maintain adequate fluid balance.

■ A combination of physical examination findings and laboratory studies is used to determine whether a patient has a volume deficit or an overload. No single laboratory study or examination finding alone is sensitive or specific enough to determine volume status.

■ A fluid challenge with direct, measurable end points may be indicated as the initial treatment for oliguria in the surgical patient. After the administration of 2 L of fluid in an undirected fashion, patients should be evaluated at the bedside.

■ Late postoperative hypovolemia is often caused by an underlying condition such as sepsis or fluid losses from a wound or fistula. These patients often need ongoing fluid replacement.

■ Hypervolemia occurs only when there is either cardiac or renal dysfunction. Once the cause of the fluid overload is determined, fluid restriction, diuresis, and dialysis are the therapeutic options.

■ MEDICAL HISTORY

If time allows, perform a preoperative evaluation in elective or semielective surgery patients for the purpose of identifying preoperative fluid status. The correction of **preoperative fluid deficit** is critical to minimizing during surgery where the induction of anesthesia produces vasodilatation, decreased systemic vascular resistance, and decreased venous return. This will cause patients who arrive at the operating room hypovolemic to become severely hypotensive during induction. Alternate agents that have less vasodilation, such as etomindate, may still result in hypotension by depressing the patient's sympathetic-adrenal mechanism.

Patients predisposed to preoperative hypovolemia include those with significant weight loss, as a result of cancer, gastrointestinal disease, or diuretic use. For at-risk patients, a **nutritional assessment** including evaluation of visceral proteins is valuable. A serum **albumin** less than 3 g/dL or serum **transferrin** less than 150 mg/dL can indicate severe nutritional and fluid derangements.

Preoperative nutritional and fluid status can also be altered by vomiting, diarrhea, diuretic use, polyuria, diaphoresis, hemorrhage, burns, and inadequate intake. **Bowel preparations** with hyperosmolar solutions can cause or exacerbate preoperative fluid losses. Prolonged periods of "nothing by mouth" prior to surgery often lead to preoperative fluid deficits. Chronically ill, hypermetabolic patients, whose operations are scheduled for the end of the day, may lose up to 2–3 L, appear stable, but develop profound hypotension with the induction of anesthesia.

Intraoperative intravascular volume is influenced by hemorrhage, loss of ascites or pleural fluid, and administration of large quantities of fluid into sites where absorption is excessive. Although intra- and postoperative fluid administrations are governed by invasive monitoring and resuscitation endpoints, anesthesiologists often use guidelines for intraoperative fluid replacements.

Postoperative fluid loss includes **blood loss**, which, in turn, is accompanied by redistribution of fluids and loss of additional extracellular and intracellular volume. To account for these shifts, a 3:1 ratio of crystalloid to blood loss is required to maintain the appropriate intravascular volume. Another fluid loss is "**third space losses**," caused by an internal translocation of sodium and water out of the vascular space into injured tissue and body cavities. Often these fluid losses exceed blood loss, especially in intra-abdominal procedures requiring extensive tissue dissection. Although it is often difficult to quantify fluid lost into these spaces, it is essential to replace the volume deficits perioperatively and immediately postoperatively, to minimize the physiologic changes induced by hypovolemia.

Urine output immediately reflects decreases in renal blood flow; thus, it is a valuable indicator of volume status. However, adequate urine output does not assure that intravascular volume is sufficient. Administration of diuretics, mannitol, or contrast agents during surgical procedures can all cause inappropriate high urine output.

Carefully review the flow sheet, anesthesia record, recovery area record, and patient-care record for **measurable losses**. Output totals should include urine, stool, vomitus, all tube drainage, and, if possible, a quantification of fluid lost in dressings. Even with a carefully documented flow sheet, net measurements of losses are not complete without consideration of the **immeasurable losses** such as fluid loss in stool, respiratory gas, and evaporation. Daily weights, laboratory tests, and invasive monitoring can be valuable tools to detect these discrepancies.

■ PHYSICAL EXAMINATION

Hypovolemia

Severe volume depletion often results in hypotension and shock, which can be easily recognized by a general examination. Modest hypovolemia is often harder to discern and may demonstrate more subtle findings. Inspect the patients for **skin changes** of cool, clammy, pale skin, with decreased or delayed capillary refill. In chronic depletion, find dry mucous membranes, loss of skin turgor, and absence of axillary sweat. Note changes in the **neurologic examination**, such as dizziness, weakness, syncope, lethargy, decreased deep tendon reflexes, or coma, all consistent with decreased cerebral perfusion. **Thirst** is another important finding which is present with as little as a 1%–2% change in serum osmolality.

Cardiovascular findings may include **tachycardia**, weak or thready peripheral pulses, narrow pulse pressure, and **hypotension**. Flat jugular neck veins may represent decreased venous filling. In addition, the patients may demonstrate anorexia, nausea, or vomiting. One of the most sensitive tests for detecting volume depletion is the evaluation of **orthostatic hypotension**. A fall in the systolic blood pressure by >15 mm Hg or an increase in the pulse by >15 beats per minute immediately after the position change suggests an intravascular volume deficit. Diabetes, Parkinson disease, antihypertensive agents, and other conditions can cause nonhypovolemic orthostasis.

Hypervolemia

In patients suspected of fluid overload, look for **edema** and **weight gain** as two of the most common presenting findings indicating excess volume. Dependent edema is often found in the lower extremities of ambulatory patients and in the buttocks and sacrum of bedridden patients. The pulmonary examination may reveal dyspnea, **crackles**, or wheezing. Recall that wheezing can be a sign of early fluid overload as the small bronchial airways swell and cause partial obstruction, a phenomenon often referred to as "cardiac asthma." Cardiovascular findings may include an S3 gallop, a **jugular vein distention**, hypertension, an increased pulse pressure, and the presence of hepatic congestion, as evidenced by the hepatojugular reflex evidenced by an increased jugular pressure induced by manual pressure over the liver.

■ LABORATORY STUDIES

Urine Studies

Order urinalysis and urine electrolytes to confirm physical findings, especially in assessing the presence and degree of volume depletion. Oliguria attributable to hypovolemia or a decrease in the effective perfusion of the kidney is termed **prerenal** failure. Oliguria attributable to disorders directly affecting the kidney, such as acute tubular necrosis, is termed **intrarenal** failure. During hypovolemia, aldosterone is secreted, which causes the reabsorption of sodium and chloride. Therefore, in volume-depleted patients, **urinary sodium** and **chloride** concentrations are usually less than 20 mEq/L. Another marker of renal perfusion or hypoperfusion is the measurement of the percentage of filtered sodium excreted in the urine, described as the **fractional excretion of sodium** (FE_{Na}). In prerenal hypovolemia, the FE_{Na} is less than 1% and may be as low as 0.5%. FE_{Na} can be used to differentiate between prerenal hypovolemia ($FE_{Na} < 1\%$) and renal causes of acute oliguric renal failure ($FE_{Na} \geq 2\%$).

Microscopic **urinalysis** may show hyaline and rare granular casts in patients with hypovolemia because of the concentration of the urine. **Urine osmolarity** greater than 500 mOsm/L or specific gravity greater than 1.020 indicates concentrated urine and may reflect hypovolemia in the presence of oliguria. Again, the renal response to volume depletion may be altered by the presence of diuretic use, solute diuresis, or acute/chronic renal failure.

Serum Studies

Order a **metabolic panel** and determine the urine **nitrogen-to-creatinine ratio** (BUN/Cr). In oliguric states, the urea absorption is enhanced, increasing the BUN level disproportionately to creatinine. Thus, a ratio of greater than 20 is often indicative of volume depletion. Caution should be used, however, in patients with liver disease or low dietary protein where the BUN may not be elevated. In catabolic states, or in the presence of gastrointestinal bleeding, the elevated BUN may signify nitrogen breakdown rather than volume depletion.

Determine the sodium level as a marker for **osmolality** or tonicity. The calculation for serum osmolality is $OSM = 2 (Na + K) + Glucose/18 + Urea/2.8$. Serum that is hyperosmolar (>300 mOsm/L) indicates hypovolemia, whereas serum that is hypoosmolar (<240 mOsm/L) may indicate fluid excess.

Determine the **base deficit** as an early indicator of the relative magnitude of intravascular volume depletion, resulting in decreased perfusion and tissue oxygen debt. Base deficit has been shown to increase with ongoing bleeding and to decrease with volume replacement. Therefore, it is used as a guide to determine the adequacy of volume administration and resuscitation. Alternatively, order a **lactate** level as the most sensitive test for poor tissue perfusion and cellular hypoxia. Lactate levels above four are abnormal, and, more importantly, a trend of rising lactate raises the concern of inadequate resuscitation.

In patients with hypervolemia, order a **beta-naturetic peptide** (BNP). An elevated BNP (above 500) may indicate active congestive heart failure, associated with fluid retention.

■ RADIOGRAPHIC AND INVASIVE STUDIES

Order a **chest X-ray** (CXR). In early stages of volume overload, there may be minimal findings on CXR. However, sequential CXRs can be useful in assessing the volume status of critically ill patients by providing information about the fullness of the pulmonary vasculature and the presence or absence of interstitial fluid in the lungs. As volume overload progresses, fluid in the interlobular septa at the lateral aspects of the lungs (Kerley B lines) may be seen. With pronounced volume overload, fluid accumulates in the alveolar spaces and frank pulmonary edema is noted (Chapter 5).

Consider **echocardiography** (ECHO) as a bedside, noninvasive test to determine volume status and ventricular performance. It can theoretically differentiate types of ventricular dysfunction (systolic vs. diastolic heart failure) and allows assessment of valvular abnormalities in a precise fashion. ECHO is not presently available on a continuous basis so that minute-to-minute changes cannot be identified. In general, if there is a question as to the adequacy of cardiac function in a patient known to be euvolemic, ECHO can provide the information more easily and accurately than pulmonary artery catheter (PAC). However, for ongoing analysis of oxygen delivery and the impact of fluid challenges on delivery and consumption, PAC may be preferable.

Determine the need for a **central venous pressure** (CVP) monitor. Central venous catheters allow direct measurement of pressures in the large central veins (Figure 6-1). CVP indirectly reflects the right atrial pressure and preload. Values between 8 and 12 mm Hg are considered "normal" filling pressures. CVP may be elevated in right ventricular infarction, pericardial tamponade, or mechanical ventilation with high intrathoracic pressure. A low CVP almost always indicates a low intravascular volume state.

Consider placement of a **PAC** for continuous determination of the **cardiac output** and **oxygen delivery** (Figure 6-3). A PAC might be appropriate if the differential diagnosis includes heart failure or sepsis with the need for inotropic support. In these cases, a patient with high filling pressures and low cardiac output can be diagnosed with myocardial pump dysfunction or failure. Conversely, a patient with low filling pressures and low cardiac output should respond to volume infusions ("preload"), with an increase in cardiac output.

The adequacy of cardiac output to provide tissue perfusion is generally measured by oxygen delivery and indirectly measured by the saturation of mixed venous blood. **Mixed venous oxygen** saturation below 60% almost always indicates inadequate oxygen delivery because of hypovolemia, poor pump function, or low hemoglobin. When mixed venous oxygen saturations are very high (>75%), oxygen utilization in the tissues is often inadequate; thus, despite adequate intravascular volume and cardiac output, patients may have oliguria and organ dysfunction. Examples include inflammatory states such as severe trauma, burns, pancreatitis, and sepsis.

■ DIAGNOSTIC PLAN

Diagnosis of fluid imbalance should focus on the deficit or excess of **intravascular** fluid. In the perioperative period, the practitioner will most often be called upon to evaluate **oliguria** alone or in association with changes in heart rate and blood pressure. On occasion, evaluation of high rates of urine flow requires the practitioner to differentiate the mobilization of fluid from true polyuria. **Hypervolemia** is typically seen later in the hospital course but can be present early in some patients such as those with primary cardiac dysfunction.

In the postoperative review, diagnostic evaluation begins with history, with special attention to the **anesthetic record**. This will provide information on the duration of the procedure, type and volume of fluid administered, blood loss, and urine output. Additional information regarding periods of intraoperative hypotension, aortic cross clamping, and medications administered (diuretics, vasopressors, and steroids) provides clues to help differentiate renal, myocardial, or endocrine disorders from hypovolemia.

If the patient presents with **oliguria**, order a **fluid challenge** consisting of 250–500 cc of normal saline or lactated ringers solution. Assure that there is a direct measurable **endpoint** for the fluid challenge and time frame for its achievement. For example, set an increase of urine output greater than or equal to 0.3–0.5 cc/kg for the next 30–60 minutes as a positive response. Consider administering no more than 2 L of undirected fluid replacement, in 500–1000 cc increments, for more than 2 hours. If the urine output does not respond, it is considered a failed fluid challenge.

A **failed fluid challenge** requires an interval history (review of all flow sheets) and a bedside examination of the patient. The examination focuses on clues differentiating intravascular volume depletion from excess. **Heart rate** can be relatively **nonspecific** in patients on beta-blockers. New-onset atrial fibrillation may suggest atrial stretch associated with volume overload or may simply reflect catecholamine surges. **Blood pressure** is not helpful as a discriminate variable unless it is abnormally low. In these cases, the practitioner is obligated to exclude shock caused by bleeding, sepsis, obstruction, or cardiac dysfunction.

Form a working diagnosis as to whether the patient is "**wet or dry**" and whether the overall clinical picture is consistent with **acute renal failure** rather than the manifestations of **hypovolemia,** because these clinical conditions necessitate different treatments. Adjunctive laboratory studies are indicated for any patient with hypotension and oliguria and are strongly considered for any patient who is anuric despite diagnostic fluid challenges.

Recall that there is no single laboratory test that, by itself, provides a high level of sensitivity or specificity for the diagnosis of volume depletion or fluid overload. These tests, alone or in combination, should be interpreted along with history and physical findings. In general, for a patient in whom the diagnosis is in doubt, order a limited or basic **chemistry** profile including electrolytes, BUN, creatinine, and glucose. **Urine studies** can be sent for electrolytes and osmolarity. **Lactate levels** can also be very useful.

If the presence of intravascular fluid status remains unclear, consider performing an **ECHO** to assess preload and cardiac function. If fluid shifts continue, and a continuous monitor of fluid status is needed, consider placing a **CVP** catheter or **PAC**. Values from the CVP or PAC are trended over time to show the result of volume resuscitation.

It is important to remember that **peripheral edema** may falsely suggest the presence of volume overload when intravascular volume is actually low or normal. Major surgery, trauma, sepsis, and other inflammatory conditions promote an endocrine and immunologic environment in which the sodium and water are avidly retained. Third space losses into soft tissues, abdomen, and retroperitoneum account for increased volume requirements in these patients.

■ DIFFERENTIAL DIAGNOSIS AND TREATMENT

Early Postoperative Hypovolemia

This is a group of potential diagnoses that include bleeding, third-space losses, and inadequate volume replacement during surgery. These conditions are most commonly encountered in the early postoperative period, although bleeding could be encountered at any time. In an oliguric postsurgical patient, fluid challenge of 2–3 L normal saline or lactated ringers may be administered without adjunctive testing. If the patient has not responded toward the end of this challenge and/or is experiencing additional symptoms, adjunctive testing is mandatory. Rule out significant **blood loss** as a cause of hypovolemia. Review the hemoglobin trend and assure that coagulopathies have been corrected. Check surgical drains and wounds for evidence of bleeding or ecchymosis formation around wound sites.

Late Postoperative Hypovolemia

Vomiting, diarrhea, excessive nasogastric (NG) losses, free water deficits secondary to tube feeding, ascites formation, and wound losses, all contribute to fluid loss days or weeks after surgery. Such patients might be oliguric on the third to fifth postoperative day, perhaps even later if diarrhea has developed or an NG has been reinserted.

As with early postoperative oliguria, begin treatment with an initial **fluid challenge**. Reviewing the clinical course may reveal a history of recent diarrhea or large-volume NG losses. The presence of a large, draining wound will be obvious, and, in the case of negative pressure dressings, output can be quantified. Order replacement intravenous fluids to balance chronic outputs such as urine, NG, wound, or rectal losses.

Unlike the early postoperative patient where normal saline or lactated ringers are infused indiscriminately, review the **electrolytes** to guide the choice of fluid replacement and need for supplementation. Patients with excessive NG losses may develop a **contraction alkalosis** through the loss of hydrogen from the stomach and a compensatory loss of potassium from the kidney. NG losses should be replaced with half-normal saline and potassium. **Diarrhea** may produce low serum bicarbonate and a compensatory increase in chloride. Lactated ringers will replace lost bicarbonate and facilitate excretion of chloride. In patients receiving **tube feeds,** a free water deficit is associated with hypovolemia and oliguria; serum sodium is elevated, and a free water deficit should be calculated and replaced with quarter normal saline or 5% dextrose in water. The deficit should be replaced within 48–72 hours, and only half the deficit should be replaced in the first 24 hours.

In patients with **complex wounds,** losing large volumes of protein-rich serum, fluid replacement may contain colloid solutions such as **albumin** or hetastarch. No independent benefit from albumin administration can be demonstrated for routine volume replacement, but patients with an albumin <1.0 and ongoing protein losses may benefit from albumin administration.

Patients who have a history of **ascites** formation prior to surgery will be more predisposed to reaccumulation of ascites in the postoperative period. The hormonal environment in the immediate postoperative period favors retention of sodium and free water. Examples of patients who may have ascites, or may be predisposed to form ascites, are patients with cirrhosis, intra-abdominal malignancy (particularly ovarian cancer), pancreatitis, portal vein thrombosis, and severe malnutrition. Attempt to **minimize salt load** while balancing free water against declining serum sodium. Thus, frequent checks of electrolytes may be helpful. Consider **colloid solutions** that are suspended in saline but contain a large volume of oncotically active solutes relative to salt concentration. The reformation of ascites is usually demonstrable on physical examination and may amount to many liters of fluid. If in doubt after more than 3–4 L of crystalloid have been given, and the patient remains oliguric, abdominal ultrasound may be helpful to confirm the formation of ascites. Only after adequate volume replacement is established by CVP should diuresis be attempted to augment urine output. Administration of diuretics in cirrhotic patients who have low intravascular volume may precipitate a hepatorenal syndrome that is difficult to reverse and leads to acute renal failure.

Relative Hypovolemia

This occurs when there is an increase in the effective blood volume such as **vasodilatation**. A group of conditions can produce this finding including sepsis, pancreatitis, severe trauma associated with systemic inflammatory response syndrome, and neurogenic vasodilatation as a result of epidural catheter use or spinal shock. Vasodilatation occurs in these conditions for complex reasons related to inflammatory mediators or neuroendocrine dysfunction so that a given volume of blood is now distributed through a larger circulatory capacity. Thus, blood pressure and renal perfusion pressure fall, producing oliguria. Patients may present with this clinical picture at any time in the pre- and postoperative continuum.

Look for obvious conditions in the **history,** such as trauma, an active infection, or recently diagnosed pancreatitis. The **physical examination** findings are often warm, well-perfused extremities with bounding pulses, while patients with typical hypovolemia are usually cool with thready pulses. The presence of a fever or hypothermia is also suggestive of sepsis or SIRS. **Laboratory** findings are usually abnormal; elevated or depressed white blood cell count is suggestive but nonspecific; and an elevated lactate level indicates a more severe or decompensated condition. Oliguria in sepsis or SIRS responds initially to fluids because the circulatory capacity is expanded so there is both a relative and absolute hypovolemia. Unlike patients with isolated volume deficits, volume alone often does not correct oliguria and hypotension in patients with sepsis and SIRS. Use caution not to be overaggressive in providing volume resuscitation alone in these patients, without more invasive monitoring and assessment of CVP and mixed venous oxygen saturation. No more than 2–3 L of crystalloid should be given without additional monitoring.

Neuroendocrine causes of oliguria include **spinal shock** associated with trauma and vasomotor dysfunction associated with **epidural catheters.** These disorders are included in the section with inflammatory disorders because they are also characterized by relative and actual volume deficits for which IV fluids are the best initial therapy but are usually inadequate as an isolated therapy. Both neurogenic shock and **vasomotor paralysis** are characterized by loss of sympathetic tone in precapillary arteriolar sphincters, leading to vasodilatation, drop in blood pressure, and decrease in effective arterial blood volume perfusing the kidney. Clinical trials of volume infusion are usually ineffective in elevating blood pressure; discontinuation of the **epidural catheter** may be ineffective if the medications are long acting and the benefits of the catheter will be lost. A low dose of a weak vasopressor such as phenylephrine is usually effective in raising blood pressure and renal perfusion pressure.

Neurogenic shock because of **spinal cord injury** presents with hypotension and patients are often bradycardic, if the level of injury is mid-thoracic or higher owing to interruption of sympathetic outflow to the heart. The skin is also warm and well perfused, provided no other injuries that produce blood loss exist. Again, isolated volume supplementation is rarely helpful and potentially harmful, as it may lead to increased swelling in the injured spinal cord. Vasopressors are almost always effective in these cases.

Relative or absolute **adrenal insufficiency** has been recognized with increased frequency in recent years. A history of recent steroid use should prompt consideration of this diagnosis. Sepsis, trauma, and other critical illnesses may precipitate relative adrenal insufficiency in patients with no antecedent history. Relative insufficiency is defined by the inability to mount an appropriate adrenal response in the setting of increased physiologic stress. Patients may be hypotensive, bradycardic, and hypothermic and may demonstrate electrolyte abnormalities including hyponatremia, hyperkalemia, and hypoglycemia. The condition is defined by a low **baseline cortisol** level, particularly in stressed patients, or failure to respond to a provocative dose of adrenocorticotrophic hormone (cosyntropin stim test).

Hypervolemia

Cardiac

Relative fluid overload occurs when there is inappropriate retention of fluid. In general, a patient with healthy kidneys and a normal heart will excrete excess fluids and will not present with hypervolemia. Thus, the presence of hypervolemia will prompt a search for a cardiac or renal dysfunction.

Disturbances of **cardiac pump** function, including congestive heart failure, acute myocardial ischemia or infarction, and pericardial tamponade, produce oliguria by **decreased perfusion** of the kidney. Perioperative cardiac ischemia events occur most commonly following major procedures, particularly those that are emergent, and usually between the third and fifth postoperative day. Any history of intra- or postoperative hypotension should elicit suspicion. Known history of preoperative ventricular dysfunction with an ejection fraction below 35% or treatment for congestive heart failure is associated with the possibility of exacerbation after surgery.

Patients may appear anxious and in cases of **CHF** will almost always complain of shortness of breath. The skin is often cool, and peripheral pulses may be thready. Important studies include a 12-lead EKG and laboratory tests including troponin and BNP. A normal BNP virtually excludes CHF, whereas a value above 600–800 is highly suggestive of active heart failure. ECHO is extremely helpful in the setting of suspected pump dysfunction and excludes **pericardial tamponade** if no effusion is seen.

Renal

Abnormal **excretory function** represents a common group of disorders producing oliguria with euvolemia and normal pump function. Urinary excretion may be impaired anywhere from the urethral meatus to the kidneys, caused by mechanical or pathophysiologic processes. Common mechanical obstructions include prostatic hypertrophy in males or obstructed Foley catheters. Physical examination reveals a restless, distressed patient with a distended lower abdomen. If available, a bladder scan confirms the diagnosis, otherwise a catheter should be placed for diagnosis.

Acute renal failure that occurs in the perioperative period is most often caused by **acute tubular necrosis (ATN)**. Determine if there is a history of previous renal insufficiency or chronic nonoliguric renal failure. Advanced age, diabetes, hypertension, and peripheral vascular disease are common associations with acute and chronic renal failure. Search for evidence of perioperative hypotension, aortic clamping proximal to the renal arteries, history of rhabdomyolysis, intravenous contrast, and certain nephrotoxic medications such as aminoglycosides and NSAIDS increases the suspicion of acute renal failure.

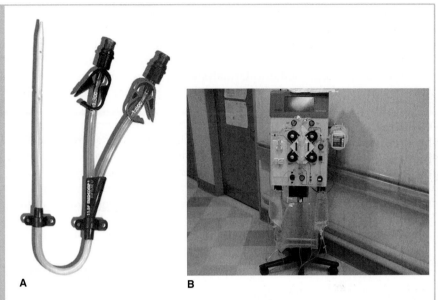

A   B

FIGURE 7-1
Continuous Renal Replacement Therapy

Continuous renal replacement therapy (CRRT) is indicated for patients who meet the criteria for HD but cannot tolerate traditional HD because of hemodynamic instability. CRRT prevents abrupt shifts in fluid balance, acid–base balance, and electrolytes by slowly adjusting fluid removal, electrolytes, and pH for a 24-hour period. Candidates for CRRT include unstable patients with volume overload and acute renal failure, life-threatening electrolyte imbalance, or drug overdose. CRRT can be administered through two options: an arteriovenous or a venovenous circuit. The venovenous technique is used most commonly in the intensive care unit. A dual lumen large bore (11.5–13.5 French) catheter is inserted into a large central vein, similar to a standard central line placement (A). The most common sites are the internal jugular, subclavian, or femoral veins. Ideal site selection is similar to site selection for central line placement. Blood is then removed via one lumen, run through the CRRT machine, and returned via the second lumen (B).

There are four types of dialysis utilized for CRRT, depending on the treatment goals. **Slow continuous ultrafiltration** (SCUF) is a method for removing fluid only and is indicated for patients with volume overload without uremia or significant electrolyte imbalance. Fluid is typically removed at the rate of 100 cc/h or more, depending on the hemodynamic status of the patient. **Continuous venovenous hemofiltration** (CVVH) uses replacement fluid to remove large solutes and is indicated for patients with severe pH or electrolyte disturbances with or without fluid overload. **Continuous venovenous hemodialysis** (CVVHD) is similar to CVVH but uses dialysate to remove small- to medium-sized molecules. **Continuous venovenous hemodiafiltration** (CVVHDF) uses both dialysate and replacement fluid to effectively remove solutes with minimal or positive net fluid balance for the patient.

Typically, there are no specific findings on **physical examination** suggesting acute renal failure in the absence of fluid overload that produces pulmonary edema. **Laboratory** findings include a rise in creatinine and BUN, where the ratio of BUN to creatinine remains below 20, and hyperkalemia; urine electrolytes demonstrate high urine sodium. **Urinalysis** may show tubular casts consistent with a diagnosis of acute tubular necrosis. In the presence of normal to slightly increased volume as measured by a CVP above 12–15 and normal pump function assessed by PAC or ECHO, a trial of **diuresis** is warranted.

In oliguric patients, determine if there are indications for acute **hemodialysis** (HD) including hyperkalemia, metabolic acidosis, volume overload, severe uremia, and pericardial effusions. In hemodynamically unstable patients, consider CRRT as an option (Figure 7-1). CRRT effectively removes volume and solute but does so at a slower rate and over a longer time frame as compared to standard HD.

Selected Readings

Bendjelid K, Romand JA. Fluid responsiveness in mechanically ventilated patients: A review of indices used in intensive care. *Intens Care Med.* 2003;29:352–360.

Cohen AJ. Physiologic concepts in the management of renal, fluid and electrolyte disorders in the intensive care unit. In: Irwin RS, Ripple JM, eds. *Intensive Care Medicine.* Philadelphia: Lippincott Williams & Wilkins; 2003.

Goodrich C. Endpoints of resuscitation: What should we be monitoring? *AACN Adv Crit Care.* 2006;17(3):306–316.

8

Changes in Mental Status

Eileen Maloney-Wilensky, MSN, APRN, BC ■ *Joshua M. Levine, MD*

Key Points

- Consciousness (*mental status*) is defined by the components of wakefulness and awareness. The components of consciousness involve higher cortical functions and include all the mental tasks at the cerebral level.

- Disturbances of arousal and wakefulness imply dysfunction of either the bihemispheric cortex or the brainstem and thalami.

- Documentation of the time intervals between changes in mental status will enable the practitioner to determine if a change is rapid or slow and which symptoms varied over time.

- Sedation may cloud the assessment of the patient and should be stopped or decreased when evaluating mental status.

- Neurologic examination of the coma patient focuses on four elements: determination of the patient's level of arousal (wakefulness), examination of the eyes, elicitation of motor responses and abnormal reflexes, and observation of breathing patterns.

- Focal neurologic signs or abnormalities of the pupillary light reflex suggest a structural cause of coma.

■ Brain death refers to irreversible cessation of whole-brain activity and is a clinical diagnosis. The three cardinal features of brain death are coma, absence of brainstem reflexes, and apnea.

■ MEDICAL HISTORY

Review the **medical record** for clues to the etiology of altered mental status. Especially pertinent are a recent onset of atrial fibrillation that could account for a new embolism and cerebrovascular event, new medications orders such as narcotics or benzodiazepines (BDZ) that may have caused lethargy and somnolence, or a new anticoagulant medication that leads to a cerebral hemorrhage.

Clarify the **history of present illness** to establish the time course and tempo of the mental status change. A rapid onset of deep obtundation could be characteristic of an embolism or thrombosis; a slow onset of lethargy and confusion may be related to electrolyte imbalances or intensive care psychosis.

Perform a thorough review of the **past medical history**. Neurologic conditions such as Parkinson's disease, multiple sclerosis, and amyotrophic lateral sclerosis (ALS) are uncommon causes of mental status changes. Survey the history for nonneurologic diseases such as cancer (metastasis), heart disease (embolism), peripheral vascular disease (carotid occlusion), and drug and alcohol abuse (withdrawal syndrome).

Review all **medication orders**, including confirmation of the actual time and dose administered by reviewing the nursing medication log. In every patient, consider a medication reaction as a reason for change in mental status. Review the home medication list for additional, possible contributors to mental status change. For patients in the outpatient or emergency department setting, note the date and time of the most recent ingestion of **alcohol** or other recreational drug use. For patients who are admitted, always consider surreptitious ingestion of recreational substances while in the hospital.

■ PHYSICAL EXAMINATION

Start the physical examination by assessing the **level of consciousness**. Patients who exhibit spontaneous opening of the eyes, verbalization attempts, moaning, tossing, reaching, leg crossing, yawning, coughing, or swallowing have a higher level of consciousness than those who do not.

Assess the patient's response to a series of stimuli that escalate in intensity. First, look for a **verbal response** by calling the patient's name loudly. If there is no response, stimulate the patient by gentle shaking. If the patient does not respond, attempt to elicit a **pain response** by using a noxious stimulus, such as pressure to the supraorbital ridge, nail beds, or sternum. Possible responses to painful stimuli, in the order of the most obtunded to most alert, are no response, grimacing, eye opening, grunting, nonpurposeful movements, purposeful actions, and verbalization.

Checking the **motor responses** provides information about not only sensation and limb strength but also level of consciousness. The highest function is seen when stimuli produce **purposeful** movements, such as reaching for an endotracheal tube with the intent to pull it out. **Localization** is defined as a nonstereotyped limb movement, such as reaching toward the site of stimulation, which implies a degree of intact cortical function. Sometimes such movements can resemble stereotypical or reflex movements. A noxious stimulus may need to be applied above and below the limb to differentiate reflex from purposeful and localization movements. **Nonpurposeful** responses, which could include stereotyped limb movements, are generally mediated by brain and spinal reflexes and do not require cortical input. Examples include extension and internal rotation of the limbs (**decerebrate** posturing), upper extremity flexion (**decorticate** posturing), and flexion at the ankle, knee, and hip (**triple flexion**). Movement of a limb toward a noxious stimulus is usually reflexive and may assist in the assessment of mental status.

Use the **Glasgow Coma Scale** (GCS) (Table 8-1) as a global measure of consciousness. The GCS is a quick, reliable, and widely accepted tool for evaluation of consciousness and predicting survival and neurologic outcome in the general

TABLE 8-1.
The Glasgow Coma Scale

Motor response	
Follows commands	6
Localizes pain	5
Withdraws to pain	4
Flexion	3
Extension	2
None	1
Verbal response	
Oriented	5
Confused speech	4
Inappropriate words	3
Incomprehensible	2
None	1
Eye opening	
Spontaneous	4
To command	3
To pain	2
None	1

Adapted from Teasdale G, Jennett B. Assessment of coma and impaired consciousness. A practical Scale. Lancet. 1974;2:81–84.

critically ill population. Limitation of the GCS includes its insensitivity to subtle variations in mental status or some signs of a major stroke without loss of consciousness, such as hemiplegia. In addition, the GCS has limited utility in patients with aphasia, with significant facial trauma, or who are sedated or intubated. Despite its limitations, the GCS is a mainstay of clinical assessment that aids in communication, prognostication, and research on mental status.

Ascertain the patients' **orientation** by having them state who they are, where they are, and the date. Patients who can answer all three are said to be alert and oriented by three parameters, or "A/O × 3." As orientation becomes impaired, patients generally forget the date (A/O × 2) and location (A/O × 1) before their name (A/O × 0).

If patients are awake and alert, then the testing of higher cortical function is undertaken. Test immediate, short-term, and long-term **memories**. Ask the patients to recall the examiner's name, once introduced (immediate); name their primary physician or a specific fact related to current medical event (recent); and state a long-term memory fact such as naming the sitting president, wedding/anniversary date, or telephone number. **Attention** and **concentration** are assessed by asking the patients to spell or count backward, count by serial 7s, or, if too difficult, serial 3s. Also, it is worthwhile to observe the patients' responses to distractions in the environment.

Language is one of the highest levels of function and can provide clues to the subtle cortical dysfunction. Observe the patient for clarity, fluency, quantity, tone, content, and pace. Note spontaneity of speech and patient response, and the patient's awareness of any deficit. **Aphasia** is an inability to communicate and can be expressive (impaired language output) or receptive (impaired language input). **Dysarthria** is impaired movement of speech musculature, leading to loss of clear articulation, phonation, and breath control.

The **eye examination** is extremely important in neurologic assessment because it can provide substantial information on neurologic function and pathologic causes of mental status disturbances. The eye examination starts with a **pupillary examination** where pupillary size, shape, and reactivity to light are assessed. Abnormalities of the pupillary **light reflex** suggest a structural abnormality. Although certain drugs may also affect the pupillary light reflex, metabolic causes of coma do not typically affect the pupils. The pupils are normally round, have equal diameters, and briskly constrict when illuminated. When unequal pupils (anisocoria) are observed, establish whether it is the larger or the smaller pupil that is abnormal. Examine the eyes both in the light and in the dark. When the lights are extinguished, an abnormally small pupil will fail to dilate fully and the degree of anisocoria will increase. When the abnormal pupil is the larger one, the degree of anisocoria will be maximal under full illumination when the larger pupil fails to constrict fully.

In the intensive care unit (ICU), the most important cause of a unilaterally dilated pupil is a compressive lesion of the oculomotor nerve complex, such as an **uncal herniation** or intracranial aneurysms. Complete **third nerve palsy** results in ipsilateral mydriasis, inferolateral deviation of the eye, and a severe ipsilateral ptosis. The most important cause of unilateral small pupil is the **Horner's**

syndrome, which includes miosis, mild ipsilateral ptosis, and occasionally ipsilateral hemianhidrosis. Bilaterally **fixed and dilated** pupils are seen in the terminal stages of brain death or with the use of anticholinergic medications, such as atropine. **Hyperadrenergic** states such as pain, anxiety, and cocaine intoxication produce bilaterally large and reactive pupils. Reactive **pinpoint** (<1 mm) pupils are observed with opioid and barbiturate intoxication or after extensive pontine injury. Occasionally, a magnifying lens may be needed to appreciate reactivity with such small pupils.

Observe the resting eye **position** and eye **movements**. Horizontal or vertical misalignment of the eyes implies ocular muscle injury or disease; spontaneous roving or rhythmic and repetitive movements can be seen in inner ear dysfunction and intoxication. The frontal lobe cortex (frontal eye fields) mediates **conjugate deviation** of the eyes toward the contralateral side. Lateral deviation of both eyes indicates either a destructive lesion in the ipsilateral (side to which eyes are directed) frontal lobe or an excitatory focus (seizure) in the contralateral hemisphere. In the critically ill comatose patients, there is a high incidence of nonconvulsive seizures, and jerking movements of the eyes may be the only evidence of seizure activity. If spontaneous eye movements are absent, then an **oculocephalic response** (doll's eyes) should be sought by turning the head horizontally and vertically. Normally, the eyes move in the opposite direction of head turning. If an oculocephalic response cannot be elicited or is contraindicated because of possible cervical spine instability, then an **oculovestibular** (cold caloric) response is sought.

The retina should be examined by performing a fundoscopic examination, looking for signs of intracranial hypertension. For example, **papilledema** is swelling of the optic nerve head from increased intracranial pressure. It is almost always bilateral and may be accompanied by retinal hemorrhages, exudates, and cotton wool spots, and ultimately by enlargement of the optic cup. Papilledema develops over hours to days, and its absence does not imply normal intracranial pressure, especially in the acute setting. **Terson's syndrome** is vitreous, subhyaloid, or retinal hemorrhage associated with subarachnoid hemorrhage.

Test the **corneal reflex** by gently touching the cornea of each eye with a drop of saline or a cotton wisp and observe for eyelid closure. Failure of unilateral eyelid closure suggests facial nerve dysfunction on that side. Failure of bilateral eyelid closure usually implies pontine dysfunction.

The symmetry of **motor responses** and **reflexes**, and the presence of abnormal movements, often allows discrimination between structural and systemic etiologies of altered mental status. Observe the patient for any abnormal or spontaneous movements. **Asterixis** implies a metabolic disturbance such as uremia or hepatic encephalopathy. **Twitching** or jerking of the face or limbs, even if subtle, raises the suspicion for seizures. **Asymmetry** of resting limb position is frequently a subtle sign of weakness. For example, a paretic leg will lie externally rotated. To further evaluate the patient, stimulate the patient and observe for asymmetry in the patient's face (grimace) and appendicular motor responses. A less vigorous response on one side of the body may indicate a contralateral structural lesion involving the motor pathways above the level of the caudal medulla. **Paraparesis** or **paraplegia** raises the possibility of spinal cord injury, especially in the trauma setting.

Disturbances in breathing patterns are often seen in neurologic injury and illness, although they are often obscured by the use of sedatives, paralytics, and mechanical ventilation. **Apneustic** respirations are characterized by a prolonged end-inspiratory pause. This pattern may be seen after focal injury to the dorsal lower half of the pons (e.g., stroke) but may also be observed with meningitis, hypoxia, and hypoglycemia. **Cluster** breathing consists of several rapid, shallow breaths followed by a prolonged pause and localizes to the upper medulla. **Apnea** may be seen in a variety of neurologic and nonneurologic disorders and is of no localizing value. **Kussmaul's respirations** are rapid, deep breaths that usually signal metabolic acidosis, but may also be observed with pontomesencephalic lesions. **Cheyne–Stokes respiration** refers to alternating spells of apnea and crescendo–decrescendo hyperpnea. It has minimal value in localization and is seen with diffuse cerebral injury, hypoxia, hypocapnea, and congestive heart failure.

■ LABORATORY STUDIES

Order a **CBC** to determine if there is a leukocytosis that may indicate an active infection. A very low hemoglobin level may cause lethargy and mental status change. Evaluate the **electrolyte panel**, with special attention to the blood glucose. Both hyperglycemia and hypoglycemia can cause neurologic symptoms. Patients who are acutely obtunded should have a finger-stick glucose checked immediately to identify and treat hypoglycemia. **Serum electrolytes** are examined for evidence of hyponatremia, hypercalcemia, hyperkalemia, and severe hypophosphatemia. Examine the **liver function tests** to exclude the presence of liver disease that may lead to hyperammonimia. If indicated, an ammonia level is ordered. Elevations in the **blood urea nitrogen** and **creatinine** are evidence of uremic encephalopathy. Consider ordering **thyroid function tests**. Hypothyroid conditions can lead to a slow progression of lethargy, whereas hyperthyroid states can produce hyperactivity or delirium-type states.

Consider an **arterial blood gas** in patients with respiratory symptoms or those with obtundation of unclear etiology to rule out hypercapnea and hypoxemia. Obtain a **toxicology screen** since intoxication from opioids, alcohol salicylates, barbiturates, BDZ can all cause significant neurologic symptoms.

For patients suspected of having infection as a cause of the mental status change, perform an infection workup. Order blood, urine, and sputum **cultures**. In cases where meningitis or encephalitis is suspected, obtain **CSF cultures**. This is crucial in patients who present with altered mental status, fever, and seizures. Always consider **occult infections**, such as intra-abdominal abscesses, sinusitis, prostatitis, and infection related to foreign bodies, such as orthopedic prosthesis or artificial heart valves.

■ RADIOGRAPHIC AND DIAGNOSTIC STUDIES

A **head CT** (HCT) is the gold-standard radiographic test for mental status changes. The HCT is the initial test because of its widespread availability, the rapidity with which images may be obtained, and the ease with which critically ill patients may be monitored during scanning. Although the HCT is ideal for detecting intra- and extra-axial blood, skull fractures, intracranial air, hydrocephalus, and metallic foreign bodies, it is less sensitive for detecting brain infarction, edema, and other structural abnormalities.

Consider a **magnetic resonance imaging** (MRI) for better visualization of neuroanatomic structures, particularly the brainstem and cerebellum. MRI is more sensitive than CT for detecting ischemia or infarction, edema, diffuse axonal injury, brain tumors, infection, abscesses, and cerebral venous sinus thrombosis. Both HCT and MRI have limitations, and some significant disease states can be present even with negative studies. These include metabolic processes, status epilepticus, hypoxic–ischemic encephalopathy, and diffuse axonal injury.

Investigate the **cerebral vasculature** as necessary with CT angiogram, MR angiogram, or conventional cerebral angiography. MR angiogram provides anatomical information about carotid and cerebral vessels without the need for nephrotoxic intravenous dye. Conventional angiogram has the advantage of possible therapeutic interventions such as embolization and carotid stenting.

Electroencephalography (EEG) is ordered when there is a suspicion of seizure activity. Continuous monitoring may be necessary to establish evidence of seizure and status epilepticus in patients who are obtunded or chemically sedated. Consider **transcranial Doppler** (TCD) studies for the detection and monitoring of intracranial stenosis, vascular occlusion, and vasospasm. TCD studies can provide adjunct data in diagnosing brain death and evaluating intracranial hypertension. A brain flow scan is performed by injecting technicium-99 labeled patient's blood back into the circulation to look for evidence of cerebral blood flow (Figure 8-1). A scan that fails to shows blood flow confirms a diagnosis of brain death.

■ DIAGNOSTIC PLAN

Determine if the mental status change is acute or progressive. Often agitation and anxiety can be symptoms of organic disease, such as hypoxia, and should be considered as seriously as a depressed mental status.

For patients who are acutely obtunded, determine the need for airway protection with **endotracheal intubation**. If intubation is to be performed, quickly perform a neurologic examination before the patient receives the typical rapid sequence of intubation medications. Some patients can have their airway maintained with less invasive adjuncts such as a **nasopharyngeal airway** and supplemental oxygen.

Consider the five Hs in treating patients with acute mental status changes. **Hypoglycemia** can occur in a patient with or without a history of diabetes. Consider obtaining a finger-stick glucose or empiric administration of a concentrated

DETERMINATION OF BRAIN DEATH

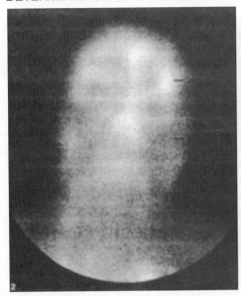 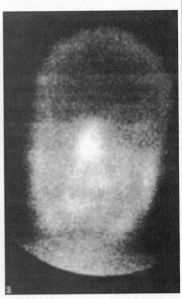

FIGURE 8-1

Showing a Techicium-99 Cerebral Blood Flow Scan in a (A) Normal and (B) Brain Dead Patient.

An individual who has sustained irreversible cessation of all functions of the entire brain, including the brain stem, meets the criteria for the diagnosis of brain death. The only spontaneous activity of an individual who meets brain death criteria is cardiovascular in nature. Apnea persists despite hypercarbia, and the only reflexes present are those that are mediated by the spinal cord. Comorbid medical conditions that may confound the clinical findings should be investigated and ruled out, including severe electrolyte or acid–base aberration, drug intoxication or pharmacologic therapy (sedatives, hypnotics, barbiturates), poisoning, hypothermia, shock, hyperosmolar state, or hepatic/renal encephalopathy.

Each patient considered for brain death must have a confirmatory physical examination that confirms the lack of brain activity. This includes the absence of motor and autonomic responses to noxious stimuli, lack of spontaneous respirations, and the absence of brainstem reflexes. The pupillary examination will show loss of spontaneous eye movements, no response to bright light, presence of fixed pupils (dilated or midposition), no evidence of oculocephalic (Dolls eyes), or oculovestibular (cold calorics) reflexes. In addition, it will show absence of the corneal, gag, cough, or sucking reflexes. In addition to the physisial examination, other confirmatory studies can be used to collaborate the evidence for brain death. The apnea test is used to demonstrate unresponsive medullary center despite a high carbon dioxide tension. Conventional angiography demonstrates no intracerebral filling above the level of the carotid bifurcation or circle of Willis. Electroencephalography shows no electrical activity during at least 30 minutes of continuous recording. Transcranial Doppler ultrasonography shows small systolic peaks in early systole without evidence of, or with reverse diastolic flow, indicative of extremely high vascular resistance associated with severe intracranial hypertension. A technetium-99m hexamethylpropylene-amineoxime brain scan shows no uptake of isotope into the brain parenchyma ("hollow skull" phenomenon). Somatosensory evoked potentials demonstrate bilateral absence of N20-P22 response with stimulation of the median nerve.

After brain death is determined, legal death is documented and the cardiovascular support is withdrawn. If the family agrees to organ donation, this process is delayed until the time of organ harvest.

dextrose solution. **Hypoxemia** is a common cause of agitation and anxiety but can cause depressed mental status in later stages. Place a **pulse oximeter** or determine the PO_2 by obtaining an arterial blood gas. **Hypotension** can cause decreased cerebral perfusion and lethargy. Check a full set of vital signs on each patient and record the values over time. **Hypercapnea** occurs with inadequate ventilation and is most often seen in obese patients or those in a weakened condition in the ICU. **Hypothyroid** conditions can cause depressed mental status, whereas acute **hyperthyroid** states can cause agitation and combativeness.

Use the initial **neurologic examination** to help narrow the list of etiological possibilities. Focal or asymmetric findings increase the odds of a structural lesion, whereas a nonfocal examination makes a metabolic, toxic, or infectious cause more likely. Guide the radiographic and laboratory workup toward the etiology most likely as determined from the history, presenting findings, and clinical situation.

Serial examinations of the comatose patient over time are essential and provide information about efficacy of treatment, worsening of the primary process, and prognosis.

■ DIFFERENTIAL DIAGNOSIS AND TREATMENT

Idiopathic Coma

Defined as a patient who presents with a depressed mental status with an unclear reason, idiopathic coma is seen in new patients arriving in the emergency department and hospital patients who have an unexpected change in the neurologic examination. Initial therapy of the comatose patient is, therefore, empiric. Administer **dextrose** if serum glucose is less than 60 mg/dL or if it cannot immediately be measured. In patients with very low thiamine stores, glucose administration may theoretically precipitate acute thiamine deficiency. Therefore, glucose should be administered after thiamine.

Thiamine deficiency alone may cause profound alterations in consciousness, and it is recommended that all comatose patients with unknown etiology should receive intravenous thiamine. Administer **naloxone** empirically to reverse any opioid effects. Although coma can be caused by the effects of BDZ, the empiric administration of the reversing agent **flumazenil** is controversial. Rapid reversal of BDZ effects may precipitate seizures and, thus, should be used with caution.

If the patient has a clinical picture of **increased ICP** or herniation, consider the administration of mannitol. **Hyperventilation** causes cerebral vasoconstriction that reduces cerebral blood volume and, hence, lowers ICP. While extremely effective, the effect on ICP is short lived and hyperventilation may cause cerebral ischemia. Hyperventilation should only be used emergently for a short period of time as a bridge to more definitive (usually surgical) therapy.

If a **toxic ingestion** is suspected, then consider gastric lavage and activated charcoal if indicated. Bacterial **meningitis** and herpes simplex **encephalitis** are associated with high mortality rates if not treated expeditiously. When brain infection is suspected, treatment with antibiotics should occur immediately, even if empiric. If a head CT and lumbar puncture cannot be performed immediately, then antibiotic administration should precede these diagnostic tests.

Iatrogenic Coma

Administration of anesthetic and analgesic medications is the most common cause of iatrogenic coma. Although overdoses do occur, each patient reacts to these medications differently and mental status changes can occur with doses well below what are deemed safe. **Airway control** and **resuscitation** take precedence over drug-reversal agent administration. Ensure an adequate airway, assist ventilation if necessary, and confirm systemic perfusion. Use intravenous fluids to treat hypotension and consider vasopressors for refractory hypotension. Immediately stop all narcotic and BDZ infusions. **Epidural infusions** often contain narcotics that can be absorbed systemically, causing narcotization. Often the analgesic effects are equally effective with a local anesthetic in the mixture, and the narcotic can be removed. Survey the chest and abdomen for **transdermal** narcotic patches. It is possible that extra patches were placed inadvertently or that the patient received intravenous narcotics without realizing that the transdermal system was in place.

Patients in the immediate postoperative period may have residual narcotics, BDZs, or anesthetic agents, which cause mental status changes. This is especially true in obese patients who have anesthetic redistributed after extubation. Administer the appropriate reversal agent. Naloxone is the reversal agent of choice for opioid overdose. Flumazenil is the reversal agent for BDZ overdose. Consider transferring the patient to intensive care to monitor and support physiologic and hemodynamic systems.

Cerebral Vascular Accident

Acute strokes have several etiologies including small-vessel lacunar infarction, cardioembolism, and carotid/vertebral/basilar thrombosis or embolism. Cerebral vascular accident (CVA) in surgical patients can occur at any time in the perioperative period and are often not related to the type of surgery that was performed (see Chapter 17).

Make the diagnosis by observing unilateral weakness, numbness, dysphasia, dysarthria, diplopia, or new ataxia. Order an HCT immediately to rule out acute hemorrhage. The hypodensity seen with infarctions increases with time, and thus CVAs may take 12–24 hours to become apparent on HCT. In the immediate period, consider MRI of the brain, since diffusion-weighted images reveal acute lesions within 1 hour of infarction. T2-weighted images will demonstrate increased signal intensity within 6–24 hours of infarct. Chronic lesions have low intensity on T1-weighted images. Transfer the patient to the ICU for close monitoring.

Treatment is most often **supportive care** with aggressive management of hypo- and hypertension. **Aspirin** provides a modest benefit when used within the first 48 hours. Consider, when appropriate, **antiplatelet agents**, long-term anticoagulation, carotid endarterectomy (see Figure 17-9), or angioplasty/stenting. **Thrombolytic** therapy can be considered, but it is seldom used perioperatively owing to the high risk of hemorrhage in the surgical patient.

Hypoxic–Ischemic Encephalopathy

Patients who suffer a prolonged period of hypoxia may develop irreversible axonal injury, even after reestablishment of cardiorespiratory function. The etiologies are varied and include suffocation, choking, near-drowning, cardiac arrest, carotid obstruction by hanging, strangulation, and shock from systemic hemorrhagic, embolic/thrombotic disorders, fat embolism, and disseminated intravascular coagulation (DIC). If appropriate, make the diagnosis of coma or persistent vegetative state. **Coma** is a total absence of awareness of self, environment, and ability to produce a response. **Persistent vegetative state** occurs with massive bilateral hemispheric damage with intact reticular activating system (RAS). A functioning RAS allows behavioral arousal and sleep–wake cycles without cognition; thus, patients are "awake" but "unaware." These patients are devoid of speech, comprehension, or purposeful movement. In addition, they have impaired motor function with spasticity, contractures, and posturing. Brainstem-level functions may be intact, such as reflex eye movements, orientation to noise, yawning, sneezing, bruxism (teeth grinding), and meaningless smiles. These functions can confuse the family into thinking that the patient is purposeful and aware.

Selected Readings

Bader MK, Littlejohns LR. *AANN Core Curriculum for Neuroscience Nursing.* 4th ed. St. Louis, MI: Saunders, an Imprint of Elsevier Science; 2004.

Campbell WW. *DeJong's the Neurologic Examination.* 6th ed. Philadelphia, PA: Lippincott Williams & Wilkins; 2005.

Jennett B, Bond M. Assessment of outcome after severe brain damage. *Lancet.* 1975;1:480–484.

Kruse JA, Fink MP, Carlson RW. *Saunders Manual of Critical Care.* Philadelphia, PA: Saunders, an Imprint of Elsevier Science; 2003.

Levy DE, Caronna JJ, Singer BH, et al. Predicting outcome from hypoxic-ischemic coma. *JAMA.* 1985;253:1420–1426.

Nolan JP, Morley PT, Vanden Hoek TL, et al. Therapeutic hypothermia after cardiac arrest. An advisory statement by the Advanced Life Support Task Force of the International Liaison Committee on Resuscitation. *Circulation.* 2003;108:118–121.

Plum F, Posner JB. *The Diagnosis of Stupor and Coma.* 3rd ed. Philadelphia: FA Davis; 1980.

Report of the Quality Standards Subcommittee of the American Academy of Neurology. Practice parameters for determining brain death in adults (summary statement). *Neurology.* 1995;45(5):1012–1014.

Stevens RD, Bhardwaj A. Approach to the comatose patient. *Crit Care Med.* 2006;34(1):31–41.

Teasdale G, Jennett B. Assessment of coma and impaired consciousness. A practical scale. *Lancet.* 1974;2:81–84.

The Hypothermia after Cardiac Arrest (HACA) Study Group. Mild therapeutic hypothermia to improve the neurologic outcome after cardiac arrest. *N Engl J Med.* 2002;346:549–556.

Wijdicks EF, Hijdra A, Young GB, et al. Practice parameter: Prediction of outcome in comatose survivors after cardiopulmonary resuscitation (an evidence-based review). *Neurology.* 2006;67:203–210.

9

Sepsis

Ruth M. Kleinpell, PhD, RN, FAAN, FCCM ■ *James S. Krinsley, MD, FCCM, FCCP*

Key Points

- The systemic inflammatory response syndrome (SIRS) is an exaggerated response of the normal immune system against an insult. It can occur in reaction to infection or non-infectious causes such as trauma or burns.

- Sepsis, defined as a SIRS response to infection associated with acute organ dysfunction, is common among surgical patients and is a major cause of morbidity and mortality.

- Alterations in respiratory function is one of the most common manifestations of organ system dysfunction in sepsis and a common clinical antecedent of acute respiratory distress syndrome (ARDS).

- In addition to the SIRS criteria, signs of sepsis include chills, hypotension, decreased skin perfusion, decreased urine output, significant edema or positive fluid balance, decreased capillary refill or mottling, hyperglycemia in the absence of diabetes, and unexplained change in mental status.

- Severe sepsis represents progression of sepsis and is characterized by organ dysfunction with hypoperfusion or hypotension.

- Septic shock occurs when hypotension is persistent despite adequate fluid resuscitation and signs of perfusion abnormalities are evident, including lactic acidosis, oliguria, or acute alteration in mental status.

- When severe sepsis and septic shock progress to multiple organ dysfunction syndrome (MODS), mortality rates can be 28%–50% or more.

- Early initiation of appropriate antimicrobial therapy is essential for the adequate treatment of sepsis. Culture and sensitivity testing early in the diagnostic process is important in ensuring effective antimicrobial coverage.

- Evidence-based guidelines for the management of sepsis highlight early goal-directed resuscitation, empiric antibiotics, and aggressive source control.

■ HISTORY

Inflammatory responses and sepsis are common causes of acute clinical deterioration in the surgical patient. Systemic inflammation may occur from a wide variety of insults such as surgery, trauma, ingestions, or burns. The term sepsis is indicated when there is a suspected or confirmed infection associated with an inflammatory response.

Common **presentations** in patients developing an inflammatory response include mental status changes, fever, respiratory compromise, malaise, or frank hemodynamic instability. Specific complaints are often related to the inciting process, such as abdominal pain patients with pancreatitis, or tachypnea after a recent aspiration event.

Determine if the patient has **risk factors** for occult infection, which include extremes of age, compromised-immune status, chronic illness, recent surgical or invasive procedures, malnutrition, or recent broad-spectrum antibiotics use. Review the medical record for **recent infection**, such as urinary tract infection or upper respiratory tract infection, which may predispose the surgical patient to developing a septic response. Common infections that increase the risk of severe sepsis include influenza and pneumonia, meningitis, abdominal perforations, wound infections, and blood stream infections.

Consider the contribution of surgically related infections that can lead to sepsis, especially anastomotic leaks and intra-abdominal abscesses. Also consider wound infection, early necrotizing fasciitis, biliary obstruction, or urinary obstruction as less common causes.

■ PHYSICAL EXAMINATION

Perform a physical examination with attention to determine whether or not the patient is exhibiting signs of sepsis. Review the **fever curve**; note any diaphoresis, tachycardia, hypotension, decreased capillary refill, decreased skin perfusion, or significant edema. Since respiratory dysfunction is a common early indicator of sepsis, look for an **increased respiratory rate** or labored breathing. Evaluate the patient's **mental status** since changes are also frequently seen in sepsis and can be confused with narcotic overdose, strokes, and psychiatric disorders.

Perform a complete examination of all **surgical wounds**, intravascular line sites, all drainage systems and surrounding tissue, and extremities. Look for signs of deep vein thrombophlebitis, which may also initiate a systemic inflammatory response that mimics sepsis. Perform a **rectal** and a perineal examination for pelvic, perirectal, prostatic, or decubitus infection. Assess **pain** location and quality. Surgical site pain that increases or fails to resolve in the 7–10 days following surgery may indicate underlying infection.

■ LABORATORY STUDIES

Order a **CBC** with differential. An abnormal WBC > 12,000 cells/mm^3, or <4000 cells/mm^3, or >10% immature (band) forms is associated with SIRS. Determine the **hemoglobin** and **platelet** counts to rule out acute blood loss as a cause of hemodynamic instability or thrombocytopenia associated with systemic infection.

Order a **lactate level** within the first 6 hours of the diagnosis of severe sepsis or septic shock. An elevated serum lactate level identifies tissue hypoperfusion in patients who may not necessarily be hypotensive. If the baseline lactate is elevated, serial lactate levels will help assess the adequacy of resuscitation. Order a chemistry panel and replete **electrolytes** as needed. Review the **amylase** and **lipase** to rule out pancreatitis as common cause of the SIRS response. Check for elevated **glucose levels** and treat appropriately. Consider the possibility of disseminated intravascular coagulopathy (DIC). The diagnosis of DIC is made by noting a decreased fibrinogen level and platelet count, with elevation of the fibrin split products and D-dimer.

Draw two or more **blood cultures,** with one drawn percutaneously and one drawn through each vascular access device. Cultures of other sites such as urine, cerebrospinal fluid, wounds, respiratory secretions, or other body fluids are guided by the suspicion of infection at each site. Whenever possible, obtain cultures that can be quantified and gathered without contamination, such as bronchioalveolar lavage (BAL) of the lungs or clean catch urine specimens. Appropriate cultures should be obtained prior to initiation of antimicrobial therapy.

■ RADIOGRAPHIC AND INVASIVE STUDIES

As respiratory dysfunction is common in sepsis, order a **chest X-ray** (CXR) for suspected pulmonary alterations. **ARDS** commonly occurs with severe sepsis and should be suspected with increasing respiratory distress, respiratory dysfunction requiring intubation, and mechanical ventilation with bilateral CXR infiltrates. Use **ultrasonography** or **computed tomography** liberally to rule out deep infections or abscesses. If deep infection or abscesses are identified, immediate decisions are made whether to treat with percutaneous drainage or surgery.

Consider **echocardiography** as a convenient bedside test for cardiac function and volume status. Cardiac dysfunction is often depressed in severe sepsis, and the ECHO may show global dyskinesis. If ongoing resuscitation is required, consider placing a central venous catheter to measure preload, or a continuous mixed venous catheter to help guide goal-directed therapy (see Chapter 6). With continued hemodynamic instability, consider placement of a pulmonary artery catheter (PAC) to measure continuous preload and cardiac output determination (see Figures 6-2 and 6-3).

■ DIAGNOSTIC PLAN

Prompt diagnosis of infection is paramount since once sepsis progresses to severe sepsis with organ system involvement, mortality rates increase significantly. Diagnosis and resuscitation must occur concomitantly, since delay in treatment can be fatal. Thus, the management of SIRS and sepsis is a true emergency that will prompt the practitioner to perform diagnostic tests in a rapid fashion.

Make the diagnosis of **SIRS** by confirming two or more of the following conditions: temperature $> 38°C$ or $< 36°C$, a heart rate > 90 beats/min, respiratory rate > 20 breaths/min or $PaCO_2 < 32$ mm Hg (<4.3 kPa), and WBC $> 12,000$ cells/mm^3, <4000 cells/mm^3, or $>10\%$ immature (band) forms. Assess for additional signs and symptoms including those associated with low perfusion such as decreased capillary refill or mottling, decreased urine output in the context of significant edema, or positive fluid balance. In addition, be aware that hyperglycemia (plasma glucose > 120 mg/dL) in the absence of diabetes and an unexplained change in mental status are possible additional indicators of early sepsis.

Sepsis is defined as a SIRS response initiated by a source of infection Thus, resuscitation is started and a search for the infectious cause ensues. Laboratory tests and cultures are sent immediately and CXR is performed. Higher-order radiographic tests are then considered in consultation with the surgeon. As diagnostic maneuvers continue, start antibiotics geared to the most likely source of infection. Common sources in hospitalized patients include pulmonary, urinary tract, wounds, abdomen, and blood stream.

Severe sepsis represents progression of sepsis and is characterized by organ dysfunction with hypoperfusion or hypotension. Patients who have progressed to severe sepsis need immediate source control and require advanced monitoring to determine fluid and cardiac status. If the patient is not in an intensive care unit, plans are made for transfer. Perform a survey of all organ functions and provide support as needed. Common treatment adjuncts for severe sepsis include ventilatory support and hemodialysis.

Septic shock occurs when hypotension is persistent, despite adequate fluid resuscitation and signs of perfusion abnormalities. Without proper treatment, there is a substantial risk of death. Resuscitation for these patients requires inotropic support and consideration of advanced therapies such as activated protein C and steroids for adrenal insufficiency.

■ DIFFERENTIAL DIAGNOSIS AND TREATMENT

Systemic Inflammatory Response Syndrome

The SIRS is an exaggerated response of the **normal immune system** against an insult. It can occur in reaction to infection or noninfectious causes such as trauma or burns. During SIRS, there is stimulation of the innate immune system, white blood cell activation, and endothelial cell response, which leads to the release of a number of mediators or cytokines. This activation causes a variety of physiologic changes, including vasodilation, enhanced expression of adhesion molecules, increased capillary permeability, increased clot formation, and decreased fibrinolysis. While the immune system response is protective in nature, aimed at combating infection in sepsis, overactivity of mediators has been cited as a causal factor in contributing to endothelial cell damage, microcapillary permeability changes, capillary leak, and profound vasodilation and hypotension.

Search for the **common conditions** that cause SIRS, such as pancreatitis (see Chapter 10), inflammatory bowel disease (see Chapter 11), trauma, burns, or autoimmune disease. The clinical presentation of SIRS can be varied and involve virtually every organ system. Look for changes in the **mental status**, from confusion and agitation to obtundation. The heart rate is often elevated, with the possible development of arrhythmias. **Tachypnea** and low oxygen saturation are common. **Fever** and **leukocytosis** are hallmarks of SIRS, making the diagnosis of associated infection difficult.

Sepsis

The diagnosis of SIRS changes to sepsis when an infectious source of the immune response is a suspected or confirmed infection. Start empiric **antibiotics** within the first 2 hours of recognition of sepsis, after appropriate cultures have been obtained. Initial empiric antibiotic therapy should include one or more agents that have activity against the likely pathogens (bacterial or fungal), based on the clinical situation.

Source control is indicated as soon as possible. Patients are evaluated for the presence of an infection source amenable to control measures such as abscess drainage, debridement of necrotic tissue, or removal of a potentially infected device.

Prompt diagnosis and initiation of treatment are important aspects in the management of sepsis in the surgical patient. The goals of treatment are based on the **Surviving Sepsis Campaign guidelines**, a set of evidence-based guidelines for the management of sepsis advocated by a partnership of the Society of Critical Care Medicine, the European Society of Intensive Care Medicine, and the International Sepsis Forum (Figure 9-1).

THE SURVIVING SEPSIS CAMPAIGN

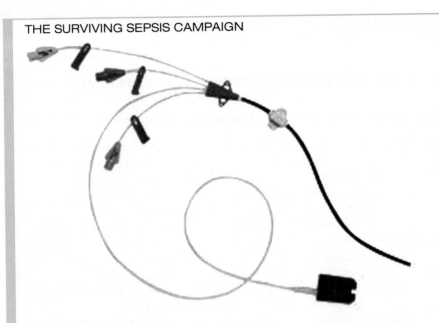

FIGURE 9-1
The PreSep® Continuous Mixed Venous Oximetry Catheter

The Surviving Sepsis Campaign guidelines outline evidence-based recommendations for targeting treatment of patients at risk of developing severe sepsis and septic shock, based on existing research evidence. The Surviving Sepsis Campaign guidelines were developed by critical care and infectious disease experts representing 11 international organizations.

The focus of the Surviving Sepsis Campaign guidelines is aimed at providing resuscitation for sepsis-induced hypoperfusion and enhancing perfusion. Central to the recommendations is the concept of **goal-directed therapy** (GDT). This is a protocol of providing hemodynamic support that bases the treatments on measurable end points of resuscitation. Thus, fluid resuscitation is guided by a goal central venous pressure, oxygen-carrying capacity is guided by a goal hemoglobin level, and tissue perfusion is gauged by the mixed venous saturation. Specific technologies make GDT possible such as continuous mixed venous saturation oximeters that can directly measure peripheral tissue perfusion such as the PreSep catheter (Edwards Life sciences, Irvine, Ca) (In Spectra™, Hutchinson technologies, MN).

Other tenets of the surviving sepsis campaign are early empiric antibiotic administration, followed by source control and therapeutic agents guided by cultures to identify the source of infection. Guidelines are also provided for mechanical ventilation to optimize oxygenation, strict glucose control, steroid use for adrenal insufficiency, prophylaxis measures for deep vein thrombosis, stress ulcer prevention, renal replacement therapies, use of recombinant human activated protein C (rhAPC), blood product administration, sedation and analgesia, and consideration for limitation of support in critically ill patients.

Awareness of the guidelines is essential for clinicians managing patients at risk of severe sepsis and septic shock.

Control the **glucose** to maintain blood glucose level <150 mg/dL. Several clinical trials in different ICU populations have demonstrated improvements in survival when continuous insulin infusion was used to maintain glucose level between 80 and 140 mg/dL. Include a **nutrition** protocol with the preferential use of enteral nutrition. Provide additional measures for deep vein thrombosis and stress ulcer prophylaxis. Discuss end-of-life care for critically ill patients when appropriate and promote family communication to discuss use of life-sustaining therapies.

Severe Sepsis

A systemic inflammatory response to infection associated with **acute organ dysfunction** is defined as severe sepsis. In addition to the diagnostic maneuvers outlined previously, begin immediate resuscitation to reverse cardiopulmonary failure. Establish **vascular access** and begin **aggressive fluid resuscitation** as the first priority. Fluid resuscitation may consist of crystalloids or colloids. In patients with suspected hypovolemia, a fluid challenge may be given at a rate of 500–1000 mL of crystalloids or 300–500 mL of colloid for more than 30 minutes to repeat based on response.

Assess the need for endotracheal intubation, since **mechanical ventilation** is indicated for sepsis-induced acute lung injury or ARDS. Use of low tidal volume (6 mL/kg of predicted body weight) is a goal along with maintaining end inspiratory plateau pressures <30 cm H_2O. Sedation, analgesia, and neuromuscular blockade should be provided during mechanical ventilation for comfort and monitored to avoid prolonged sedation.

Initiate hemodynamic assessment and **goal-directed therapy**. The Surviving Sepsis Campaign (Figure 9-1) guidelines outline initial resuscitation goals for sepsis-induced hypoperfusion as **fluid resuscitation** to a central venous pressure of 8–12 mm Hg, and a **central venous oxygen saturation** ($S_{CV}O_2$) of ≥70%. Consider packed red blood cell **transfusion** to achieve a hematocrit of ≥30%. If volume resuscitation is inadequate, start **vasopressor** and **inotropy** therapies. Inotropic therapy is indicated for patients with low cardiac output despite adequate fluid resuscitation. If an inotrope is used in the presence of hypotension, consider combined with vasopressor therapy.

Septic Shock

Septic shock occurs when **hypotension is persistent** despite adequate fluid resuscitation and signs of perfusion abnormalities being evident, including lactic acidosis, oliguria, or acute alteration in mental status.

In addition to the resuscitation steps outlined above, consider **adrenal insufficiency** for patients in septic shock who require maximum vasopressor therapy despite adequate fluid resuscitation. Order a random **cortisol** level and adrenocorticotropin hormone stimulation testing. A low random cortisol level or a failure of the cortisol to elevate after stimulation indicates relative adrenal insufficiency. Intravenous **corticosteroids,** such as hydrocortisone, have been advocated for patients with adrenal insufficiency during septic shock.

Assess the need for **renal replacement therapy** for acute renal or management of fluid and electrolyte balance, especially in the setting of intractable hyperkalemia, volume overload, acidosis, or clinical manifestations of uremia. If dialysis is needed, offer hemodynamically unstable patients continuous renal replacement therapy (CRRT) as an alternate to intermittent hemodialysis (see Figure 7-1).

Multiple Organ Dysfunction Syndrome

Unabated, severe sepsis and septic shock can lead to a progression of multiple organ failure. Make the diagnosis of MODS by having at least two organ system failures in the context of a critical illness. The most common involved systems are neurologic, pulmonary, cardiac, and renal. MODS is associated with and often complicated by the adult respiratory distress syndrome (see Chapter 5). Mortality for patients in MODS from sepsis has been reported to be from 28% to 50%. Therefore, early detection and treatment of sepsis are important for promoting the best outcome in surgical patients. There is no specific treatment for MODS other than for the care outlined above for SIRS and sepsis syndromes.

Selected Readings

Balk RA. Optimum treatment of severe sepsis and septic shock: Evidence in support of the recommendations. *Dis Mon.* 2005;50:168–213.

Dellinger RP, Carlet JM, Masur H, et al. Surviving Sepsis Campaign guidelines for management of severe sepsis and septic shock. *Crit Care Med.* 2004;32:858–872.

Evans DC, Meakins JL. Clinical and laboratory diagnosis of infection: Approach to diagnosis of surgical infection. http://www.medscape.com/viewarticle/525765. Accessed September 4, 2006.

Hotchkiss RS, Karl IE. The pathophysiology and treatment of sepsis. *N Engl J Med.* 2003;348:138–150.

Lowry SF, Awad S, Ford H, et al. PROWESS Surgical Evaluation Committee. Static and dynamic assessment of biomarkers in surgical patients with severe sepsis. *Surg Infect.* 2004;5:261–268.

Townsend S, Dellinger RP, Levy MM, Ramsay G. *Implementing the Surviving Sepsis Campaign.* Society of Critical Care Medicine, the European Society of Intensive Care Medicine, and the International Sepsis Forum, 2005.

Section II

SURGICAL PROBLEMS

10

Acute Abdominal Pain

Rita Rienzo, MMsc, PA-C ■ *Adam D. Fox, DPM, DO*

Key Points

- Any abdominal pain that last for more than 6 hours is concerning for a serious, surgical pathology.

- Radiation of visceral pain is determined by the anatomic location of the disease, with foregut organs radiating to the epigastrum, midgut to the umbilicus, and hindgut to the suprapubic region.

- The diagnosis of acute abdominal pain is primarily made by the history and physical examination.

- Peritonitis, as evidenced by generalized pain, rebound tenderness, and nonvoluntary guarding, suggests a true surgical emergency.

- For cases where the diagnosis is unclear, the abdominal CT scan is the most sensitive and specific diagnostic test for intra-abdominal disease.

- Cholecystitis is distinguished from simple biliary colic by the persistence of pain and associated fever and leukocytosis.

- Pancreatitis has a spectrum of presentation from mild abdominal pain to a systemic inflammatory response with shock.

- Adhesions from previous surgery and incarcerated hernias are responsible for the vast majority of bowel obstructions.

- Most cases of diverticulitis will respond to bowel rest and antibiotics. If conservative therapy fails, the patient often will need a segmental colon resection with colostomy.

- The hallmark of acute mesenteric ischemia is pain that is out of proportion to the physical findings, often associated with bloody diarrhea.

- Acute volvulus is reduced by colonoscopy and stented with a long rectal tube. Surgery with colon resection during the same admission is indicated to prevent recurrence.

■ MEDICAL HISTORY

Abdominal pain encompasses a vast array of possible pathological conditions ranging from the benign to the catastrophic. Abdominal pain is also a common complaint, which causes patients to seek medical attention. Despite advances in diagnostic testing including radiographic images, the history and physical findings will lead to an accurate diagnosis of abdominal pain in the great majority of cases.

Perform a thorough and accurate **history** to determine which organ system is involved and the severity of the presenting illness. **Pain** is characterized to location, duration, quality, quantity, and aggravating and alleviating factors. Abrupt onset of significant pain in a previously asymptomatic patient warrants serious evaluation, as does pain, which has progressed in severity over a period of hours. A complaint of acute abdominal pain which has persisted and then suddenly eased, is not dismissed without further assessment. Abrupt cessation acute abdominal pain may be due to a process that has progressed to the point of vascular infarction or subsequent perforation.

Review elements of the **presenting illness** that lend clues to the eventual diagnosis. Have the patients describe in their own words the **progression** of symptoms, starting from a point when they felt normal to the time they came to seek medical attention. During this interview, look for clues from the **pain character** as to whether it is constant, intermittent, worsening, or improving. Ascertain if the pain was followed by nausea, such as in appendicitis, or nausea was followed by pain, such as in gastroenteritis. Elicit **precipitating events**, such as heavy alcohol consumption causing pancreatitis or a fatty meal instigating biliary colic. The character and frequency of **stools** can lead to a diagnosis of colitis and constipation. Determining recent **ingestions** will help to rule out poisoning or allergic reactions.

Perform a thorough review of the **past medical history**, especially if the history includes previous episodes of similar pain. Often **chronic conditions**, such as peptic ulcer disease, can present with an acute exacerbation, such as a

perforation. Patients with diabetes, coronary disease, peripheral vascular disease, and autoimmune disorders are particularly prone to intra-abdominal catastrophes, such as perforations or mesenteric occlusions. Review **medications**
that can be responsible for abdominal complications, such as nonsteroidal anti-
inflammatory agents and coumadin.

Consider the underlying anatomical structures, as the patient describes the location or migration of the pain. Typically pain from abdominal viscera radiates to
the epigastrum, mid-abdomen, or suprapubic region, depending on pain stimulus emanating from the foregut, midgut, or hindgut, respectively. The boundary
of the foregut and midgut is the duodenum, whereas the demarcation of the
mid- and hindgut is at the cecum.

The **foregut** organs include the esophagus, stomach, liver and pancreaticobil-
iary structures, and duodenum. Thus, right upper quadrant (RUQ) or epigastric
pain may be caused by gallbladder inflammation, pancreatitis, or cholecystitis.
Epigastric pain may suggest a peptic ulcer, particularly if the pain is gnawing in
nature and radiates to the back. Subxiphoid pain can be caused by an occult
cardiac pathology, such as an acute myocardial infarction. An abrupt onset of
knifelike mid-epigastric or midline abdominal pain, particularly in the presence
of hypovolemia, hemodynamic instability, suggests a diagnosis of abdominal
aneurysm.

Midgut abdominal pain is almost exclusively caused by pathology involving
the small bowel and cecum. Periumbilical pain may herald the onset of appendicitis, although eventually the patient's pain will migrate to the right lower
quadrant (RLQ), as the peritoneal irritation becomes more localized over the
appendix. Other surgical conditions, which present with central abdominal or
poorly localized pain, include small bowel obstruction, mesenteric ischemia,
volvulus, intussusception, and Meckel's diverticulum.

Hindgut pain radiates to the suprapubic area and is almost exclusively caused
by colonic pathologies, such as diverticulitis, colonic volvulus, colitis, and constipation. Lower abdominal pain also occurs with diseases of the pelvic organs,
especially the female reproductive system. Etiologies include ectopic pregnancy,
ovarian torsion, and ovarian cyst rupture. Pain from ureteral obstruction may
migrate from the flank to the lower quadrants, as the stone progresses down the
ureter.

In addition, the **character of pain** can help narrow the differential diagnosis
substantially. Pain from any obstructed hollow viscous tends to be intermittent
and crampy, termed "colic." Thus, a colic-type pain radiating to RUQ narrows the
possible causes to the biliary tree or ureter. Pain from the retroperitoneally placed
organs often radiates to the back, such as in aortic aneurysms or pancreatitis. Pain
that is relieved by vomiting is suggestive of bowel obstruction.

■ PHYSICAL EXAMINATION

Begin with **general examination** of the entire patient. Patients who have peritonitis lie rigidly, intolerant of any movement of the stretcher. Conversely, patients

with colic or retroperitoneal pain writhe in pain, continually moving to try and get comfortable. Pallor suggests occult bleeding, whereas jaundice is indicative of hepatobiliary disease. Poor skin turgor and dry mucosa are suggestive of dehydration, often owing to the prolonged vomiting or diarrhea.

Inspect the patient's abdomen. Look for surgical scars suggesting previous abdominal surgeries, which can lead to the formation of intra-abdominal adhesions or opportunities for herniation and, thus, subsequent small bowel obstruction or incarceration. Congenital hernias most often occur at the umbilicus without the presence of a prior incision. Inguinal hernias may also progress to an extent that bowel has become incarcerated. A distended abdomen suggests ileus, obstruction ascites, or an undetected pregnancy. Pain with coughing indicates peritoneal irritation.

Auscultate the abdomen to detect the presence or absence of bowel sounds. High-pitched or "tinkling" bowel sounds are suggestive of obstruction, whereas the complete absence of bowel sounds suggests ileus. A midline bruit, particularly in conjunction with a history of abrupt knifelike central abdominal pain, is strongly suggestive of a dissecting aortic aneurysm.

Palpate the abdomen to localize the source of the pain and differentiate between localized inflammation and a more diffuse or advanced process. If possible, have the patients bend their knees and flex at the hips while lying flat, to facilitate a maximally flaccid abdominal wall. This will help enable adequate palpation by relaxing tension on a potentially inflamed peritoneum. Start with **light palpation** over all areas. Localized tenderness is exhibited in conditions where the infectious or inflammatory process is still contained within the effected organ, such as left lower quadrant pain in diverticulitis. Generalized tenderness or a tense, **rigid abdomen** suggests peritonitis. **Rebound tenderness** is elicited by slowly pressing on the abdominal wall and abruptly releasing the pressure. Pain on release causes the peritoneum to bounce and will cause acute pain if the peritoneum is inflamed. **Nonvoluntary guarding** is a spinal reflex that causes the muscles overlying an area of peritoneal inflammation to become rigid and is pathonomonic of peritonitis. Nonvoluntary guarding can occur unilaterally and will not abate with pain medicine or even anesthesia.

Search for **abdominal wall weakness** in surgical incision sites, periumbilical region, midline, and groins. The presence of a hernia, even if reducible, in the setting of nausea, vomiting, abdominal distention, or cessation of flatus or bowel movement, is considered a strangulated hernia until proven otherwise (Figure 10-1). If peritonitis is not present, **percuss** the abdomen to elicit tympany, suggesting a distended viscous as a result of bowel obstruction or free intraperitoneal air after a perforation. Inspiratory arrest during deep RUQ palpation (Murphy's sign) suggests gallbladder inflammation, or possibly Fitz–Hugh–Curtis syndrome. A palpable, pulsatile abdominal mass indicates an aortic abdominal aneurysm. A **rectal examination** and a **complete internal pelvic** examination are considered in every patient with acute abdominal pain. Bright red blood per rectum suggests a lower gastrointestinal (GI) bleed, and darker blood or melena is suggestive of an upper GI source, such as peptic ulcer. The presence of stool in the rectum does not rule out a bowel obstruction.

INGUINAL HERNIA REPAIR

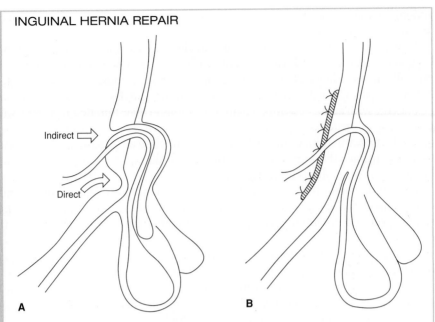

Indirect

Direct

A

B

FIGURE 10-1
A) Inguinal hernia occuring in the direct and indirect spaces and,
B) Mesh repair.

In a supine position, the penis and scrotum are included in the prep. Local anesthesia is infiltrated along the incision line, and an incision is made somewhat transversely along a skin fold line just above the inguinal ligament. The incision is then carried down using electrocautery through the subcutaneous tissue layers until reaching the external oblique fascia, which is then opened in the direction of its fibers to the external inguinal ring, revealing the inguinal canal. Here the spermatic cord and vessels are dissected from muscle fibers (cremaster) that emanate from the floor of the inguinal canal. The hernia sac is then identified and dissected from the cord structures. The sac is usually ligated and pushed back into the hernia defect.

Attention is then turned to repairing the hernia. A direct hernia is a weakness in the floor of the inguinal canal. (A) An indirect hernia is a weakness around the internal inguinal ring, where the spermatic cord and vessels exit the abdominal cavity to pass into the scrotum. (A) Both defects are repaired by sewing a mesh patch (nonabsorbable) to cover the floor of the canal and internal inguinal ring. (B) In addition, some surgeons will use another piece of specially designed mesh to "plug" the internal ring before placing the mesh on top (plug and patch technique). After the mesh is secured, the incision is closed layer by layer.

■ LABORATORY STUDIES

Review the **CBC** for elevations in the white blood cell count suggesting infections or anemia suggesting a process associated with blood loss. In patients with suspected liver disease or those on coumadin, check the **prothrombin time** and decide if reversal is indicated. All patients who are being evaluated for acute abdominal pain have blood sent for a **type and cross** in anticipation of the need of emergency surgery.

Evaluate the **serum chemistry** to rule out electrolyte abnormalities, renal function, and serum glucose levels. Patients with prolonged bowel obstructions will typically have evidence of dehydration, and metabolic acidosis must be corrected before surgery. Consider liver function tests, serum **amylase**, and **lipase** level on all patients with acute abdominal pain. Elevations in **liver function tests** may suggest biliary obstruction or primary liver dysfunction as a result of a gallstones, cystic duct obstruction, or hepatitis. Elevated **amylase** and **lipase**, usually greater than three times the upper limit of normal, are the most commonly occurring laboratory abnormalities in acute pancreatitis.

Urinalysis is required on all patients with abdominal pain, in order to rule out an infectious cause, such as cystitis or pyelonephritis and to assess the patient's level of dehydration. The presence of hematuria suggests the possibility of nephrolithiasis.

A **pregnancy test** is performed in all female patients of child-bearing age, from menarche through menopause, regardless of history given as to contraceptive use, sexual abstinence, timing of last menstrual period, history of tubal ligation, or perceived perimenopausal status. History of a tubal ligation, in fact, increases the risk of ectopic pregnancy as much as 27-fold.

■ RADIOGRAPHIC STUDIES

Order an **abdominal series** as the first radiographic test in any patient with abdominal pain to look for obstructive patterns, ileus, or free peritoneal air. Order an **abdominal CT** as the definitive test for anatomic diagnosis in the abdomen, with an understanding of the limitations. The CT is very sensitive and specific for the diagnosis of solid organ disease, such as pancreatitis or liver masses. The modality is now considered for the diagnosis of appendicitis. Also use CT to define bowel pathology, such as obstruction, volvulus, diverticulosis, and ischemia. Consider an **upper GI series** with small-bowel follow through (SBFT) if information about the stomach and small-bowel anatomy and function are needed. Order a **barium enema** to evaluate for diverticulosis, colon cancer, intussusception, and volvulus.

In patients suspected of having a biliary tract disease, consider an **abdominal ultrasound** (US). While US results are highly operator dependent, a simple US can identify biliary or gallbladder pathology without the need for further imaging. Consider a bile excretion study such as a **HIDA scan** to determine cystic duct obstruction. A "positive" HIDA scan is one in which radiographic tracer enters the duodenum but fails to reflux into the gallbladder, suggesting cystic duct obstruction.

In patients with suspected mesenteric ischemia, use CT angiogram, MRI, or conventional angiogram to rule out vascular occlusion or spasm. The **CT** and **MRI** have the advantage of allowing visualization of the bowel and being noninvasive, while the formal **angiogram** allows for concurrent therapeutic maneuvers, such as angioplasty and stenting.

■ DIAGNOSTIC PLAN

Using the **history** and the **physical examination**, determine if the patient may have an acute abdominal crisis that needs immediate treatment. Although it is surgical dictum that patients with peritonitis do not require any further testing, some diagnostic testing may be indicated for planning the operation or ruling out potential nonoperative diseases (pancreatitis and ruptured ovarian cyst).

Order laboratory studies to prepare the patient for surgery, with special attention to **electrolyte** and **coagulation** abnormalities. Review the CBC to determine the need for blood transfusion, platelet transfusion, or blood product availability. Specifically review values that can suggest a nonoperative source of severe abdominal pain. Check the **urinalysis** for evidence of blood suggesting nephrolithiasis, the **amylase** and **lipase** for pancreatitis, and the vaginal smear for evidence of pelvic inflammatory disease.

For the vast majority of patients, the radiographic study of choice is an **abdominal CT** with PO and intravenous contrast. If cholecystitis is suspected, order an abdominal **US** as the test of choice. Consider MRI as an alternate for those patients who are pregnant.

If several radiographic tests fail to reveal a source of the pain, consider **consultation** with gastroenterology, infectious disease, or general medicine, as the situation dictates. If no pathology is found after multiple examinations and consultations, some patients are considered for **diagnostic laparoscopy** as a final attempt to make an anatomic diagnosis (see Figure 21-1). Patients are extensively counseled that diagnostic laparoscopy may not find a source and rarely is a therapeutic maneuver.

■ DIFFERENTIAL DIAGNOSIS AND TREATMENT

Acute Appendicitis

Obtain a **chief complaint** of abdominal pain that starts periumbilical and then migrates to the RLQ. The pain will change in character from intermittent and dull to sharp and constant. Nausea will develop after the pain begins, and a low-grade fever may be reported. Despite this "classic" presentation, there are many variants, and thus, the disease is considered in the differential diagnosis of any patient with acute abdominal pain. Prompt diagnosis and treatment are necessary to prevent perforation, since this disease increases significantly 48–72 hours after onset of the symptoms.

On examination, find RLQ tenderness with rebound, often centered at a point two thirds the distance from umbilicus to anterior superior iliac spine (**McBurney's point**). Additional findings might include right-sided pain with palpation of LLQ (**Rovsings sign**), tenderness with flexion and medial rotation of the right leg (**obturator sign**), or pain on extension of right thigh (**psoas sign**). A rectal examination may demonstrate right-sided tenderness.

Order a **CBC** to demonstrate leukocytosis. Obtain a **urinalysis** to rule out the possibility of nephrolithiasis, which can mimic appendicitis. A **pregnancy test** is obtained in any woman of child-bearing years. Check **electrolytes** if there is a history of prolonged vomiting or period of poor PO intake.

Although the diagnosis of appendicitis can be made purely on clinical grounds, radiographic imaging is frequently used in an attempt to decrease the false-negative appendectomy rate. If **plain radiographs** have been performed, search for a hardened piece of feces in the RLQ (appendicolith). **Abdominal CT** is now considered valuable in establishing a diagnosis of appendicitis. Consider **US** in children and women who are pregnant. US is specific in making the diagnosis if the appendix is seen, but not specific in excluding the diagnosis if the appendix is not seen.

Patients with acute appendicitis are offered immediate appendectomy. Consider a delayed operative approach in the patient who presents with a perforation and abscess on CT that appears localized. Since rupture has already occurred, immediate appendectomy will not alter the disease process. Manage these patients with prolonged intravenous **antibiotics** and **percutaneous drainage**. Offer surgery when the inflammation is resolved (interval appendectomy).

The **appendectomy** is performed by either a laparoscopic or an open approach (Figure 10-2). The techniques are similar in the effectiveness, complications, and patient care issues, such as pain and time back to work. Laparoscopy has the advantage of being able to view the entire abdomen in patients where the diagnosis is not clear, and the open approach has the advantage of using less resources.

Cholecystitis

Intermittent obstruction of the cystic duct by a stone or inflammation can result in distention of the gallbladder and pain described as biliary colic (see Chapter 11). When the obstruction becomes constant, the distention of the gall bladder wall can become ischemic and infected, resulting in cholecystitis. Thus, differentiate acute cholecystitis from biliary colic from a history of nonremitting abdominal pain, associated with fever and possibly nausea and vomiting. **Pain** typically begins soon after a fatty meal initially and is described as a dull ache. The location of the pain may be variable, from the midepigastric region to RUQ, with radiation primarily to the right shoulder or back.

The focused physical examination will demonstrate mild abdominal distention, abnormal hypoactive bowel sounds, and RUQ tenderness. Look for cessation of inspiration upon palpation of the RUQ **(Murphy's sign)** as a sensitive indicator of gallbladder inflammation.

Order a CBC to document **leukocytosis**, which is often present typically between normal and 15,000. Obtain **electrolytes** and replete as necessary, especially in patients who have had significant vomiting. Review the liver function tests along with a mild elevation in **bilirubin** and **alkaline phosphatase**. Significant elevation of these parameters suggests a common bile duct obstruction (choledocholithiasis). Obtain the **amylase** and **lipase** to rule out concomitant pancreatitis.

Use the abdominal US to make the diagnosis and assess the common bile duct for associated obstruction. Look for the classic US findings of a thickened

OPEN AND LAPAROSCOPIC APPENDECTOMY

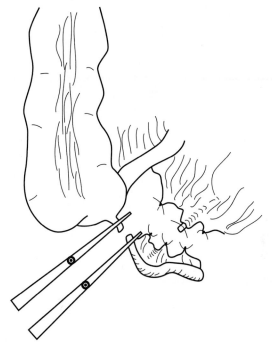

FIGURE 10-2
Ligation of the appendix and mesentery during open appendectomy

Open technique: The patient is placed in a supine position and an incision is made in the RLQ. The muscles are divided in the plane of the fibers as not to transect any muscle. Entry into the abdomen is made, and the appendix is identified at the base of the cecum. The mesentery, which contains the blood supply, is identified and ligated. Once the blood supply to the appendix has been ligated, the appendix is tied and ligated at its base (A). The site is inspected for adequate hemostasis, irrigation is performed, and the bowel is placed back in the abdomen. The abdominal wall is then closed in layers, and the skin is closed with either absorbable suture or skin clips.

Laparoscopic: Again in the supine position, a Foley catheter and a nasogastric tube are placed prior after induction of anesthesia to decompress the bladder and stomach. The abdomen is inflated either by placing a small needle into the peritoneal cavity (Veress technique) or by incising the skin and dissecting a hole into the peritoneal (Hassan technique). A camera port (umbilical) and two smaller (5 mm) ports are placed usually in the suprapubic region or left lower abdominal area. Using the appropriate instrumentation, the bowel is gently manipulated to expose the cecum and appendix. The appendix is then gently retracted to reveal its mesentery, which is then ligated. An endovascular stapling device is then used to transect the base of the appendix. The appendix is then placed in a bag and delivered from the abdomen through the umbilical site. Removal of the ports under direct visualization after examination of the cecum for hemostasis and adequacy of the staple line, irrigation, and suctioning of the abdomen. The port sites are then closed and dressings applied.

LAPAROSCOPIC CHOLECYSTECTOMY

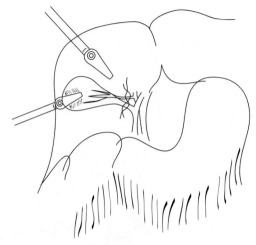

FIGURE 10-3

Laparoscopic cholecystectomy with ligatures shown around the cystic artery and cystic duct.

After an incision is made in or around the umbilicus, a Veress needle or Hasaan trocar is used to gain entry into the abdomen. Carbon dioxide is then insufflated into the abdomen to expand the peritoneal cavity for visualization. Additional ports are placed in the RUQ to provide access for instruments. The gallbladder is identified and grasped at its dome and retracted in a cephalad fashion. The cystic duct and artery are carefully dissected while avoiding any manipulation of the common bile duct (CBD). This is the most crucial part of the operation, since injury to the CBD can result in significant morbidity. The cystic artery and cystic duct are ligated and the gallbladder is dissected free from the liver bed. The freed gallbladder is placed in a bag for delivery out of the abdomen. The placement of a drain in the RUQ is at the discretion of the surgeon. While removing the ports, every attempt is made to decompress the abdomen, as retained CO_2 might add to discomfort postoperatively. The incision sites are then closed and dressed.

gallbladder wall (>3 mm), pericholecystic fluid, and gallstones. Additionally, document pain associated with placing the US probe in the RUQ (a sonographic Murphy's sign). If the diagnosis is in question after the US, order a **HIDA scan** as the definitive physiological test of cholecystitis.

Acute cholecystitis will, most often, require urgent surgery. Admit the patient to the hospital, order NPO, and start broad-spectrum antibiotics. Offer **laparoscopic cholecystectomy** as the procedure of choice to remove the gallbladder (Figure 10-3). Advantages to the laparoscopic cholecystectomy compared with the traditional open approach are smaller incisions with less pain, earlier mobilization, and discharge from the hospital. Patients who are found to have a high bilirubin level or a dilated CBD on US are offered **endoscopic retrograde cholangiopancreatogram** (ERCP) for possible CBD stone removal before proceeding with cholecystectomy.

Bowel Obstruction

Intestinal obstruction is a common problem that may occur anywhere along the GI tract. There are many possible causes of obstruction, which can be divided into mechanical and nonobstructive etiologies. The problem can further be classified, based on location (small or large bowel) and how the bowel is being obstructed (extrinsic, intramural, or intraluminal).

The most common causes of small bowel obstruction are **postoperative adhesions** and **abdominal wall hernias** (Figure 10-1). Other less common causes include tumors, inflammatory bowel disease, radiation enteritis, gallstone ileus, and intussusception.

While the presentation of a small bowel obstruction varies depending on location of the obstruction and duration, the most common **chief complaint** is abdominal pain with nausea and emesis. Characterize the pain as intermittent (colic) and centered around the umbilicus for a small bowel (midgut) process or suprapubic area (hindgut) etiology. Establish a **time course** of symptoms in the history of the present illness, including onset of symptoms, ability to sleep with pain, and recent food ingestion or travel. Determine the recent bowel movement pattern, including any failure to pass stool (constipation) or flatus (obstipation), or diarrhea. Diarrhea can sometimes precede constipation and obstipation in evolving obstructions.

The **physical examination** will also vary, depending on severity and duration of the obstruction. Observe abdominal distention, auscultate high pitched or tinkling bowel sounds, percuss tympany, and elicit diffuse tenderness to palpation.

Obtain a **CBC** for leukocytosis and anemia. Uncomplicated bowel obstruction should not cause an increased white cell count, and leukocytosis should raise the suspicion of bowel ischemia or perforation. Anemia may be an indicator of a tumor or inflammatory condition, which has caused a low-grade GI bleed. Review the **electrolyte panel** for signs of dehydration, hypokalemia, and hypochloridemia. A decreased bicarbonate level, acidosis on an ABG, or an elevation in the serum lactate all prompt concern for associated bowel ischemia.

Order an **abdominal series**, which includes a flat and upright abdominal film with a chest X-ray. Review the films in regard to the bowel gas pattern and caliber of the bowel wall and for the presence of free intraperitoneal air. Radiographic signs of small bowel obstruction include dilated loops of bowel with absence of air distally and *air fluid* levels on upright images.

Order an **abdomen CT** scan with oral and IV contrast to diagnose and stage bowel obstruction. In addition to revealing a transition point, the CT scan show internal and abdominal wall hernias, masses, and signs of bowel ischemia such as thickened wall, pneumatosis, and abscesses. Alternatively, consider a **small bowel follow through** as a dynamic examination to further define the exact point of obstruction along the bowel segment.

In patients who present with a partial small bowel obstruction, offer a trial of **nonoperative therapy**. Place a nasogastric tube (see Figure 13-1), start intravenous fluid resuscitation, correct electrolytes, and order NPO. Place a Foley catheter to monitor adequacy of resuscitation. In general, significant narcotics should not be needed in uncomplicated bowel obstruction. Withhold antibiotic therapy unless the patient fails nonoperative management and requires surgery. This approach can continue for 2–3 days as long as the patient begins to show signs of improvement, such as less distention, decreasing nasogastric output, and bowel movements. If no improvement is made with 72 hours, consider exploratory laparotomy.

Prepare for **immediate surgery** if the patient presents with peritoneal signs or evidence of complete bowel obstruction. In the operating room, a full exploration is performed, resecting all nonviable bowel and performing a lysis of adhesions (Figure 10-4). Postoperatively, resuscitation with fluid and blood

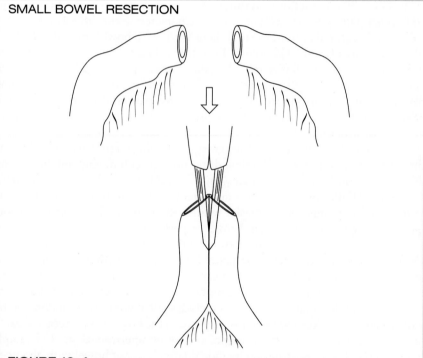

SMALL BOWEL RESECTION

FIGURE 10-4
Bowel anastamosis after lysis of adhesions and bowel resection.

Once the margins of the resection are identified, the mesenteric–bowel border is identified and entered, creating a window that will allow one limb of the stapler through. This should be repeated at the other margin. Once the windows have been created, a "gastrointestinal anastamosis" (GIA) stapler is used to transect the bowel at either margin. The mesentery of the transected portion is then divided by clamping and tying mesenteric vessels. With the pathologic specimen resected, the bowel is then placed together in a side-to-side fashion and anastomosed using another GIA stapler with a limb placed on either segment. The resultant opening in the bowel is then closed with another stapler or by suturing. Defects in the mesentery need to be addressed and closed, in order to prevent internal hernias. The abdomen should then be irrigated and closed. There is no need for external drainage.

products is continued as needed. Continue NG decompression and NPO status until bowel function returns.

Perforated Duodenal Ulcer

Patients with a perforated duodenal or gastric ulcer typically have a **dramatic presentation** with severe peritonitis and shock. The history often reveals a sudden onset of severe epigastric pain, sometimes followed by a short period of relief, and then a crescendo increase in the pain until medical attention is sought.

Although there may not be a specific history of ulcer disease in the past, most patients will relate long-standing reflux symptoms or chronic epigastric pain. The examination is dramatic, with cool clammy skin, agitation, and tachycardia. The abdominal examination reveals peritonitis, with the maximal tenderness in the epigastric region. Look for **free air** on the abdominal series, although appreciate that 30% of perforations will not show free air on plain radiograph. If the diagnosis is in doubt, an abdominal CT will show air in the periduodenal region with free fluid and possibly edema of the duodenum.

Begin fluid resuscitation immediately for the profound third space losses associated with a perforated ulcer (see Chapter 7). In preparation for surgery, **replete electrolytes** and **correct coagulopathy**. The most common surgical procedure for a duodenal perforation is the Graham patch duodenoplasty (Figure 10-5). In very unique cases, patients may present several days after a perforation has occurred. If there is evidence that the perforation has sealed, nonoperative management is possible; however, this is a complex decision that is made by experienced clinicians.

Pancreatitis

Acute pancreatitis occurs when parenchymal or ductal damage leads to pancreatic enzyme leakage with autodigestion of peripancreatic tissues. The most common causes of pancreatitis in the United States are common **bile duct stones** (blocking the pancreatic duct) and excessive **alcohol ingestion**. Multiple other etiologies including hypertriglyceridemia and medication reactions exist. Patients often present with severe and **unremitting epigastric pain**, with radiation to the back. Associated symptoms may include nausea, vomiting, and fever. The abdominal examination findings include mild-to-moderate distention with hypoactive bowel sounds. Depending on the severity of disease, tenderness could be mild to severe pain with rigidity and guarding.

Patients with severe disease may manifest all of the signs and symptoms of the **systemic inflammatory response syndrome** without a true infectious source (see Chapter 9). Thus, determining simple pancreatic necrosis from superinfection (infected necrosis) is difficult.

Order an **amylase** and **lipase** as the diagnostic laboratory values. The level of elevation of enzymes does not always correlate with the severity of the inflammation. Order an **abdominal CT** as the radiographic test of choice to evaluate the anatomical changes. By showing areas of nonuptake of intravenous contrast, the CT scan will reveal the amount of necrosis present, as well as associated

GRAHAM PATCH DUODENOPLASTY

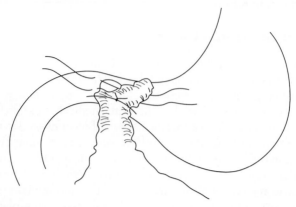

FIGURE 10-5
A tongue of omentum is secured over the ulcer site to 'patch' the ulcer.

With the patient in a supine position, a midline incision is made. If frank pus is found upon opening the abdomen, some surgeons will perform cultures of the peritoneal fluid. The stomach and duodenum are then examined for the site of perforation. Simple closure of the ulcer is not warranted, since the tissue is extremely friable and attempts to place and tighten sutures through the ulcer often result in tearing and enlargement of the ulcer. Thus, the concept of the Graham patch is to "plug" the hole with viable tissue that will let the ulcer heal.

Sutures are placed in an interrupted fashion from one side of the ulcer to the other, leaving a long tail on each side. A tongue of omentum is then placed over the closure as a means of filling the defect. The omentum is then tacked to the site with the long tail of the suture material. The site is then inspected, and the abdomen is copiously irrigated and suctioned until clear. A drain is sometimes left next to the repair. The abdominal incision should then be closed in the standard fashion.

---

retroperitoneal hemorrhage. If the inciting event is thought to be choledo-cholithiasis, perform an **abdominal US** to look for stones in the common bile duct.

Once the diagnosis of pancreatitis has been made, admit the patient to the hospital for supportive care. Pancreatitis causes significant third space fluid loss; thus begin **resuscitation** with intravenous fluids and provide hemodynamic support as needed (see Chapter 7). Seek to identify and **correct the cause** of the pancreatitis. There is controversy of when and how to manage common bile duct stones associated with severe pancreatitis. In these patients, consult a gastroenterologist for possible endoscopic retrograde cholangiopancreatogram. In severe cases, start **antibiotics**, including medications that have documented penetration into the pancreas.

Consider **surgical debridement** for infected pancreatic necrosis or in patients who have sterile pancreatic necrosis but do not improve and/or have fulminant disease. The goal of surgery is to drain infected tissue and debride necrotic tissue. Standard approaches include an upper midline laparotomy or a chevron-type bilateral subcostal incision. Once debridement is completed, the abdomen may be closed over drains (closed technique) or left open with the plan to perform intermittent dressing changes in the wound (open technique).

Diverticulitis

Diverticular disease of the large bowel is common among older patients in the United States. The anatomic hallmark of **diverticulosis** is false (or pulsion) diverticula, which develop at weak points along the bowel wall where blood vessels penetrate the muscular layers of bowel. It is felt that a typical Western diet low in fiber results in altered bowel function, with elevated intraluminal pressures causing the disease. Simple diverticulosis is often asymptomatic. Clinical syndromes occur when the diverticuli become infected (diverticulitis) or bleed (see Chapter 14).

Elicit a **chief complaint** of left lower quadrant pain and fever. Although the sigmoid colon is by far the most site of disease, occasionally the right colon is affected, causing RLQ pain. The pain is steady, described as a pressure, or crampy. Often, patients will describe a sensation that they need to have a bowel movement (tenesmus). Other complaints might include nausea, emesis, constipation, and dysuria. Ask about previous similar attacks and other bowel problems in the past. Diverticulitis is not associated with ingestion of any single food or food type.

Physical examination findings can be variable, depending on the severity of the disease. The **abdominal examination** demonstrates tenderness, which may range from mild to severe with peritoneal signs. It is important to recognize and distinguish localized from diffuse peritonitis as management may differ. A lower abdominal mass may be palpated if an abscess is present.

Laboratory studies include a **CBC** to look for elevation in the white blood cell count seen in diverticulitis and a chronic anemia often presenting long-term diverticulosis.

Order a **plain radiograph** of the abdomen to identify abnormal bowel gas patterns (ileus) or the presence of free air in cases of perforation. Use the **abdominal CT** scan as the gold standard for diagnosis and staging of diverticular disease. Presence of a mass or phlegmon next to the colonic wall, with stranding of mesenteric fat or localized free air, is a sign of diverticulitis.

Treatment for diverticulitis depends on the severity. In cases of **mild disease**, offer outpatient treatment with oral antibiotics and closely follow. With moderate to **severe disease**, admit the patient, order **NPO**, start intravenous **hydration**, and begin intravenous **antibiotics**. If there is evidence of a fluid collection on CT scan, consult interventional radiology for possible **image-directed drainage**. Once the clinical picture improves as evidenced by decreasing pain, normalizing temperature, and normalizing white count, the patient is started back on a diet. Antibiotics should be continued for a specific time frame, dictated by the severity of the disease.

Patients with diffuse peritonitis, or who fail to improve with nonoperative therapy, are offered Colon Resection (see Figure 14-3). The diseased segment of colon is completely resected. The surgeon then has three options for **reconstruction**. The Hartman's procedure involves exteriorizing the proximal colon as a colostomy, leaving the rectal stump. Alternatively, the colon can be anastamosed alone or with a proximal diverting loop ileostomy (protective ileostomy). In most cases of acute diverticulitis taken for surgery, a Hartman's procedure will be performed. Subsequent surgery is then planned for reversal of the Hartman's or the protecting ileostomy.

Volvulus

A volvulus is defined as a twisting of bowel, usually as a result of a redundant mesentery. This can ultimately result in ischemia to the affected segment with subsequent perforation. While most commonly seen in the sigmoid colon, the process can also occur in the cecum and transverse colon.

The signs and symptoms of colonic volvulus are same as those of **GI obstruction**. Elicit a chief complaint of distention, abdominal pain, nausea and emesis, obstipation, and constipation. The **distention** may be profound and, in the elderly or demented patients, may be the only significant finding. Enquire about items in the history that are associated with volvulus, such as chronic constipation, excessive laxative use, or long-term confinement to bed.

Laboratory values are unrevealing for the diagnosis. However, if there is a history of vomiting, consider obtaining a **CBC** and **electrolyte** panel to look for evidence of dehydration and anemia.

Inspect the plain abdominal film for the **bent inner tube** sign that is highly suggestive of a sigmoid volvulus. An image that appears with a **coffee bean-shaped** pattern is consistent with a cecal volvulus. If there is suggestion of volvulus on plain film, perform a water-soluble **enema** contrast study, which may show a **bird's beak sign**, indicating an abrupt cutoff of the contrast flow.

Medical management includes prompt resuscitation and repletion of electrolytes. Place a nasogastric tube to help avoid aspiration and a Foley catheter to measure urine output as an indicator of resuscitation.

Offer **endoscopic decompression** of a sigmoid volvulus unless hemodynamic instability or peritonitis is present. The advantage of colonic decompression is that once untwisted, a bowel prep can be performed prior to the needed colon resection. A **rectal tube** is placed at the time of decompression and left in place until the patient is brought to the operating room. After sigmoid decompression, offer a sigmoid colectomy to all patients who are surgical candidates on account of the high likelihood of recurrence without surgery. If sigmoid decompression fails, or the patient is found to have a cecal or transverse colon volvulus, consider immediate resection in the operating room.

Acute Mesenteric Ischemia

Acute mesenteric ischemia can involve either the small or the large bowel. Ischemia can be acute or chronic (see Chapter 11) and further classified into embolic, thrombotic, or nonocclusive.

Consider mesenteric ischemia in any patient with a sudden-onset mid-abdominal pain. Probe the past medical history for **risk factors**, including atrial fibrillation, previous myocardial infarction (with aneurysm or mural thrombus), mitral valve disease, aortic atherosclerosis, or previous embolic disease. Determine if the patient has peripheral vascular disease of the extremities (see Chapter 16).

Abdominal tenderness is distinctly absent during the early stages of the disease. The **perceived pain** is severe, however, leading to the axiom that the "pain is out of proportion to the physical examination." Peritoneal signs indicate that the ischemia has become full thickness or that a segment has been perforated, causing generalized spillage of enteric contents.

There is no specific laboratory study to diagnose ischemic bowel. Indirect evidence for bowel ischemia is the development of a lactic acidosis. Obtain an electrolyte panel, with special attention to the **bicarbonate** level. Obtain serial **lactate** levels to follow the trend and to judge adequacy of resuscitation. If the patient is taking anticoagulants, determine the prothrombin time, partial thromboplastin time (**PTT**), and **platelet** level. Consider reversing coagulopathy only after consultation with the vascular surgeon.

Use the **CT angiogram** to identify occlusion of the more proximal mesenteric vessels, such as the celiac axis and superior mesenteric artery. In patients with renal failure, consider an **MR angiogram** to avoid nephrotoxic contrast used in CT or conventional angiogram. Despite the rapidly advancing technology found in CT and MR, **contrast angiography** remains the gold standard, since it can detect disease at all locations of the vascular tree, not just the major branching points, and can offer therapeutic options. Therapeutic options available during angiogram include local injection of papaverine for spasm, balloon angioplasty, and endovascular stent placement.

Regardless of the etiology, prompt intervention is warranted. Admit the patient to an intensive care unit with proper cardiac monitoring. Start resuscitation with **intravenous fluids** and provide **pain relief** with analgesics. At the discretion of the vascular surgeon, a **heparin drip** may be started until definitive diagnosis and treatment is possible. Consider intravenous **antibiotics** in all patients with potential bowel ischemia.

Definitive therapy will depend on the exact etiology of the ischemia. **Nonocclusive mesenteric ischemia** is a primarily spasmodic condition that responds to aggressive fluid resuscitation and an intra-arterial infusion of the smooth muscle relaxant papaverine. **Embolic disease** should be managed with the goal of restoring normal pulsatile flow to the involved vessel, followed by resection of full-thickness ischemic portion of bowel. This is possible by a combined operative embolectomy and bowel resection or endovascular embolectomy followed by exploratory laparotomy. **Thrombotic disease** is treated most often with surgical bypass (see Figure 11-4).

Nephrolithiasis

Consider nephrolithiasis in patients who present with severe, colicky flank, groin or lateral abdominal pain. The onset is often abrupt, followed by nausea and vomiting. Urinalysis will show hematuria. See **Chapter 23** for a full discussion of nephrolithiasis.

Ectopic Pregnancy

Depending on the implantation site, symptoms of ectopic pregnancy can manifest anywhere from 6 to 16 weeks' gestation. In addition to abdominal pain, there may be associated vaginal bleeding. Tubal rupture may ensue, accompanied by hemodynamic instability. See **Chapter 21** for a full discussion of ectopic pregnancy.

Selected Readings

Cameron JL, ed. *Current Surgical Therapy.* 8th ed. New York, NY: Mosby; 2004.

Sabiston DC, ed. *Atlas of General Surgery.* Philadelphia: Saunders; 1994.

Silen W, ed. *Cope's Early Diagnosis of the Acute Abdomen.* 20th ed. New York: Oxford University Press; 2000.

11

Chronic Abdominal Pain

Ruby A. Skinner, MD, FACS, FCCP ■ *Terri R. Martin, MD, FACS*

Key Points

- Unlike in acute abdominal pain syndromes, patients with chronic abdominal pain have a lengthier past medical history.

- Patients with chronic pain syndromes can have acute abdominal catastrophes. Look for signs of peritonitis to distinguish acute problems from ongoing chronic issue.

- The most helpful radiographic studies are abdominal computed tomography, abdominal ultrasonography, and an upper GI series.

- Peptic ulcer disease is a common cause of chronic pain. Direct the treatment toward eliminating *Helicobacter pylori* infection and decreasing acid secretion.

- Gastric ulcers have a much greater potential for harboring a malignancy than duodenal ulcers. Thus, obtain biopsies to rule out gastric cancer.

- Although gastroesophageal reflux disease (GERD) is treated symptomatically, an esophagogastroduodenoscopy (EGD) is considered to examine the extent of esophageal mucosa damage and to rule out premalignant (Barrett's esophagus) or frank cancer at the gastroesophageal junction.

- Consider antireflux surgery in patients with severe reflux by physiologic tests, intractable symptoms, or evidence of severe mucosal inflammation on EGD.

- Biliary colic is distinguished from acute cholecystitis in that biliary colic is intermittent, recurring, and not associated with evidence of infection, such as fever and leukocytosis.

- The sine quo non of chronic mesenteric ischemia is the history of postprandial diffuse abdominal pain, weight loss, food fear, and associated peripheral vascular disease.

- Inflammatory bowel disease includes Crohn's disease and ulcerative colitis (UC). Both are chronic, remitting, and recurring inflammatory syndromes, characterized by diarrhea and abdominal pain.

- Functional abdominal pain syndrome (FAPS) is related to abnormal intestinal motility and alterations in pain perception. Irritable bowel syndrome (IBS) is a disorder of intestinal motility in addition to abnormal pain processing. Both are difficult to diagnose and treat.

■ HISTORY

Chronic abdominal pain is defined as pain or abdominal discomfort that reoccurs and is distinguished from acute abdominal pain, which is discussed in the previous chapter. It is a common chief complaint for emergency department and outpatient visits, and it has been estimated that up to 30% of Americans suffer from chronic pain at some point in their lifetime. There are several structural (organic) causes that are very familiar to the general surgeon as well as functional causes that must be considered once organic causes have been ruled out.

Unlike acute abdominal pain syndromes, patients with chronic abdominal pain often have multiple previous admissions and visits to physicians, and thus, often have a lengthy past medical history. Start by clearly defining the **chief complaint**, taking care to distinguish a new complaint from a chronic complaint that is ongoing. Chronic conditions can get suddenly worse, such as a perforation of an ulcer that had been the source of chronic pain. In other situations, the symptoms may not be new, but the patient now seeks medical attention for other reasons. Determine the type and quality of **pain**, as discussed previously (see Chapter 10).

Determine the **changes in symptoms** evident in the history of the present illness. In patients with Crohn's disease or ulcerative colitis, determine new patterns in diarrhea or if there are new possible areas of enterocutaneous fistulas.

In patients with gastric reflux disease, elicit changes in pain control with medication or new food intolerances. Inquire whether patients with known ulcer disease ever completed a course of treatment for *H. pylori*.

Perform a thorough **past medical history**, medications, family history, substance abuse history, surgical history, recent travel history, and occupational history. Many patients will have previous examinations and diagnostic tests, which have already been performed. Take time to review all **old records** and radiology reports. This will decrease duplication of the diagnostic workup and provide clues to narrowing the differential diagnosis. Often times when a surgical consult is obtained on a patient with chronic abdominal pain, the consulting physician will present the patient as if the workup is complete and the only alternative is surgical intervention. Take care to review all of the diagnostic data so that an informed decision can be made about the need for surgical intervention.

■ PHYSICAL EXAMINATION

The abdominal examination begins with a **general observation** of the patient's behavior, body positioning, and visual abdominal inspection. One can usually easily exclude peritonitis, which causes patients to appear uncomfortable and often lie still, as any movement will exacerbate the pain. Patients with mesenteric ischemia may complain of severe pain, which is out of proportion to the physical findings, unless they have associated intestinal necrosis. A patient with renal colic may writhe in pain and complain of back pain radiating to the groin but have a soft abdomen. An acute process is often associated with abnormal vital signs, including tachycardia, fever, altered mental status, and tachypnea. Patients with chronic disorders most commonly have no significant changes in the vital signs.

Auscultate the abdomen to focus on the presence or absence of bowel sounds as well as the character of intestinal peristalsis. Hypoactive or absent bowel sounds are often owing to an ileus, whereas high-pitched sounds with tinkles and rushes indicate a possible obstruction. The presence of a vascular bruit suggests possible vascular stenosis, which may be related to mesenteric ischemia.

Palpate all quadrants of the abdomen to determine localized tenderness, which can help limit the diagnosis. Young patients with chronic pain and tenderness to palpation, primarily in the right lower quadrant, may have inflammatory bowel disease, such as Crohn's ileitis. A patient who presents with right-sided flank pain that radiates to the groin associated with episodes of hematuria most likely has chronic pain associated with nephrolithiasis. Lastly, if a patient has a soft abdomen with no specific area of tenderness but reports severe pain, which is at times related to eating, then one should consider mesenteric ischemia.

Functional disorders such as fibromyalgia and irritable bowel syndrome are usually associated with diffuse pain, which is difficult to localize. These patients may be extremely hypersensitive to pain, and, although the abdomen is soft, palpation may cause an exaggerated response. The pain at times may be described as crampy in nature, which may be associated with alternation of constipation and diarrhea. These patients on occasion have associated psychological disturbances; thus, a sensitive approach is warranted in examining them.

Abnormal abdominal **masses** should be noted, as they may represent benign or malignant neoplasms. Enlargement of the liver or spleen are commonly associated with portal hypertension, sickle cell anemia, infections such as hepatitis, and some malignancies. Patients with severe liver disease often are jaundiced and may have altered mental status because of encephalopathy. Renal failure patients when they are uremic can have altered mentation as well.

A surgical physical examination is not complete without proper evaluation for groin and ventral **hernias**. Inspect for less common lateral abdominal wall hernias (Spigelian) and obturator hernias. Patients with obturator hernias may present with nonspecific abdominal pain, with a mass in the upper medial thigh or obturator canal. Pain may be elicited in the medial thigh upon internal rotation of the limb and is called the **Howship–Romberg** sign.

Perform a **rectal examination** as an essential component of the physical examination. The perianal area is inspected for abnormal lesions, fistulas, fissures, and evidence of hemorrhoids. The rectum is palpated for the presence of rectal lesions, and anal tone is noted. The prostate is palpated in men and the ovaries in women. Consider a vaginal or bimanual examination in all women as well to feel for masses or tenderness over the ovary or fallopian tube areas, which may reveal masses or sites of infection.

■ LABORATORY STUDIES

Order a **CBC** to look for elevations in the white blood cell count suggesting infections and to determine the hemoglobin level. Evaluate the **serum chemistry** to rule out electrolyte abnormalities, renal function, and serum glucose levels. Patients with chronic bowel obstructions will typically have evidence of dehydration, and metabolic acidosis must be corrected before surgery. Elevations in **liver function tests** may suggest biliary obstruction or primary liver dysfunction as a result of a gallstones, cystic duct obstruction, or hepatitis. Order an **amylase** and **lipase** in patients suspected of having pancreatitis, although elevations of these parameters are not always seen in cases of chronic pancreatitis.

In patients with suspected peptic ulcer disease, determine whether there is infection with *H. pylori*. Order a serum **H. pylori titer** or, alternatively, have a tissue biopsy obtained during EGD tested for *H. pylori* activity. Consider obtaining a serum **gastrin** level in patients with intractable or recurrent peptic ulcer disease to rule out gastrin-secreting tumors.

Perform a **urinalysis** to rule out cystitis or pyelonephritis and to assess the patient's level of dehydration. The presence of hematuria suggests the possibility of nephrolithiasis.

A **pregnancy test** is performed in all female patients of child-bearing age, from menarche through menopause, regardless of history given as to contraceptive use, sexual abstinence, timing of last menstrual period, history of tubal ligation, or perceived perimenopausal status.

■ RADIOGRAPHIC STUDIES

Radiography is often a key adjunct to the history and physical examination in the diagnostic process. In all patients, order an upright chest X-ray (**CXR**) to look for the presence of free air, an elevated left diaphragm because of a process in the LUQ, such as a subphrenic abscess, spleen pathology, or a dilated stomach owing to peptic ulcer disease. Also use the CXR to rule out pulmonary processes, such as pneumonias, which may result in referred pain to the abdomen. Order an **abdominal series** to rule out abnormal gas patterns as seen in obstruction, ileus, or mass effect due to an intra-abdominal tumor or inflammatory process.

Consider an abdominal **ultrasound** for the diagnostic of choice for biliary disease, such as cholelithiasis. Ultrasound is also considered in the diagnosis of abdominal or pelvic masses or to document presence or extent of abdominal ascites. **Ultrasound duplex** of abdominal vessels is considered in patients who are suspected of having portal or hepatic vein obstruction or abdominal aortic aneurysms causing abdominal pain.

In patients with symptoms consistent with biliary colic or recurrent cholecystitis, consider a radionuclide excretion study, such as a **HIDA scan**, to determine whether the cystic duct is obstructed. The examination involves the administration of a radiotracer and following its excretion from the liver into the biliary system by scintigraphy. If tracer does not fill the gallbladder retrograde, there is evidence for cystic duct obstruction, which is consistent with biliary colic and cholecystitis.

Order an abdominal CT as the definitive diagnostic test for most abdominal disease processes. The evolution of CT scan technology has revolutionized the precise identification of hepatobiliary, intestinal, vascular, and abdominal wall pathology. Consider oral contrast to enhance the identification and differentiation of hollow visceral structures. Administer intravenous contrast to aide in the enhancement of areas of inflammation (such as abscess cavities) and allow diagnosis of abdominal vascular lesions. Use caution in the administration of IV contrast in patients with a known allergy or in the context of acute or chronic renal failure. Often radiology departments will have specific protocols for certain potential diagnoses, such as appendicitis. Thus, provide accurate patient information and potential clinical diagnosis to help the radiologist plan the appropriate CT protocol. In patients with an IV contrast allergy, those with a suspected abdominal mass, or patients who are pregnant, consider an abdominal **MRI** as an alternative to a CT scan to make an anatomic diagnosis.

In patients with chronic intestinal obstructions, suspected bowel mass/stricture, or suspected ulcer disease, obtain an **upper GI series** with small bowel follow through (SBFT). Alternatively, consult a gastroenterologist to perform an **EGD** in selective cases in patients suspected of intestinal disorders such as peptic ulcer disease, inflammatory bowel disease, or malignant neoplasms.

■ DIAGNOSTIC PLAN

Using the **history** and the **physical examination**, determine if the patient may have an acute abdominal crisis that needs immediate treatment (see Chapter 10). For all others, guide the radiographic workup toward the most likely diagnosis. Thus, if cholelithiasis is suspected, order an abdominal ultrasound. Avoid the practice of ordering a standard "battery" of tests for every patient, for this is impractical, uncomfortable for the patient, and not cost effective.

If several radiographic tests fail to reveal a source of the pain, consider **consultation** with gastroenterology, infectious disease, or general medicine, as the situation dictates. If no pathology is found after multiple examinations and consultations, some patients are considered for **diagnostic laparoscopy** as a final attempt to make an anatomic diagnosis (see Figure 21-1). Patients are extensively counseled that diagnostic laparoscopy may not find a source and rarely is a therapeutic maneuver.

Patients who have had extensive workup and still have no source of pain are entered into a **pain management** program and are followed for changes in their clinical situation. Referral to **psychiatry** is considered for ruling out psychosomatic disorders and to deal with the very real depression that often accompanies chronic pain syndromes.

■ DIFFERENTIAL DIAGNOSIS AND TREATMENT

Peptic Ulcer Disease

Peptic ulcer disease, including duodenal and gastric ulceration, is a common disorder causing chronic abdominal pain. The history will reveal intermittent dull or gnawing epigastric pain, often becoming worse several hours after eating. Many patients have temporary relief of symptoms with antacid or additional food intake. Physical examination will often include tenderness to deep palpation of the epigastrum, without an associated mass. The symptoms and examination are similar to, and are often confused with, the symptoms of cholelithiasis or cholecystitis.

Make the diagnosis by obtaining a barium or gastrograffin **upper GI series**. In cases where the upper GI is equivocal, or there is a suspicion of malignancy, consult a gastroenterologist to perform **EGD** (see Figure 13-2) as the definitive diagnostic modality. EGD has the advantage of the ability to biopsy suspicious ulcers and provides treatment in cases of acute bleeding.

Treatment depends on the location and likely cause of the ulceration. Since duodenal ulcers are most often associated with gastric acid hypersecretion and *H. pylori* infection, medical management includes antacids, H2 blockers, and antibiotic therapy against *H. pylori*. With eradication of *H. pylori* infection, ulcer recurrence drops to approximately 5%. With the success of medical management for peptic ulcer disease, the need for surgical intervention has become very uncommon. For patients with intractable symptoms, or complications from long-term disease such as pyloric stricture, the most common surgical option is the **vagotomy and antrectomy** (Figure 11-1A). Complication of duodenal ulcer includes perforation (see Chapter 10) and acute upper GI hemorrhage (see Chapter 13).

Patients with **gastric ulcers** often have symptoms indistinguishable to those with duodenal disease. The etiology is more related to the loss of the mucosal barrier, as opposed to acid over secretion. Gastric ulcers have a much greater potential for harboring a malignancy. Thus, arrange for an EGD to make the definitive diagnosis and to obtain biopsies to rule out **gastric cancer** (see Chapter 18). Direct medical management at re-enforcing the mucosal barrier by having patients avoid nonsteroidal anti-inflammatory medications, smoking, alcohol, and steroids. Provide a full course of antibiotics to eliminate *H. pylori* infection similar to duodenal ulcer disease. Large ulcers, those that have an associated cancer, or ones that acutely bleed or perforate are resected by performing a partial gastrectomy (Figure 11-1B).

Gastroesophageal Reflux Disease

Elicit the hallmark complaint of **epigastric burning** pain that radiates into the chest (heartburn). Determine if symptoms are exacerbated by meals and recombinant position. Ask about foods that cause the symptoms such as caffeinated products or chocolate.

Although the diagnosis of GERD is primarily made by the history, characterization of the extent and severity of disease is important when determining the type of treatment indicated. Arrange for an **EGD** to examine the extent of damage to the esophageal mucosa and to rule out premalignant (Barrett's esophagus) or frank cancer at the gastroesophageal junction. Consider a **physiologic test** to determine the extent of reflux. Esophageal **manometry** is used to measure esophageal peristalsis and lower esophageal sphincter (LES) function. The more severe the reflux, the lower the LES resting pressure, and the slower the esophageal peristalsis becomes. **Continuous pH monitoring** involves a probe, which is placed within the esophagus for a 24-hour period while the patients perform their normal activity. The probe measures pH changes in the esophagus, which indicates the severity of reflux from the stomach. Results are reported in percentage of time the probes measure a pH < 4.0, with a normal value being around 4%.

Direct the **medical management** toward decreasing symptoms by avoiding large meals before sleeping, encouraging positional changes such as sleeping at 30 degrees, and using prokinetic medications such as metoclopramide.

Consider surgery in patients with severe reflux by physiologic tests, intractable symptoms, or evidence of severe mucosal inflammation on EGD. The surgical correction of GERD involves correction of the gastroesophageal junction anatomy to bolster the LES function. The most commonly performed procedure is the **Nissen fundoplication**, by either open or laparoscopic technique (Figure 11-2). In patients who have been diagnosed with Barrett's esophagus or frank carcinoma, begin a workup for metastatic disease and consider esophagectomy for cure or palliation (see Chapter 12).

SURGERY FOR ULCER DISEASE

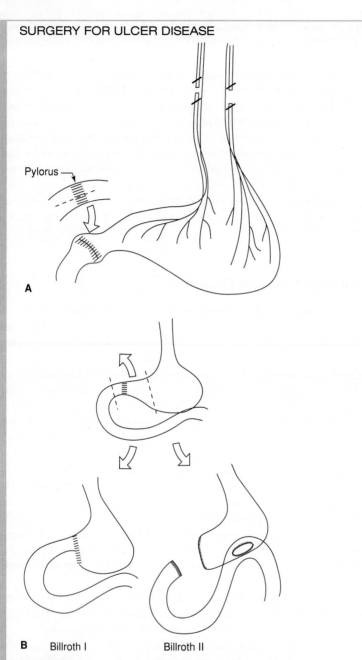

FIGURE 11-1
(A) Vagotomy and Pyloroplasty, (B) Antrectomy with a Billroth I and Billroth II reconstruction

On account of the success of medical management, surgery is rarely indicated for ulcer disease and is reserved for patients with complicated disease or intractable symptoms. The parietal cells of the stomach are under positive feedback from the vagus nerve to produce acid. A

vagotomy is a procedure to sever the vagus stimulation to the stomach, decreasing the production of acid, in an attempt to allow ulcer healing. (A) The vagotomy is performed via a midline laparotomy or by laparoscopy. After mobilization of the hiatus of the stomach, the two main branches of the vagus nerve are found and small sections are cut from each one. The sections are sent for frozen section to confirm that the vagus nerve has indeed been severed. A side effect of performing the vagotomy is that the pylorus function will be impaired, which can cause a functional gastric outlet obstruction. To prevent this, a **pyloroplasty** is performed, which involves transecting the pyloric muscle and reapproximating it to make the sphincter incompetent (A). This will result in free flow of chime through the pylorus, despite loss of vagal function. Alternatively, a **selective vagotomy** can be attempted where only the branches of the vagus innervating the antrum are severed, leaving the branches to the pylorus intact, obviating the need for a pyloroplasty (not shown).

In cases of severe duodenal ulceration and gastric obstruction from scarring, a **vagotomy and antrectomy** (V&A) is considered. (B) The goal of the V&A is to remove the ulcer, remove the acid-producing cells of the stomach antrum, and sever the vagal stimulation to the stomach. It is performed via a midline laparotomy. The duodenum is mobilized and transected in the first portion. The stomach is transected in the mid body. A vagotomy is performed as described above. There are then two options for restoring continuity of the bowel. Either the distal stomach is anastamosed to the duodenum (Billroth I) or a loop of small bowel is brought up to perform a gastroenterostomy (Billroth II).

Cholelithiasis

Biliary colic is distinguished from acute cholecystitis in that biliary colic is intermittent, recurring, and not associated with evidence of infection such as fever and leukocytosis. Elicit a history of right upper quadrant pain that radiates to the back in a band-like fashion. The crampy pain often occurs a few hours after a meal and remits within a few hours after symptoms start. Determine if there is associated nausea and vomiting, which are commonly present.

Confirm the diagnosis by obtaining a right upper quadrant **ultrasound** with special attention to the presence of cholelithiasis. Presence of a thickened gallbladder wall or pericholecystic fluid is suggestive of acute cholecystitis. Biliary duct dilation is not seen in uncomplicated biliary colic and prompts a concern for choledocholithiasis or a pancreatic head mass causing obstruction of the common bile duct.

Uncomplicated biliary colic is self-limiting. For patients with recurrent attacks of biliary colic, consider offering elective cholecystectomy for relief of symptoms and to avoid progression of the disease to acute cholecystitis. The vast majority of elective cholecystectomy is performed by a laparoscopic technique (Figure 10-3).

Chronic Mesenteric Ischemia

As opposed to acute mesenteric occlusion, chronic ischemia is a progressive disorder, characterized by generalized abdominal pain that occurs after meals, leading to **avoidance of eating** (food fear) and **weight loss**. The etiology is progressive stenosis of the celiac and superior mesenteric arteries (SMA) to the

NISSEN FUNDOPLICATION

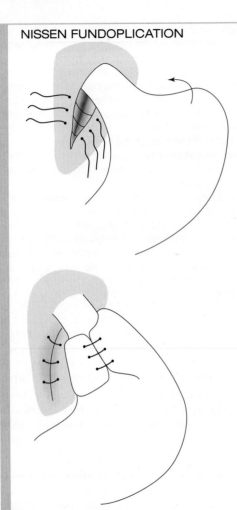

FIGURE 11-2
The Nissen Fundoplication for the Treatment of GERD

The goal of the Nissen fundoplication is to restore the proper anatomy of the gastroesophageal hiatus, allowing normal swallowing and deterring esophageal reflux. The procedure can be performed as an open technique but is most often performed in the United States, now by the laparoscopic route. In either type of approach, the stomach is mobilized at the hiatus. The crux is sling of muscle around the esophagus, as it enters the abdominal cavity. The first objective is to tighten the crux around the esophagus by suture ligature. A bougie is often placed in the lumen of the esophagus to assure that the esophagus is not strictured during this maneuver. Next the short gastric vessels running from the stomach to the spleen are ligated, and the fundus of the stomach is wrapped around itself at the hiatus, creating a collar at the GE junction. The "wrap" is secured, again with the boogie in the esophageal lumen. Sutures are then used to bolster the collar to the underside of the diaphragm, to prevent the wrap from slipping. Some surgeon may add a **gastrostomy** tube for early postoperative feeding in debilitated patients or to further anchor the stomach.

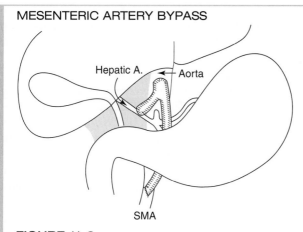

FIGURE 11-3
Mesenteric Bypass from the Aorta to the SMA and Celiac Trunk

The procedure starts with a midline laparotomy, and the aorta near its entrance to the abdomen is exposed and prepared for grafting. In general, both the celiac axis and the superior
mesenteric artery are bypassed for every patient needing revascularization. This is due to the
high proportion of patients with disease in both arteries and the fact that, with two arteries
revascularized, bowel perfusion can continue if one became thrombosed in the perioperative
period. A bifurcated PTFE graft is sewn into the aorta in an end-to-side fashion, and the distal
ends are typically anastamosed to the common hepatic artery and SMA. The common hepatic
artery is often used because it is a direct branch of the celiac axis and easier to expose and
work with the celiac axis proper. At the conclusion of the anastamoses, the bowel is inspected
for viability and the abdomen is closed.

point where a chronic low-flow state exists in the visceral vessels. Any stress,
such as food ingestion, causes ischemia and pain.

The diagnosis is suggested by the distinctive history along with the finding
of weight loss, especially in patients with known history of peripheral vascular
disease. Order an anatomic test such as **CT angiogram** or **MR angiogram** to
determine the exact location and extent of vascular stenosis. Formal invasive
angiogram is reserved for situation where a concomitant therapeutic angioplasty
or stenting is planned as part of the overall management.

Arterial bypass is considered in patients who are at acceptable operative risk
and have continuous symptoms that are resulting in morbidity such as continued weight loss. The most common procedures are aortoceliac and aorto-SMA
bypasses with vein or synthetic graft (Figure 11-3).

Chronic Pancreatitis

Patients who have had multiple episodes of acute pancreatitis can develop a
chronic pancreatitis. The chronic disease is an inflammatory process of the pancreas, which results in severe structural changes of the gland. Pain distribution
is similar to that of pancreatic cancer, which involves the epigastrum often ra-

diating to the back. The pain can be incapacitating, and narcotic abuse may be associated with this disorder. Make the diagnosis by noting an uneven **distension of the pancreatic duct** on CT scan ("chain of lakes"), pancreatic **calcifications**, and **pseudocyst** formation.

Therapy is directed at restoring pancreatic function in addition to pain control. The medical management is directed at providing **enzyme replacement** as well as **insulin** therapy for endocrine insufficiency. Initial **pain control** is narcotic therapy, although many patients develop dependency problems with long-term use. When medical therapy by traditional means fails, then more invasive pain control measures are used. This includes **chemical ablation** of the periceliac splanchnic innervations of the pancreas via endoscopic, intra-abdominal, percutaneous, and thoracoscopic routes. Success rates with this technique have been reported to be as high as 70% for significant pain relief.

Surgical resections for chronic pancreatitis are used in severe cases of untreatable symptoms. Procedures are based on removing or draining the portion of the pancreas that is diseased. Diseases of the head may be managed by local head resection (Frey procedure) or more aggressive therapies such as a Whipple procedure (see Figure 18-4). Disease involving the body and tail may require a Puestow procedure, which provides wide drainage of the pancreatic duct (Figure 11-4).

Inflammatory Bowel Disease

Both Crohn's disease and UC are remitting and recurring inflammatory syndromes that can cause significant morbidity and mortality. **Crohn's disease** is characterized by small bowel involvement, strictures, and enterocutaneous fistula formation. **UC** is associated with rectal and variable colonic involvement, with a significant risk of subsequent mucosal carcinoma.

Obtain a history of **diarrhea** as the hallmark sign of both disorders. The diarrhea can be continuous or intermittent and is more likely to be bloody in cases of UC. The character of the **pain** in Crohn's disease is colicky mid to lower abdominal, signifying the watershed involvement of the mid–hind gut boundary. UC most often involves the rectum and sigmoid, with variable involvement of the rest of the colon. Thus, the pain is typically isolated to the hindgut and radiates to the suprapubic region. Perform a thorough examination, including a rectal examination, looking for new sites of induration, suspecting new fistula formation.

Order an **SBFT**, with barium as the diagnostic test of choice for Crohn's disease. Typical findings on SBFT include thickened bowel wall with strictures (string sign), cobble stoning, and enterocutaneous fistula formation. In patients suspected of UC, obtain a **barium enema** study, which may show the classic shortening and loss of haustral markings, giving the colon a "lead pipe" appearance. Consider **CT scan** of the abdomen when perforation or localized abscesses are suspected, and in cases of new enterocutaneous fistula formation.

SURGERY FOR CHRONIC PANCREATITIS

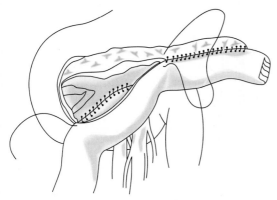

FIGURE 11-4
The Puestow Procedure

The pain from chronic pancreatitis is most likely a result of ductal dilation and inflammation of the surrounding nerve plexus. The goal in surgical procedures for chronic pancreatitis is to remove inflamed tissue, provide ductal drainage, or obliterate nerve function. The simplest procedure involves CT-guided or, rarely, operative injection of the **celiac plexus** with concentrated ethanol. This provides substantial pain relief in a majority of patients. The **Berger** procedure is a formal pancreatic head resection with preservation of the bile duct (unlike the Whipple procedure where the bile duct and duodenum are resected with the pancreatic head). The **Puestow** and the **Frey** procedures are variations of the same concept. After a midline laparotomy, the pancreas is exposed and the usually large pancreatic duct is opened longitudinally and then anastamosed to a segment of small bowel. This provides wide drainage of the pancreatic duct, decreasing ductal pressure and pain. Rarely, a **total pancreatectomy** is the only option for recurrent of intractable pain. Obviously, this leaves the patient totally dependent on oral exocrine replacement and insulin therapy for induced diabetes mellitus.

Treatment is suppressive and supportive, since there is currently no cure for either disorder. Direct the **medical management** toward relieving outside stress, providing adequate nutrition, and controlling inflammation with steroids or sulfasalazine. Consider surgical intervention for complications of Crohn's disease and UC such as perforation, stricture, intractable disease, or cancer. New-onset Crohn's disease is always considered in the differential diagnosis of **right lower quadrant pain** in young patients, and it is common for the disease to be diagnosed at appendectomy.

The most common indication for surgery is complete **bowel obstruction** from either strictures or local perforations with abscess formation and scarring (see Chapter 10). Surgical options include resection of effected bowel segments and colectomy for effected UC segments of colon. Since UC most often affects the rectal mucosa all the way to the anal verge, many patients will require total **proctocolectomy** with an ileoanal pouch reconstruction (Figure 11-5).

PROCTOCOLECTOMY

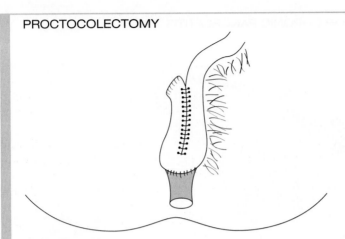

FIGURE 11-5
Proctocolectomy with Ileoanal Pouch for Ulcerative Colitis

Since UC invariably involves the rectal mucosa, and there is a risk of cancer in any affected mucosa left behind, the procedure of choice when patients need resection is total protocolectomy with reconstruction. The patient is positioned in the modified lithotomy position to give access to the abdomen and perianal region. A midline laparotomy is performed, and the entire colon and rectum are resected. Via the perianal approach, the distal rectal mucosa is resected, leaving a cuff of rectal muscle above the anal sphincters. Next a continent pouch is formed to act as a surrogate rectum to allow for less frequent bowel movements. This is performed by looping the small bowel back on itself to form a "J"- or "S"-shaped pouch. The distal ileum is then brought down through the defect left from the rectal resection and anastamosed to the anal muscle through the perianal region.

Endometriosis

Of the many disorders that can cause chronic pelvic pain in women, endometriosis is the most common. The disorder is caused by the deposition of normal endometrial tissue in abnormal locations, such as the ovaries, pelvic cavity, and peritoneal cavity. The hallmark of chronic pain from endometriosis is that the severity coincides with the menstrual cycle. See **Chapter 21** for a full discussion of endometriosis.

Functional Abdominal Pain Syndrome

FAPS is related to abnormal intestinal motility and alterations in pain perception. The pain associated with this disorder is often nonspecific and may be difficult to localize. IBS may be associated with this disorder. Elicit a history of pain that is chronic, recurrent, or continuous and associated with at least 6 months of the following symptoms: (1) continuous or nearly continuous abdominal pain, (2) no or occasional association of pain with physiologic events (menses, defecation, and eating), (3) the pain is not due to malingering, (4) insufficient criteria for other functional GI disorders explain the pain.

FAPS is also linked to **psychological disturbances** and the pain and associated symptoms causes significant impairment of quality of life. IBS may be present concomitantly with the diagnosis; however, patients with IBS do not have the severe incapacitating symptoms as patients with FAPS. Determine if psychological disturbances are associated, such as a history of depression, anxiety, or possible sexual abuse.

The symptoms associated with FAPS are incapacitating, and pain medication has little benefit. **Nonsteroidal agents** are generally not useful, and **narcotics** are used cautiously as to avoid dependence and narcotic-induced constipation. Consider central acting agents, such as **tricyclic antidepressants**, and selective serotonin uptake inhibitors. Also consider behavioral therapy and psychotherapy as key elements in treatment. Irritable bowel syndrome can coexist with FAPS. These patients have disorders of intestinal motility, in addition to abnormal pain processing. Consider bulk agents (fiber) and antispasmodic agents to improve stool consistency. Antidepressants, serotonin reuptake inhibitors, behavioral modification, and dietary modifications are commonly used adjuncts.

Selected Readings

Silen W, ed. *Cope's Early Diagnosis of the Acute Abdomen*, 20th ed. New York, NY: Oxford Press; 2000.

Talamini MA. Crohn's disease of the small bowel. In: Cameron JL, ed. *Current Surgical Therapy*. 6th ed. New York, NY: Mosby; 1998.

Murayama KM, Joehl RJ. Chronic pancreatitis In: Cameron JL, ed. *Current Surgical Therapy*. 6th ed. New York, NY: Mosby; 1998.

Cullen JJ, Martin RF, eds. Current management of inflammatory bowel disease. *Surg Clin North Am*. 2007;87:575–785.

Cooperman AM, Chamberlain RS. The pancreas revisited. *Surg Clin North Am*. 2001;81:259–482.

12

Chest Pain

Susan Baker-Sample, RN, MSN, CRNP ■ *Jeffrey Cope, MD*

Key Points

- ■ Chest pain can be a clinical symptom of many different organ systems.

- ■ The specific characteristics of chest pain have clinical significance in the formulation of differential diagnoses.

- ■ Stable angina is predictable and treatable. Unstable angina is a prelude to myocardial infarction and requires prompt investigation.

- ■ Acute cardiac ischemia is treated with oxygen, aspirin, beta blocker, and possibly heparin.

- ■ Patients with unstable angina or acute myocardial infarction are considered for emergent coronary catheterization or coronary artery bypass grafting (CABG).

- ■ Significant diseases that cause chronic chest pain include abdominal, pulmonary and esophageal masses.

■ HISTORY

Perform a complete **cardiac history** assessment. Patients with chest pain caused by a cardiac event will often have symptoms that correlate with cardiac ischemia, such as radiation of pain to arm or jaw, shortness of breath, palpitations, nausea/vomiting, paroxysmal nocturnal dyspnea, orthopnea, and fatigue. Assess the **time course** of symptoms. Acute myocardial infarction may present with sudden dramatic symptoms, whereas chronic cardiac failure usually presents with long-term, vague symptoms.

Obtain any history of **pulmonary disease**, both chronic and acute. Excessive coughing or use of accessory muscles can produce pain in the chest area, caused by muscle strain. A history of spontaneous pneumothorax is important, as this condition has a propensity to recur. A history of **autoimmune disease** may be a key finding in the symptoms of chest pain. Many autoimmune diseases can affect either the cardiovascular or pulmonary systems, leading to symptomatic chest pain.

Perform an assessment of **gastrointestinal** (GI) symptoms including bowel habits and eating patterns. Many GI symptoms, especially gastroesophageal reflux, can manifest as chest pain (see Chapter 11). A history of an esophageal motility disorder or hiatal hernia is also important in defining the differential diagnosis.

A complete **social history** is elicited from the patient or family members to determine if alcohol intoxication, drug abuse, or cigarette smoking has contributed to the patient's clinical presentation. Many times patients can have chest pain secondary to coughing, smoking, or drug abuse or withdrawal. Rare cases of alcoholic cardiomyopathy will present as chest pain or acute heart failure. Determine if the patient had any recent **foreign travel** that would preclude the potential for a viral or fungal infection, which has affected the cardiopulmonary system. Establish **familial predisposition** to cardiac disease, premature coronary artery disease, thoracic aortic disease, or Marfan syndrome.

Perform an in-depth assessment of the **chest pain**, since specific characteristics of the chest pain may lead to formulation of a differential diagnosis. Pain that can be exactly **localized** is characteristic of noncardiac causes such as muscle injury, rib fracture, or costrochondritis. Pain that increases and decreases with **inspiration** may signify a chest wall injury, a pulmonary diagnosis such as pleuritis, or pneumonia. Pain that increases with **activity** or that radiates to the entire chest area or to the arm or jaw may indicate a cardiac diagnosis. Chest pain that **radiates** to the back or abdomen will prompt a cardiac or aortic disease diagnosis. Chest or back pain that is described as **tearing** and/or the worst pain the patient has ever experienced often heralds the diagnosis of acute aortic dissection or ruptured aortic aneurysm.

Special circumstances include a history of recent **medical procedures** that should be assessed, particularly orthopedic procedures, which may increase the risk of pulmonary embolism (see Chapter 5). In addition, history of a recent upper **endoscopy** may be an important piece of information, since this is one of the most common causes of esophageal perforation. Medication history should be elicited as well as potential for **overdose** of prescription or nonprescription drugs. A history of previous **device implantation** such as a defibrillator or pacemaker should be ascertained to rule out possible causes of chest pain symptoms. A history of **trauma** to chest area or overexertion of chest and arm muscles should be assessed.

■ PHYSICAL EXAMINATION

The primary assessment should focus on **cardiopulmonary stability**. Patients who are clinically unstable with faint pulses, difficulty breathing, diaphoresis, pale and cold skin, and a low blood pressure may be suffering from cardiogenic shock (see Chapter 6). Begin immediate resuscitation until life-saving cardiac reperfusion can be established.

Patients who are hemodynamically **stable** will have a complete cardiac examination performed. Assess the heart tones for murmurs, gallops, and rubs, and the point of maximal intensity location. The presence of a **murmur** or gallop can indicate underlying valvular dysfunction, which may be contributing to the patient's symptoms. The presence of a **gallop** can also indicate congestive heart failure resulting from volume overload or left ventricular hypertrophy. A **rub** may be indicated in the presence of pericarditis, myocardial infarction, chest trauma, or autoimmune disease that may present with symptoms of chest pain.

Examine the **pulmonary** system, noting symmetry of chest excursion, respiratory rate, depth of breathing, lung sounds, and skin color. Localized findings of crackles or E to A changes point to a pulmonary process. Order **pulse oximetry** as a noninvasive and simple measurement of the oxygen saturation in the arterial blood. This test can be performed easily, and inform the clinician if the patient is oxygenating adequately.

The **abdominal** examination will include palpation and auscultation for pulsatile masses often seen in aortic aneurysms or an enlarged liver that can result from right heart failure. Last, perform a **vascular** examination including assessment of the carotid arteries for bruits and palpation of peripheral pulses. Asymmetric pulses can be a sign of a thoracic aneurysm. Weak thready pulses in all extremities signify a low cardiac output and cardiac failure.

■ LABORATORY STUDIES

Order a cardiac panel to measure cardiac enzymes levels. **Creatinine phosphokinase** (CPK) is nonspecific for skeletal, cardiac, or smooth muscle injury. The CPK enzyme can be fractionated into different subtypes, and the CPK-MB subtype is specific for myocardial ischemia or infarction. Elevation of the total CPK and the CPK-MB in a series of tests for more than 24 hours is evidence for myocardial infarction. The **troponin** measurement is viewed clinically as the most reliable laboratory test to detect myocardial injury. Ideally a troponin I level should be between 0.00 and 0.15 NG/mL. Those with troponin I levels greater than 1.50 NG/mL have the maximum specificity for cardiac diagnosis and warrant further cardiac diagnostic testing. Troponin levels can remain artificially elevated in patients with renal failure.

Order a **complete blood count**. An elevated WBC may indicate an infectious process, such as pneumonia. A low hemoglobin may indicate a chronic or acute bleeding event contributing to cardiac stress. Obtain a complete **electrolyte** panel to determine electrolyte imbalances, which may be a result of an underlying pathology or the cause of the current clinical presentation. Aggressively correct potassium, magnesium, and calcium disorders, since they all can cause or exacerbate cardiac dysfunction. Order a **beta naturetic peptide** if heart failure is suspected. The beta naturetic peptide is substantially elevated in the presence of fluid overload with acute heart failure or acutely decompensated chronic heart failure. Consider the need for **coagulation** studies to determine if the patient has a preexisting coagulopathy that may be contributing to the clinical presentation or may influence diagnostic procedures or treatment options.

Consider an **arterial blood gas** if there is a question as to the cardiopulmonary circuit is adequately oxygenating the patient. The results of this test may indicate if the patient is acidotic and if the acidosis is of respiratory or metabolic origin.

■ RADIOGRAPHIC AND DIAGNOSTIC STUDIES

Order a **chest X-ray** as initial radiographic diagnostic tool to determine abnormal anatomy of heart or lungs, fluid accumulation in lungs or pleural spaces, enlarged heart silhouette, or a chest mass. Order a **computed tomography** (CT) scan of the chest and abdomen if a pulmonary embolism, pulmonary neoplasm, or aortic dissection/aneurysm is suspected.

Order an **echocardiogram** to assess the heart valves, filling, pulmonary hypertension, and cardiac function. Results of this test may provide valuable information regarding congenital defects, valvular disorders, and overall heart function. Consider **cardiac stress testing** in a patient presenting with stable chest pain who is in no acute distress. A stress test is a **physiologic** measure of cardiac ischemia or signifies the presence of coronary disease that may warrant medical treatment or further diagnostic evaluation.

Cardiac viability testing, such as a thallium stress test, is considered to delineate what sections of heart muscle are viable, infracted, or at risk for infarction. Viability testing is particularly important when a high-risk coronary bypass is anticipated, since it may determine if restoring blood flow to areas of cardiac muscle will improve heart function. **Cardiac catheterization** is the gold standard diagnostic procedure for evaluating the **anatomic** presence of coronary artery disease.

Additional test may include **pulmonary function testing** if the differential diagnosis is trending toward a pulmonary problem. If the history and physical examination point to a GI cause of the pain, consider an **esophagogastroduodenoscopy**. This study will rule out inflammation and/or ulceration of the stomach or esophagus, which may be causing chest pain symptoms.

■ DIAGNOSTIC PLAN

Determine if the patient is hemodynamically **unstable**. Unstable patients are assessed for the emergency intubation and resuscitation. Rapid assessment is made of their cardiac function. Many of these patients will require immediate transfer to the cardiac catheterization laboratory for an emergent coronary angiogram with subsequent coronary angioplasty or stenting. It is important to consult **cardiac surgery** immediately in case of a need for emergent surgery.

Perform a **12-lead electrocardiogram** as the initial diagnostic procedure. This test may provide insight into the presence or regional distribution of cardiac ischemia and the age of the event, whether it is acute or chronic. Leads that have **S–T segment** changes can predict the area of the heart that is ischemic due to coronary occlusion or stenosis. These changes may be obvious or vague, and the extent of S–T segment changes does not always correlate with the degree of myocardial injury. **Q waves** usually occur days after S–T segment changes and usually indicate a completed myocardial infarction. Identify any rhythm disturbances such as atrial fibrillation, premature complexes, bradyarrhythmias, or tachyarrhythmias.

In stable patients who do not qualify for immediate **catheterization** based on history, examination and EKG findings will have an **echocardiogram** performed. Based on these findings, determine if **stress testing** is warranted. If the stress is concerning for myocardium at risk, **coronary angiogram** for delineation of the anatomy is a prerequisite for any possible coronary **reperfusion procedures**.

■ DIFFERENTIAL DIAGNOSIS AND TREATMENT

Angina

Reversible ischemic chest pain is often described as pressure or squeezing sensation in the chest, jaw, neck, or arm and may be accompanied by other symptoms such as shortness of breath, palpitations, syncope, nausea, or diaphoresis. Angina is typically a symptom of coronary artery disease but could also be a symptom of valvular disease, hypertension, cardiac arrhythmias, and congenital heart defects. All patients being seen for chest pain symptoms should be evaluated for cardiac ischemia.

Angina can be classified as stable, unstable, or variable. **Stable angina** is the most common type of angina, which usually occurs with exertion or when there is an increased workload on the heart and the supply cannot meet demand. There is usually a regular pattern to stable angina with repeated and predictable symptom presentation. Treatment consists of rest when symptoms appear and/or nitrates such as sublingual or transdermal nitroglycerin.

Unstable angina is less common and can be an extremely dangerous condition that requires emergent medical treatment. This unstable type of angina does not follow any pattern and is usually unpredictable in nature. Frequently unstable angina does not respond to rest or medications and, therefore, can progress to myocardial infarction quickly if not treated. Treatment can include sublingual or oral nitrates and pain medications.

Variable angina or Prinzmetal's angina is very rare. It classically occurs with rest, usually during the nighttime hours. Variant angina usually responds to medication therapy, such as nitrates and calcium channel blockers, with relief of the anginal pain.

Cardiac Ischemia

Ischemia of the cardiac muscle occurs when there is an inadequate amount of oxygenated blood flow to the heart. This is most commonly the result of atherosclerotic coronary artery disease with total or partial obstruction of the coronary arteries. Other causes of cardiac ischemia that affect the entire heart may include cardiac arrhythmias or low cardiac output states. Symptoms of cardiac ischemia can include any combination of chest pain, neck or jaw pain, arm pain, diaphoresis, shortness of breath, palpitations, nausea or vomiting, and cool skin.

Non-life-threatening cardiac ischemia can be treated with a combination of strategies to decrease myocardial oxygen consumption and prevent further platelet function and clot progression. Regimens include **Aspirin** by mouth or rectum to inhibit platelet adherence, consideration of anticoagulation with **heparin**, and **beta blockade** to decrease heart rate and blood pressure.

Consider **thrombolytic therapy** such as tissue plasminogen activator to attempt lysis of recently formed thrombus (usually if seen within 1–2 hours of symptom onset). This therapy may assist to reestablish blood flow in a majority of cases when percutaneous intervention in not immediately available. For life-threatening cardiac ischemia, consider treatment in a **cardiac catheterization** laboratory with a percutaneous coronary intervention such as **angioplasty** with stent placement (Figure 12-1A and B). In cases of multiple coronary artery blockages or technically difficult anatomy for percutaneous intervention, consider **CABG** as a definitive procedure for revascularization (Figure 12-1C).

Pericarditis

Inflammation of the pericardium will elicit symptoms of chest pain, which is predominantly felt below the sternum or below the ribs on the left side of the chest. Pain can occasionally occur in the upper back or neck. The quality of pain with this disease can sometimes make for easy distinction between pericarditis and angina pain. Breathing will cause changes in pain intensity from the lung and heart moving within the chest. This will irritate or rub the pericardium, causing increased pain with breathing. Changes in position can also cause increased or decreased pain sensation.

Review the various **clinical conditions** that can cause pericarditis, including infection, myocardial infarction, kidney failure, metastatic disease, and radiation therapy. If none of the above is found, consider idiopathic pericarditis as a potential cause. Also review the medical record for **medications** that can trigger an immune response with secondary pericarditis such as hydralazine, procainamide, and phenytoin.

Esophageal Spasm

Esophageal spasms produce irregular contractions of the esophageal muscles, therefore, not effectively emptying food into the stomach. The cause of this disorder is unknown; however, specific foods and the extreme temperatures of food can trigger this reaction. The predominant symptoms of esophageal spasm are heartburn, pain in chest, and difficulty or pain with swallowing. Order an **upper GI series** to make the diagnosis of spasm. Patients are treated for their symptoms and seen by a GI specialist if symptoms persist.

CORONARY REVASCULARIZATION PROCEDURES

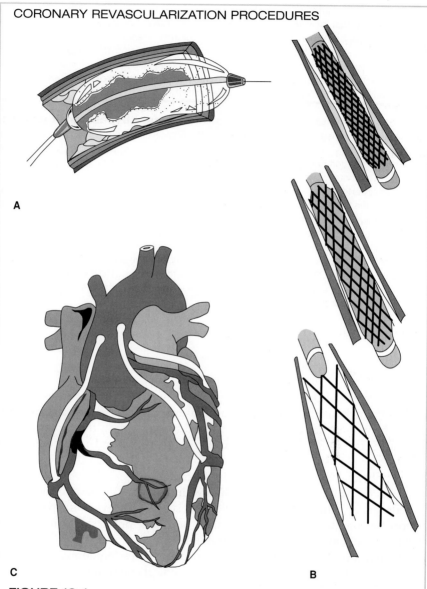

FIGURE 12-1

(A) Balloon Angioplasty, (B) Coronary Stenting, and (C) Coronary Artery Bypass Grafting

A patient presenting with chest pain, is considered for early diagnostic coronary arteriography to define the coronary anatomy and identify the presence of coronary artery disease. In general, coronary revascularization is performed by either a percutaneous or a surgical technique. A **percutaneous coronary intervention** (PCI) is performed under mild sedation and local anesthesia in the cardiac catheterization laboratory at the time of coronary arteriography. Coronary arteriography involves the insertion of wires and catheters into a peripheral artery (e.g., femoral artery), retrograde passage of these devices into the proximal ascending aorta, and subsequent cannulation of the left and right coronary arteries. **Percutaneous transluminal coronary angioplasty (PTCA)** is performed using a specialized catheter, which is advanced into the diseased coronary artery to be angioplastied (A). This specialized catheter contains a collapsible balloon, which is inflated across the coronary lesion at a specified pressure and length of time. This effectively "cracks" open the stenotic plaque to relieve the blockage. Insertion of metal **coronary artery stents** across the angioplastied lesion is then performed in selective cases (B).

When PCI is considered unsafe or inappropriate as treatment for significant coronary artery disease, the patient is often referred for **coronary artery bypass graft (CABG)**. CABG is performed under general anesthesia and may be accomplished on cardiopulmonary bypass, with the aid of the heart–lung machine (the so-called on-pump approach) or on the beating heart (off-pump approach). The operation is most frequently performed through a median sternotomy. The common conduits used in CABG include the left and right internal mammary arteries, greater saphenous veins, and radial arteries. These conduits are used to re-route the blood supply around the area of blockage to provide improved perfusion of the myocardium subtended by the diseased coronary artery (C). The internal mammary arteries are most often left attached to the respective subclavian artery to provide arterial inflow into the graft. However, other conduits (saphenous vein and radial artery) require a proximal anastomosis to another arterial source, which is most commonly the ascending aorta. Modern-day mortality rates for CABG have diminished to the 1% to 2% range. The most frequent sources of morbidity after CABG include stroke, myocardial infarction, renal failure, pulmonary insufficiency, and wound infections.

Dysphagia

Difficulty with swallowing or dysphagia can cause symptoms of chest pain and pressure, which may be mistaken for a disease of cardiac origin. Dysphagia occurs when the patient has the sensation of food being stuck in the throat or upper chest area. The pain phenomenon can be from the throat and neck area to behind the sternum. Causes of dysphagia can be discovered through thorough medical history, physical examination, and diagnostic testing.

Assess for common **medical conditions** that may cause spasm or obstruction include anxiety, tumors, foreign bodies, and strictures. Review the past **medical history** for conditions that can cause nerve or muscle problems including stroke, Parkinson's disease, multiple sclerosis, Huntington's disease, myasthenia gravis, muscular dystrophy, esophageal spasm, infection, and scleroderma. Direct treatment for dysphagia toward the underlying medical condition.

Pulmonary Neoplasms

Malignant tumors of the lung can be classified as either small cell or non-small cell. Patients with pulmonary neoplasms may experience such symptoms as chest pain, shortness of breath, hemoptysis, wheezing, loss of appetite, weakness, and difficulty swallowing. Order a **chest CT** as the imaging test of choice to identify a pulmonary mass. Chest CT will also provide information on lymph node involvement and associated pleural effusion. Depending on the particular case, offer **bronchoscopy** (Figure 12-2) or **mediastinoscopy** (Figure 12-3) to provide

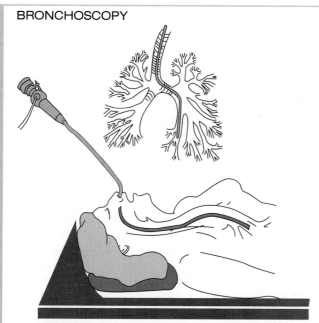

BRONCHOSCOPY

FIGURE 12-2
Insertion of the Bronchoscope into the Bronchial Tree

The procedure entails visualization of the upper and lower airways of the lungs through a rigid or fiberoptic bronchoscope. The structures visualized during this procedure can include the larynx, trachea, mainstem bronchi, and segmental bronchi. This procedure can also be used to collect specimens such as sputum for culture, tissue samples, or bronchial cell washing. This diagnostic procedure can also be used to visualize obstruction of the airway such as in lung tumors. This procedure can be used to assist in diagnosis of such pulmonary disorders as lung infections, lung cancer, lung deformity, excessive secretions, hemoptysis, tuberculosis, and foreign body identification and removal.

further diagnosis. Treatment plans include a combination of **radiation, chemotherapy**, and surgery. The most common surgical procedure is a **pulmonary resection** (Figure 12-4).

Mediastinal neoplasms are tumor cells that form in the pleural cavity that separates the lungs. Organs that may be affected by mediastinal neoplasms are the heart, trachea, thymus, large vessels, and connective tissue. Order a **chest CT** as the imaging test of choice to identify a mediastinal mass. Depending on the case, treatment includes **mediastinoscopy** (Figure 12-3) or surgical exploration and resection.

Esophageal Cancer

Along with chest pain, the most common presenting symptom of esophageal cancer is dysphagia. Weight loss is another prominent feature. Laboratory values

MEDIASTINOSCOPY

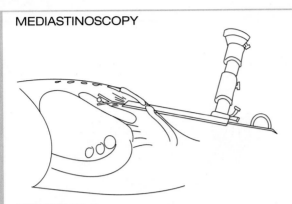

FIGURE 12-3
Placement of the Mediastinoscope into the Anterior Mediastinal Space

Mediastinoscopy is a procedure designed to biopsy masses of the middle mediastinum, the former of which most frequently represents enlarged lymph nodes. The most common indications for mediastinoscopy are the diagnosis and/or staging of lung carcinoma, lymphoma, or benign entities such as sarcoidosis or granulomatous disease. Only those lymph nodes immediately adjacent to the central airway (i.e., trachea and carina) are accessible with the mediastinoscope. Hence, neither the anterior mediastinum (e.g., thymus) nor the posterior mediastinum (periesophageal and paraspinous tissues) is approachable via this route.

The procedure is performed under general anesthesia, usually on an outpatient basis. A short transverse skin incision is made just above the sternal notch. Following division of the platysma muscle and separation of the midline strap muscles of the neck, the pretracheal plane is entered. This allows blunt dissection in the anterior pretracheal plane all the way to the carina. At this point, the mediastinoscope is inserted into the dissected space anterior to the trachea, and a thorough visual evaluation of the middle mediastinum is performed. Various lymph node basins (e.g., paratracheal, precarinal, and subcarinal) are then biopsied. At the completion of the procedure, hemostasis is ensured and the neck incision is closed in multiple layers.

The most significant complications of mediastinoscopy include tracheal injury, esophageal injury, hoarseness caused by injury to the recurrent laryngeal nerve, and massive bleeding. The latter occurs in 1% of cases and is normally due to inadvertent injury to the innominate artery, aorta, pulmonary artery, azygous vein, or superior vena cava. Such bleeding almost always requires conversion to a median sternotomy to repair the site of hemorrhage. For this reason, mediastinoscopy should not be considered a simple, innocuous procedure.

may reveal a chronic anemia from slow bleeding. Although the diagnosis can be made by **upper GI series**, arrange for an esophagogastroduodenoscopy for biopsy and possible staging using **endoscopic ultrasound**.

Offer surgical resection as the only option for cure. **Esophagectomy** is a procedure with many risks, including anastomotic leaks, cardiac dysfunction, and respiratory failure (Figure 12-5). Although patients with advanced local disease or metastatic disease to the mediastinum are not candidates for curative resection, some surgeons may consider esophagectomy for palliation. The overall prognosis remains poor, with a 5-year survival in only 10–30% of patients who have had *curative resection*.

PULMONARY RESECTIONS

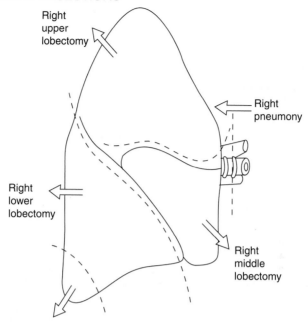

Right
upper
lobectomy

Right
pneumony

Right
lower
lobectomy

Right
middle
lobectomy

FIGURE 12-4
Delineation of the Various Pulmonary Resections on the Right Side

Pulmonary resection is a general term referring to removal of an entire lung or any portion thereof. Such a resection may be of an anatomic (pneumonectomy, lobectomy, and segmentectomy) or a nonanatomic nature (e.g., wedge resection). The most common indication for a pulmonary resection is in the surgical treatment of lung cancer.

All types of lung resections are performed under general anesthesia, utilizing a double-lumen endobronchial tube for selective ventilation of the nonoperative lung. Although a variety of chest incisions—both open and thoracoscopic—have been described for pulmonary resection, the most commonly utilized is that of a standard posterolateral thoracotomy.

A **wedge resection** is a limited pulmonary resection in which a lung mass is excised with at least a 1-cm margin of normal surrounding lung tissue. A wedge resection is most commonly employed for surgical biopsy of a previously undiagnosed lung mass.

Anatomic **segmentectomy** refers to the excision of a bronchopulmonary segment of a pulmonary lobe. Of all the types of pulmonary resections possible, segmentectomies are the least commonly performed and require the greatest degree of technical skill and experience. Most commonly, a segmentectomy is performed in the treatment of lung cancer in a patient with compromised pulmonary function who cannot tolerate removal of the entire lobe.

Pulmonary lobectomy is, by far, the most common type of resection for lung cancer. It involves the ligation and division of the lobar bronchus, pulmonary artery, and pulmonary vein supplying the lobe to be excised. A **pneumonectomy** involves removal of the entire right or left lung with ligation or division of the corresponding mainstem bronchus, pulmonary artery, and pulmonary veins. It is reserved for tumors in a central location in which a lesser resection (i.e., lobectomy) would not yield complete eradication of the tumor. As a consequence of the shear volume of lung tissue removed in a pneumonectomy, this type of pulmonary resection is attended by the highest rates of morbidity and mortality. Complications of pulmonary resection in general include a prolonged air leak, bronchopleural fistula, empyema, atrial arrhythmias, and respiratory failure.

ESOPHAGEAL RESECTIONS

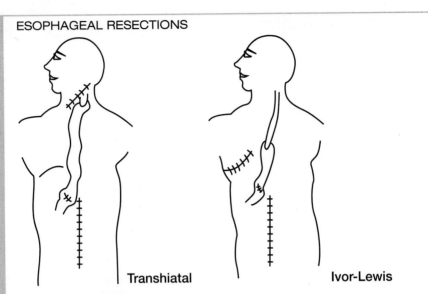

Transhiatal   Ivor-Lewis

FIGURE 12-5
Incisions and Placement of Anastamosis in the Transhiatal and Ivor-Lewis Types of Esophageal Resection

There are two popular approaches to resection of the esophagus, depending on the tumor location, the patient's clinical situation, and the surgeon's choice. The most important differences between the three are how much esophagus is resected and where the resulting anastomosis is positioned. Since the gastric–esophageal anastomosis is tenuous, with a high risk of leak, the transhiatal esophagectomy has the advantage of having the anastomosis in the neck, and not in the chest. This makes management of leaks much easier and safer.

The **Ivor–Lewis** procedure is usually performed for tumors in the distal third of the esophagus. The patient is first positioned supine, and the operation begins with a midline abdominal incision. The stomach and esophagus with the mass are mobilized through the esophageal hiatus. A pyloroplasty is considered to avoid problems with gastric emptying after the vagus nerves are cut during the subsequent resection (see Figure 11-1). With full mobilization, the midline incision is closed and the patient is then repositioned on the left lateral decubitus position to allow access to the right chest. A right thoracotomy and then further mobilization of the thoracic esophagus are performed. The distal esophagus is then resected 10 cm above the mass and at its insertion to the stomach. The stomach is then anastomosed to the remaining esophagus using either a hand-sewn or a stapled technique. The chest is drained with a chest tube.

The **transhiatal esophagectomy (THE)** starts with the patient in the supine position. A laparotomy is performed, and the stomach is mobilized in the same manner as in the Ivor–Lewis technique. A left neck incision is then made, and the proximal esophagus is mobilized into the mediastinum. From the abdomen and the neck, the surgeon then bluntly mobilizes the esophagus along its entire length in the posterior mediastinum. When fully free, the esophagus is completely resected and removed. The stomach is then pulled through the posterior mediastinum into the neck and anastomosed to the remaining pharynx cuff. A Jackson–Pratt drain is left in the neck.

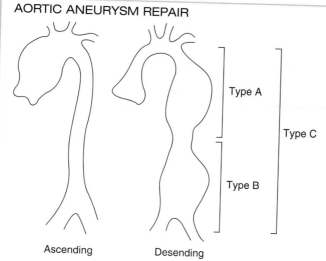

AORTIC ANEURYSM REPAIR

Type A

Type C

Type B

Ascending   Desending

FIGURE 12-6

Showing the Classification of Aortic Aneurysms

A thoracic descending aortic aneurysm is classified into three types. Type A is when the aneurysm is in the portion of the aorta from the left subclavian to T6 vertebral level. Type B is from T6 vertebral level to the diaphragm. Type C aneurysm is when the defect covers the area noted in both types A and B.

Traditional **open surgical repair** of thoracic aneurysms involves a large thoracic or sternal incision to expose the aneurismal area of the aorta. The aneurysm is dissected and replaced with a prosthetic graft material to reestablish a normal aortic blood flow. This procedure could take several hours to complete with a significant aortic cross clamping time, which poses additional risk to the patient. Morbidity can be significant with this approach, including respiratory failure, renal failure, paraplegia, stroke, and death.

Conversely, thoracic **endograft stenting** procedures are a minimally invasive approach to repair. With arterial access established via the femoral or iliac artery with a guide wire, a stent is deployed to the aneurysm site, thereby eliminating the aortic defect. This approach reduces some morbidity that is otherwise associated with the open repair.

Current treatment for thoracic aortic aneurysms has shifted in the high-risk elderly patients from the open surgical procedure to the minimally invasive stent. Only those patients who would not be candidates for the stent procedure owing to extent of aneurysm or complex anatomy would undergo surgery. This is a significant shift from less than 5–10 years ago, when most aneurysm repairs required a lengthy surgical procedure.

Hiatal Hernia

Hiatal hernia is a fairly common condition in patients older than 50 years. It is characterized by a portion of the stomach protruding upward into the chest through an opening in the diaphragm. The cause of this disorder is unknown but is a result of the weakening of the supporting muscle in the diaphragm. Obesity, smoking, and increased age can be risk factors for hiatal hernia. Assess for symptoms of chest pain, heartburn, dysphagia, and belching. Pain and discomfort

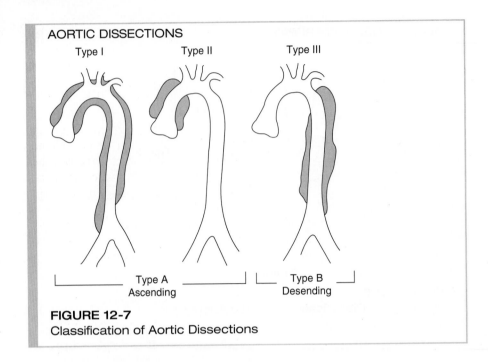

AORTIC DISSECTIONS

Type I   Type II   Type III

Type A
Ascending

Type B
Desending

FIGURE 12-7
Classification of Aortic Dissections

associated with hiatal hernia are usually associated with gastroesophageal reflux.

Make the diagnosis on upper GI series or abdominal CT scan. Treat with **histamine blockers** or **proton pump inhibitors**. Consider surgical repair of the hernia if symptoms become unmanageable or there is an indication that the hernia has become intestinal ischemia. Signs and symptoms include intractable pain, fever, elevated WBC, and shock. For such cases, the treatment is **operative reduction** and repair similar to a Nissen fundoplication (see Figure 11-2).

Aortic Aneurysm and Dissection

Disorders of the aorta can be a life-threatening emergency when presenting with chest pain. **Aortic aneurysms** are characterized by a widening or bulging of the wall of the aorta, usually in the thoracic or abdominal areas (Figure 12-6). The most common causes of this disease are atherosclerosis and long-standing hypertension. Most aortic aneurysms found incidentally in asymptomatic patients are monitored closely and surgically repaired when they reach 5–6 cm in size. Patients develop chest pain from an aneurysm when there is an acute **expansion** or **leak** of the aorta. Consider chest pain in the context of a known or newly diagnosed aneurysm as a surgical emergency. Treatment options can include an operative vascular surgical repair or endovascular stent placed at the site of the aneurysm (Figure 12-6).

Aortic dissection is when there is a tear or damage to the inner wall of the aorta, which allows blood to flow along a false lumen of the aorta. There is usually a channel created within the aorta, which abnormally shunts blood flow. This usually occurs in the thoracic portion of the aorta but could also occur in the abdominal portion. Causes of this disorder can include atherosclerois, hypertension, and Marfan syndrome.

Characterize the dissection as **type A or B** (Figure 12-7). Type A begins in the ascending portion of the aorta and typically moves to another part of the chest. Type B begins in the descending portion of the aorta and moves down the abdomen. Assess organ function (kidney, liver, bowel, and spinal cord), since aortic dissection can cause poor perfusion of various organs and ultimately lead to death if not surgically treated.

Start treatment to **lower the wall stress** in the aorta. Treatment options include beta blockers, nicardipine, and nitroprusside. Transfer the patient to the intensive care unit and monitor continuous blood pressure with an **arterial line** to titrate vasoactive drips.

Selected Readings

Edmunds LH, Cohn LH, eds. *Cardiac Surgery in the Adult.* New York: McGraw-Hill; 2003.

Hurst JW, Morris DC, eds. *Chest Pain.* Armonk, NY: Futura Company; 2001.

13

Upper Gastrointestinal Bleeding

Corinna P. Sicoutris, RN, MSN, CRNP, CCRN ■ *John P. Pryor, MD, FACS*

Key Points

■ Gastrointestinal (GI) bleeding can be slow and chronic, or fast and acute. Significant GI bleeding can cause shock and death in a span of a few hours. Do not underestimate the amount of potential blood loss because the bleeding is not visible.

■ Although blood from the rectum often indicates a lower GI source, brisk upper GI bleeding can present with bright red blood from the rectum. Thus, consider an upper GI source in all cases of rectal bleeding or melena.

■ Bleeding from gastritis, duodenal ulcer, and gastric ulcer (GU) make up 80–90% of all cases of upper GI bleeding.

■ Management priorities are fluid resuscitation, diagnosis, and control of the bleeding. Resuscitation may involve intravenous crystalloid infusion, blood transfusion, vasopressor support, and, in some cases, ventilation support.

- Have an esophagogastroduodenoscopy (EGD) performed as soon as possible for acute and subacute bleeding, since the maneuver is both diagnostic and potentially therapeutic for the most common bleeding sources.

- Chronic, slow bleeding is considered in patients who have anemia and occult blood on stool examination. Active resuscitation is not needed, and attention is concentrated on determining the exact source of blood loss.

■ HISTORY

Determine the **presenting symptom**, since it often relates to the rapidity and severity of bleeding. Patients complaining of gross **hematemesis**, with associated syncope or near syncope, suggest an acute, brisk bleeding source. In these cases, where the patient may lose consciousness or need elective intubation for airway control, a rapid review of the medical history may prove invaluable in determining the cause of the bleed.

Those with more indolent symptoms, such as **melena**, have ample opportunity to provide information relative to past diagnoses and hospitalizations, which may help in identifying the cause of the bleeding. The **acuteness** of the bleed can also lend clues to the ultimate diagnosis. Bleeding from a duodenal ulcer, a Mallory–Weiss tear, or an esophageal varix often cause significant acute bleeding, while conditions such as gastric cancer and esophagitis are more likely to manifest as chronic anemia.

Determine early on if and when the patient has had **previous bleeding**. Although some patients will not be able to give all of the clinical details pertaining to a previous episode, they can often describe the various diagnostic and treatment modalities they have experienced. If the patient received care elsewhere, obtain **medical records** from the institution where treatment was performed as soon as possible. Conditions that are most likely to cause multiple **isolated episodes** of upper gastrointestinal bleeding (UGIB) are duodenal/GUs, esophageal/gastric varices, and esophagitis/gastritis.

Clarify the tempo and **progression of symptoms** during the period of time leading up to the chief complaint. A history of forceful vomiting just before hematemesis is a classic presentation for a Mallory–Weiss tear, whereas a recent course of antiviral medication may suggest esophagitis as an inciting factor. Elicit any conditions or activities that may have contributed to the symptoms. Common examples are heavy use of nonsteroidal anti-inflammatory (NSAID) medications, systemic steroid use, or poison ingestions. All information is important, even if the significance is not immediately obvious.

Thoroughly review the **past medical history** to uncover diseases that are associated with GI bleeding, such as end-stage liver disease, heart disease with antiplatelet and coumadin therapy, end-stage renal disease, and cancer. Conduct a full **surgical history** to reveal potential problems such as marginal ulceration after gastric bypass surgery, previous duodenal ulcer surgery, and neoplasm resections that may have reoccurred or metastasized to the GI tract.

■ PHYSICAL EXAMINATION

Foremost, perform a physical examination to determine whether or not the patient is in clinical **shock**. A patient who presents ashen, diaphoretic, with mental status changes is in severe shock, and no other diagnostic test need to be considered before acute resuscitation is started. If the patient is well perfused, with acceptable heart rate and blood pressure, examine for external clues to the ultimate diagnosis.

Cachexia would suggest an underlying neoplasm, whereas stigmata of dehydration would be seen in patients with esophagitis or expanding esophageal mass. It is *not* common to find any abnormalities on abdominal examination, including tenderness, in most patients with UGIB. Note stigmata of significant **liver disease**, including a distended abdomen from ascites, telangtasias, venous malformations on the anterior abdomen (caput medusa), and scleral icterus. Perform a **rectal examination** on every patient with GI bleeding for evidence of hemorrhoids and to determine if there is frank blood or melena present in the stool.

■ LABORATORY STUDIES

Order a **CBC** with red cell indices and a blood type and cross. Use caution in the interpretation of the hemoglobin and hematocrit levels during acute blood loss, since these parameters may not change for several hours after bleeding has occurred. Obtain a **coagulation panel**, particularly in those patients who are on coumadin or have end-stage liver disease. Recall that aspirin and other platelet inhibitors will not affect the prothrombin time or partial thromboplastin time. Although the **platelet count** may be normal, conditions such as end-stage renal disease can cause significant platelet dysfunction. Although platelet function can be directly tested with a bleeding time determination, this test is impractical and rarely performed.

Inspect the **chemistry panel** for evidence of chronic blood loss, such as an increased BUN from excessive red cell turnover and a decreased mean corpuscular hemoglobin concentration. A low bicarbonate level is evidence of acidosis most often associated with under-resuscitation.

■ RADIOGRAPHIC STUDIES

Order a **chest X-ray** (CXR) as the first radiographic test for every patient with UGIB. Perform the radiograph upright if possible or, if not, obtain a second left cross table lateral film. In both cases, determine if there is evidence for pneumoperitoneum or mediastinal emphysema. **Pneumoperitoneum** most often suggests a perforated viscous duodenal or gastric ulcer as the cause of the bleed (see Chapter 10). **Mediastinal air** is associated with esophageal perforation, such as a Mallory–Weiss tear. Finally, inspect the lung fields closely in cases where patients have vomited to look for early evidence for **aspiration**.

Order additional radiographic tests on a case-by-case basis. Occasionally, a **KUB** abdominal film will add information such as showing a dilated stomach from an obstructing duodenal mass. Although the most sensitive and specific test for abdominal anatomy is the **abdominal computed tomography** (ACT) scan, the vast majority of UGIB disorders are not associated with large structural lesions and thus the ACT is not traditionally part of the acute diagnosis plan. However, in cases where mass lesions are involved, such as a gastric mass, ACT can help define the relative anatomy.

In cases of chronic bleeding, and when lesions such as duodenal or GUs are suspected, **UGI series** can be performed either in the acute care setting or as an outpatient. Order dilute **gastrograffin** if there is a concern for a perforation, since the contrast will not irritate the peritoneal lining if spilled into the cavity. In patients with altered mental status with a risk of aspiration, order **barium,** since it is better tolerated in the respiratory tract if accidentally aspirated. A properly performed UGI series can make the diagnosis of esophagitis, esophageal mass, esophageal and gastric varix, gastric and duodenal ulcer, gastric mass, and duodenal diverticulum. The test is not adequate to see minor anatomical conditions such as Dieulafoy's lesion or Mallory–Weiss tears without perforation.

■ DIAGNOSTIC PLAN

Make the diagnosis accurately and as soon as possible, since the treatment of UGIB differs considerably for the various causes. In all cases of suspected UGIB, place a **nasogastric (NG)** tube and lavage the stomach of the contents (Figure 13-1). It is assumed that there will be blood aspirated immediately after NG placement, what is more important is what the aspirate looks like after the initial lavage. If bright red blood is continually aspirated, then a brisk bleed is evident. If the NG appears brown, with a "coffee-ground" color, a subacute bleed is suspected. A clear aspirate would indicate that active bleeding has stopped or the bleeding is minor and slow.

If brisk or subacute bleeding is suspected, arrange for an **EGD** immediately. EGD is a unique procedure in that it can be both a diagnostic and a therapeutic maneuver (Figure 13-2). Determine if the patient needs elective **endotracheal intubation** to protect and maintain the airway before the EGD is performed. Although EGD can be performed under conscious sedation, some patients, especially the older people and those in clinical shock, will not be able to tolerate the procedure without a significant risk of aspiration. Emergent EGD can often be performed at the bedside in the emergency department or intensive care unit, although some practitioners prefer to perform the procedure in an endoscopy suite.

PLACEMENT OF THE NASOGASTRIC TUBE

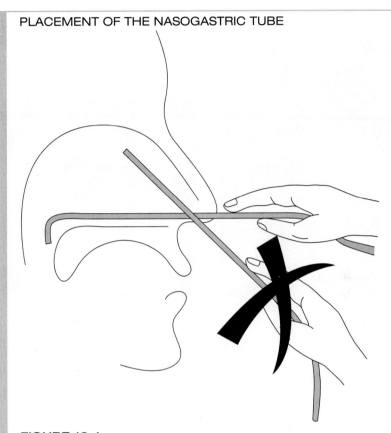

FIGURE 13-1
Proper Placement of the Nasogastric Tube Through the Nasopharynx

If possible, the patient should sit upright. The clinician assembles all equipment and ensures that adequate suction is available. Sedation for the procedure is not used, since this inhibits the patient's protective mechanisms against aspiration. The NG tube is lubricated well with water-soluble gel. The patient is handed a cup of water with a straw. The procedure is explained to the patient in detail both to relieve anxiety and to elicit the patient's cooperation during the procedure. The tube is placed into the nares parallel to the floor of the nares, which extends straight back to the nasopharynx, not upward as might be expected. As the tube is advanced into the nasopharynx, the patient will experience discomfort and the tube will meet resistance. This is caused by the angle of the nasopharynx and the true pharynx. Even slight pressure will cause the tube to make the turn, and a small pop is sometimes felt as the tube begins the descent down the true pharynx. At this point the patient may gag; thus, it is important to move the tube swiftly but gently. Also at this point, the patient can assist in directing the tube toward the esophagus by sipping water and swallowing. The tube is advanced as the patient swallows. This allows the tube to follow the natural path into the esophagus the pharynx makes during a normal swallowing reflex. Once the tube is in the esophagus, it is advanced swiftly into the stomach. To confirm the placement, the patient is asked to speak. A normal speech provides evidence that the tube is inadvertently going into the trachea. Gastric contents should be aspirated from the tube. Lastly, a loud gurgle should be heard when air is quickly insufflated into the tube while auscultating over the epigastrum. Care is taken to properly secure the tube to the nose so as not to cause nasal ischemia.

ESOPHAGOGASTRODUODENOSCOPY

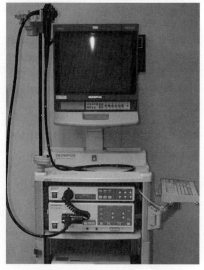

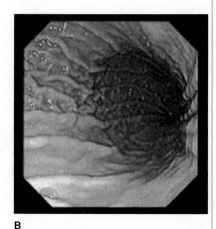

A

B

FIGURE 13-2

(A) A Traditional EGD Mobile Cart and (B) a View into a Normal Stomach

Only clinicians who have had specific training perform the procedure. Conscious sedation is given, usually with a combination of a benzodiazepine and narcotic. The patient is closely monitored with continuous ECG, pulse oximetry, and blood pressure measurements. With the patient in the lateral decubitus position, a bite block is inserted into the mouth and the scope is placed into the posterior pharynx and advanced into the esophagus. The highest risk of gagging and aspiration is at this point, so suction is readily available. In addition to visualizing the lumen, the scope is designed with the capability to insufflate air, suction fluid out, and introduce catheters and instruments through a side port (A). During the advancement of the scope, air is insufflated to expand the lumen and torque wheels on the head of the scope are adjusted to "steer"' the tip of the scope further in the lumen (B). The scope is advanced quickly into the duodenum and then withdrawn slowly to fully inspect all of the luminal walls. When a bleeding source is found, injections and electrocautery are performed by introducing special catheters through the side port. Final inspection of the gastric and esophageal lumen is performed as the scope is withdrawn.

Involve the **general surgeon** early in cases of significant bleeding, including having the surgeon present for the EGD procedure. This allows the surgery team to be familiar with the patient, and, if surgery is eventually needed, the surgeon will have a visual idea of the bleeding source from the EGD, perhaps allowing better operative planning.

In cases where the EGD fails to identify the source of bleeding, blood is refluxing from the small bowel, bleeding from a ruptured pancreatic pseudocyst is suspected, or there is evidence for hemobilia, consider using **angiography** as a diagnostic and therapeutic tool. Selective angiograms of visceral vessels such as the celiac axis and superior mesenteric artery may be able to localize the bleeding source and, in some cases, arrest hemorrhage by embolization with gel foam or coils.

In cases where very slow or intermittent bleeding is suspected, the initial diagnostic workup usually includes an **UGI series** and/or an **ACT**, as described in the radiology section. In general, if abnormalities are found on either one of these examinations, a follow-up EGD is often performed for confirmation and sometimes for further diagnosis such as obtaining tissue biopsies for GUs.

■ DIFFERENTIAL DIAGNOSIS AND TREATMENT

Resuscitation

In all cases of acute of subacute bleeding, begin **resuscitation** immediately. Continue resuscitative efforts concurrently with the diagnostic workup and in conjunction with procedures to stop the bleeding such as EGD. There is a natural tendency to underestimate blood loss when it is not externally visible. Any clinician who has seen active bleeding from a duodenal ulcer during an EGD can attest that the blood loss is impressive, and thus there must be a sense of urgency with any patient suspected of having GI bleeding. Apply the principles of resuscitation as for any other type of hemorrhage (see Chapter 6). Establish large-bore **intravenous access**: 14- or 16-gauge peripheral IVs in the antecubital fossa. If there is clinical evince of shock, infuse 2 L of **normal saline** (NS) or lactated ringers solution immediately.

If there is no change in the clinical appearance, or if tachycardia with a systolic blood pressure below 90 remains, transfuse two units of **packed red blood cells**. If at all possible, type-specific blood should be used, but if there will be a significant delay before this is available, infuse type O, Rh-negative blood.

If there is evidence of coagulopathy, either from preexisting disease (hepatic failure) or from coumadin use, infuse two units of **fresh frozen plasma** immediately. Further units of fresh frozen plasma may be needed to correct the INR to below 1.3.

Patients with a quantitative or qualitative platelet dysfunction may benefit from **platelet transfusion**. Patients with end-stage renal disease may benefit from vasopressin (DDAVP) injection to counter the renal-induced platelet dysfunction.

During acute resuscitation, **monitor** the patient closely with continuous ECG, continuous oximetry, and frequent blood pressure determinations. Place a **Foley catheter** to monitor the urine output as a guide to the adequacy of resuscitation. As discussed previously, decide early whether the patients are adequately maintaining their airway, and if there is any doubt, endotracheal intubation is performed by a certified practitioner.

Duodenal Ulcer

By far the most common etiology of UGIB is **duodenal ulcer** (DU) disease. Inspecting the duodenum during EGD or detecting the lesion on an UGI series makes the diagnosis. The condition is related to **hyperacidity** and the mainstay of medical management remains, decreasing gastric acid with histamine (type-2) receptor blockers and proton pump inhibitors.

There is now also clear evidence that a bacterium, *Helicobacter pylori*, has a contributing role to the formation and reoccurrence of ulcers. On account of successful medical management with acid reduction and antibacterial for *H. pylori*, the rate and severity of DU disease have dramatically declined during the last two decades. Either patients with bleeding DU typically have never been treated for ulcer disease and have bleeding as their first sign of having the disease or they have a known ulcer that has failed medical management.

DUs are mucosal erosions usually found in the **duodenal bulb**. Bleeding occurs when the ulcer erodes the posterior part of the duodenum into the pancreatic head. The **gastroduodenal artery** (GDA) is a major artery that passes behind the duodenum just at the bulb and is almost always the source of bleeding in DU disease.

Arrange to have an **EGD** performed as the diagnostic and therapeutic maneuver of choice. Vessel bleeding is controlled during EGD using injections of epinephrine that constricts the vessel, allowing it to clot. Alternatively, electrocautery is applied to coagulate the vessel. These maneuvers are successful in arresting the hemorrhage in approximately 80–90% of cases.

If EGD fails to stop the bleeding, or if the patient suffers recurrent bleeding after multiple attempts with EGD, consider surgical exploration. The goal of **surgery** is to stop the bleeding, not to perform an elaborate operation, especially in a patient who is mot likely in shock or just finishing a significant resuscitation. The most common surgical procedure is a **gastrostomy** with oversewing of the ulcer (Figure 13-3). Resection of the ulcer is neither practical nor prudent, since the posterior ulcer has eroded into the pancreas, making resection nearly impossible without resecting a part of the pancreas. No attempt is made to perform a classic "ulcer operation" such as a vagotomy or antrectomy (see Chapter 11). These procedures are complex, have many complications, and are generally unnecessary with the success of modern medical management of ulcer disease.

Concurrently, begin intense **medical management** to decrease the acid environment and eradicate *H. pylori*. Administer a proton pump inhibitor by continuous intravenous injection and continue for several days. Eventually, this can be transitioned to an oral medication that is continued for several months, if not indefinitely. On account of its resilience, treat *H. pylori* with a triple drug regimen including two antibiotics and bismuth. There are several different recommended combinations of medications and a few combination products that provide all three drugs in one pill. This treatment is also continued for several months.

Esophagitis and Gastritis

Erosive esophagitis and gastritis are common conditions, especially in patients already hospitalized and often in those with critical illness. It is also possible to

SURGERY FOR BLEEDING DUODENAL ULCER

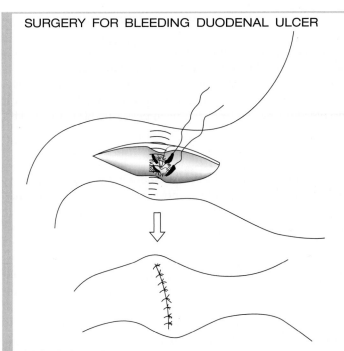

FIGURE 13-3

A Pylorotomy Made in the Area of the Ulcer, with Repair and Closure

The procedure begins with an exploratory laparotomy performed through a midline abdominal incision. The stomach is opened with a transverse incision that crosses the pylorus. The ulcer is generally seen in the posterior position overlying the GDA. Suture ligatures are placed cephalad, caudad, and medial to the ulcer. The last stitch is to control bleeding from a common branch off the GDA, which supplies blood to the pancreas. The gastrostomy is closed in a transverse manner to avoid stricture formation, similar to a formal pyloroplasty procedure (see Figure 11-1A). Drains are not typically placed, and the anterior abdomen is closed in the standard fashion.

acquire these problems from varied medical conditions and as complications to medications. **Gastritis** is differentiated from GU in that the mucosal erosion is not limited to one small area of the stomach but is present in the form of multiple small ulcerations throughout the gastric mucosa. Gastritis is caused by a breakdown of the gastric mucosal barrier that protects the gastric cells from the harsh acidity of the stomach contents. Often the causes for the mucosal breakdown are multifactorial and include relative ischemia during states of shock, shunting of blood from the visceral circulation, and complex neuroendocrine responses to certain injuries, such as burn injuries (Curling's ulcers).

Esophagitis is most often associated with a *Candida* infection, most often secondary to excessive antibiotic use. Gastritis and esophagitis can also be exacerbated by mechanical shear from tubes such as NG and feeding tubes. Make the diagnosis during EGD where large areas of the mucosa appear friable and ulcerated—bleeding often occurs from the simple rubbing of the EGD scope along the walls (scope trauma).

Attempt to prevent gastritis in hospitalized patients by prophylactically protecting the mucosal barrier with **H2 antagonist** or **sulcralfate**, a gastric mucosal buffer. If gastritis does occur, remove all unnecessary tubes to provide adequate barrier protection. Most cases are self-limiting. In very rare cases of severe gastritis that will not stop bleeding, gastrectomy has been performed (Figure 11-1B).

Gastric Ulcer

GUs have a completely different pathophysiology than DUs. Unlike DU, GU is not associated with hyperacidity, and, in fact, most patients have a lower than normal acid level. Similar to gastritis, the problem is with a breakdown of the mucosal barrier of the stomach lining. Some elements of harsh living can contribute to this breakdown, such as excessive alcohol use and smoking. More concerning are the number of patients who suffer gastric ulceration as a consequence of medical treatment for other disorders. **Medications** such as aspirin, NSAID, and systemic steroids all predispose a patient to gastric ulceration. Thus, unlike gastritis, which is mostly limited to patients already in the hospital, GU typically occurs in patients who are not hospitalized, and thus, is more likely to be seen first in the medical clinic or emergency department.

Make the **diagnosis** by inspection during EGD or by interpretation of a UGI series. For all cases where a GU is diagnosed on UGI series, perform EGD to obtain tissue biopsies on account of the significant risk of a GU being a gastric cancer (see Chapter 18).

Treat acute bleeding in a similar way to DU in that EGD is the first line of therapy, with attempts and injection and cautery to arrest bleeding. However, unlike DU, GUs are much more amendable to surgical therapy, since the vessels involved are within the actual wall of the stomach and there is no penetration into retroperitoneal structures. Thus, if surgery is necessary, the ulcer can often be **wedge resected** in total, with plenty of stomach left for normal function.

Esophageal and Gastric Varices

Varices are abnormally large veins that appear just under the mucosal surface of the esophagus and stomach in patients with significant portal hypertension. The most profound collateral drainage occurs in the veins around the stomach, causing enlargement and engorgement. At times these large varices can erode into the lumen of the stomach or esophagus causing massive bleeding.

Make the **diagnosis** by direct visualization of the varices during **EGD**. Often, the diagnosis is suspected in patients with advanced liver disease, although it should not be assumed that varices are the cause of bleeding, since other conditions, such as ulcer disease, also occur in patients with end-stage liver disease. Because the bleeding is exclusively venous, there is no role for angiography in the diagnosis of treatment. Direct treatment is intended to control the bleeding and decrease the portal pressure. Arrange for an **EGD** and consider injection of

epinephrine or other "sclerosing" agent. A unique procedure to variceal bleeding control is **banding**—a process whereby small rubber bands are deployed through the EGD scope that pinch off the vessel, allowing it to clot and heal. In addition to mechanical maneuvers, consider vasoactive therapy. **Vasopressin,** a naturally occurring hormone with vasoconstriction properties, can be given by continuous intravenous infusion to constrict vessels and halt bleeding. Care is taken with patients who have known heart disease, since vasopressin is nonselective and can cause coronary vasoconstriction. If these maneuvers fail, place a **Stengstaken–Blakemore** tube (SBT) (Figure 13-4) and consider a **transjugular intrahepatic portosystemic shunt** (Figure 13-5) to acutely relieve portal

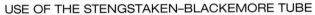

USE OF THE STENGSTAKEN–BLACKEMORE TUBE

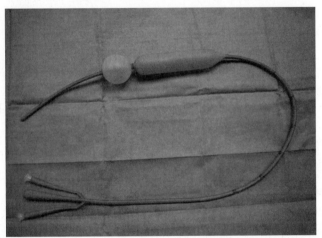

FIGURE 13-4
The Stengstaken–Blackemore Tube (SBT) Shown with both Gastric and Esophageal Balloons Inflated

Insertion of the SBT should only be performed by practitioners who have received specific training. It is mandatory to protect the airway with endotracheal intubation before the tube is inserted. The tube consists of a large distal balloon, a long proximal balloon, and an aspiration port at the tip. The concept of the device is to tamponade variceal bleeding with insufflation of the long proximal tube within the esophagus. The distal balloon is inflated as an anchor to keep the device in place.

The tube is lubricated and then introduced into the esophagus similar to placement of an NG tube. When the tube is felt to be in position, a CXR is ordered and reviewed to ascertain that the distal balloon is in the stomach. Inadvertent positioning of the distal balloon too proximal in the esophagus can lead to esophageal rupture when it is inflated. After correct position is confirmed, the distal balloon is inflated and gentle pressure issued to pull back the tube until the distal balloon is felt to abut the GE junction. Typically, the tube is then held in this position with some type of rigging; most often a football helmet is the most practical method. The proximal balloon is then gently inflated. Some devices have a manometer on the proximal balloon to make sure that the transluminal pressure in the esophagus does not become too high, risking ischemia.

TRANSJUGULAR INTRAHEPATIC PORTOSYSTEMIC SHUNT

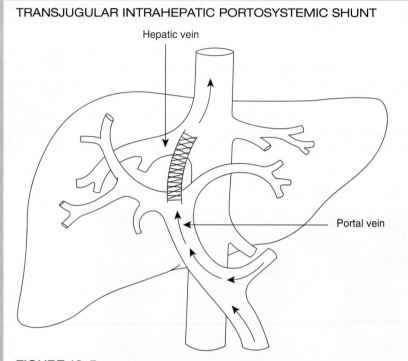

Hepatic vein

Portal vein

FIGURE 13-5
A Schematic Showing Placement of a Stent Between the Portal and Hepatic Circulations

The procedure is performed in the angiography suite by interventionist specially trained in procedure. The internal jugular vein is accessed by percutaneous Seldinger technique, and a catheter is advanced into the hepatic vein. The interventionalist then attempts to penetrate the tip of the catheter through the liver parenchyma into a branch of the portal system. Intermittent injection of contrast is used to determine when the tip has passed into a portal vein. When a fistula has been created, the tract is dilated and a flexible, expandable stent is placed to allow free flow of blood from the high-pressure portal system into the systemic venous system. The stent is permanent but does have a chance of clotting off over time. Subsequent attempts and stent placements are possible.

pressure. Consider **hepatic transplantation** as a final salvage technique for patients in whom bleeding cannot be controlled by any other means.

Mallory–Weiss Tear

A **Mallory–Weiss** lesion is a tear in the esophagus, just proximal to the GE junction most often caused by forceful vomiting. Order a **CXR** to rule out mediastinal air that would signify an esophageal perforation. If a perforation is suspected, use EGD with great caution, since the procedure could exacerbate the tear. Make the diagnosis during **EGD** by observing clot and ecchymosis in the area of the GE junction. Use similar techniques of injection and electrocautery to control bleeding at the tear. Most cases are self-limiting and require nothing per os for several days as the main treatment follow-up.

Dieulafoy's Lesion

There are several vascular abnormalities that may present with bleeding, the most common of which is **Dieulafoy's lesion:** a submucosal enlarged vein that erodes into the surface of the gastric lumen. It is distinguished from gastric varices in that it is not associated with portal hypertension. Make the diagnosis on **EGD** by observing a single area of ecchymosis with central bleeding and a visible vessel. Treat with standard **injection** and electrocautery techniques. If surgery is needed for recurrent bleeding, the area of stomach that includes the vessel can be controlled with a **wedge resection**.

Gastric and Esophageal Mass

Gastric masses are almost always neoplasms and could have bleeding as a presenting symptom. Unlike other causes of UGIB, this lesion sometimes can cause abdominal pain and demonstrate a palpable mass on physical examination. Use **ACT** to characterize the location of the mass and associated evidence for disease in the lymph nodes and liver. Perform **EGD** for diagnosis and biopsy. Bleeding control is less successful than in ulcer disease on account of the friable nature of the tumor mass; thus, surgical resection may be needed more often. See **Chapter 18** for a full discussion of gastric cancer.

Esophageal masses typically present with dysphasia and pain; bleeding often occurs in patients who already have a diagnosis made. Perform **EGD** with care, since there is a risk of perforation with larger masses as the central tissue becomes necrotic. Unlike gastric masses, which are amendable to surgery, esophageal resection is much more difficult and has higher risks. Thus, make every effort to control bleeding with endoscopic techniques. See **Chapter 12** for a full discussion of esophageal cancer.

Hemobilia (<1%)

A very uncommon cause of UGIB is bleeding from the common bile duct into the lumen of the duodenum. A hepatic vessel–bile duct communication caused by tumor, infection, or trauma, including surgical trauma, most often causes bleeding. Make the diagnosis by observing blood emanating from the ampulla of Vater during EGD. If a diagnosis of hemobilia is made, order angiography to localize the bleeding source and possibly embolize.

Selected Readings

Rockall TA. Management and outcomes of patients undergoing surgery after upper gastrointestinal hemorrhage. *J R Soc Med.* 1998;91:518.

Calam J, Baron JH. ABC of the gastrointestinal tract: Pathophysiology of duodenal and gastric ulcer and gastric cancer. *BMJ.* 2001;323:980.

Jamieson CG. Current status of indications for surgery in peptic ulcer disease. *World J Surg.* 2000;24:256.

Gerbes AL, et al. Transjugular intrahepatic portosystemic shunt (TIPS) for variceal bleeding in portal hypertension: Comparison of emergency and elective interventions. *Dig Dis Sci.* 1998;43:2463.

14

Lower Gastrointestinal Bleeding

Michael Daly, MSN, MBA, ACNP-BC ■
Oscar Guillamondegui, MD, FACS

Key Points

■ Lower gastrointestinal bleeding refers to bleeding beyond the ligament of Trietz and includes small and large bowel sources.

■ Only approximately 10% of patients who present to the emergency department with gastrointestinal bleeding have a lower gastrointestinal source. Patients will present with melena, hematochezia, or bright red blood per rectum (PRBPR).

■ Hemodynamic stability will determine the urgency and pace of the evaluation. Patients who have hematochezia or PRBPR on arrival to the emergency department or upon consultation in hospital indicate the probability of active hemorrhage.

■ Hemodynamically unstable patients require aggressive management of bleeding disorders/coagulopathies and rapid identification of the gastrointestinal pathology.

- Consider tagged red cell scan or colonoscopy as first-line diagnostic modalities in patients with acute bleeding.

- Visceral angiogram can be both diagnostic and therapeutic if selective embolization is possible.

- Hemodynamically stable patients can be managed with a methodical, efficient workup, which includes colonoscopy, angiography, or radionuclide studies to make a definitive diagnosis of the bleeding source.

■ HISTORY

Determine the characteristics of the **presenting symptoms**. Blood from a gastrointestinal source undergoes degradation as it passes through the bowel, and the type of rectal effluent will indicate the amount and time course of the bleeding. PRBPR indicates brisk bleeding, whereas melena suggests a slower bleed with a longer transit time.

Determine if the patient has ever experienced similar symptoms or a **previous diagnosis** of a cause of bleeding prior to the current presentation. If the patient has experienced these symptoms before, verify previous diagnostic studies or medical records. Elucidate if there are any **associated symptoms**, such as weight loss, changes in bowel habits, and abdominal distension, that could lead to a presumptive diagnosis. Investigate the patient's **medication history**, especially the use of anticoagulants, NSAIDs, antiplatelet medications or steroids. Determine if the patient has any **preexisting condition** that commonly leads to bleeding, such as malignancy, inflammatory bowel disease, diverticulosis, hemorrhoids, or anal fissures.

■ PHYSICAL EXAMINATION

Begin the examination by evaluating the patient's vital signs, focusing on **hemodynamic stability**. A patient who is pale, diaphoretic, hypotensive, and tachycardic must first be adequately resuscitated (see Chapter 6).

In general, examine the patient for signs of a poor **nutritional state**, possibly denoting cancer or a chronic, previously undiagnosed inflammatory bowel disease. Assess the signs of **hemorrhage**, such as amount of hematemesis or hematochezia, and the presence of orthostatic hypotension. Perform an abdominal examination for signs of **peritonitis** or **masses**. Associated abdominal tenderness may indicate active ulcer perforation or bowel infarction. Perform a **rectal examination** on all patients with GI bleeding for evidence of hemorrhoids, fissures, or anal warts and to determine if there is frank blood or melena present in the stool.

The rectal examination is particularly important if colonoscopy is used to make a diagnosis, since that procedure will miss lesions in the first few centimeters of the rectum.

■ LABORATORY STUDIES

Order a **CBC** to determine the hemoglobin and platelet level. In episodes of acute bleeding, it takes time for the hemoglobin to drop, as fluid redistributes into the vascular space. Thus, a normal hemoglobin level early in the course does not rule out active hemorrhage, and the values should be repeated in 4–6 hours.

A **prothrombin** time and a **partial thromboplastin time** are ordered, especially in patients on anticoagulation medications. Correct any coagulopathy before further diagnostic and therapeutic maneuvers. **Lactic acidosis** is a sign of poor tissue perfusion and will be evident in prolonged hemorrhagic shock. Having an up-to-date type and cross will allow appropriate, rapid transfusion, if necessary, in the resuscitation efforts. Look for abnormalities on the **chemistry panel** such as acidosis with a low bicarbonate level or an imbalance of sodium, potassium, and calcium if there has been associated diarrhea and vomiting.

A visual **stool examination** and guaiac is performed on all patients looking for occult blood. PRBPR can be mixed with stool or lining the outside of formed stool. The latter indicates a distal source that has bled onto the formed stool as it passes. **Melena** is black tarry stool, which suggests a proximal source since the blood is mixed and digested with the stool. Brown stool that tests positive for **guaiac** suggests a slow, proximal bleed.

■ RADIOGRAPHIC AND DIAGNOSTIC STUDIES

Order **abdominal X-rays** to see anatomical changes such as free intra-abdominal air with a perforated viscous or massive dilatation of the small or large bowel in cases of an obstructing mass. Consider an **abdominal CT** to rule out a colonic mass or diverticulosis. The newer, multislice CT scanner may have the ability to determine the sites of bleeding that are not associated with gross anatomical abnormalities such as arteriovenous malformations in the colon. This technology is not universally available and is still being evaluated in research studies.

Order a **radionucleotide** scan, such as the tagged red-cell scan, to localize a colonic bleeding source. These scans are very sensitive, detecting slow rates of hemorrhage less than 0.5 mL/min. Thus, the radionuclide scan is valuable in identifying the sight of bleeding that is not apparent on angiography or colonoscopy. The major disadvantage is that they localize the bleeding to a general area of the abdomen but do not diagnose the specific location and cause of the source. On account of its sensitivity, but lack of specificity, the radionucleotide study is often used as a screening tool to determine that bleeding is indeed from a lower source. Then, angiography or colonoscopy is used to determine the exact source.

Consider **angiography** in patients with severe GI bleeding or in those patients who have had a positive radionucleotide study. Extravasation occurs when the rate of bleeding exceeds 0.5 mL/min. Successful identification of the hemorrhage source depends on the presence of active arterial bleeding at the time of the study. Failure to identify the bleeding point may be due to cessation during the time of the study and does not rule out the lower GI tract as the hemorrhage source.

Barium enema is a procedure used in cases of chronic bleeding. The barium will alter the viewing of other tests such as colonoscopy and angiography. Although it may define a mass or diverticulosis, it will not define small lesions such as an arteriovenous malformation (AVM). There is little role for barium enema in patients with acute active bleeding. **Small bowel barium** study can be performed if no colonic source of a lower hemorrhage is identified after an exhaustive search. The small bowel may have pathology that can be seen on barium examination, such as a neoplasm, Meckel's diverticulum, or other inflammatory disease.

Perform **anoscopy** as a mandatory examination for all patients with lower GI bleeding. This is performed at the bedside with a clear plastic speculum, which allows inspection of the anus and very distal rectum. This will rapidly rule out rectal or anal sources of hemorrhage, such as hemorrhoids, anal fissures, or malignancy at or below the dentate line.

Colonoscopy is useful when injection or cauterization of the pathologic process is necessary (Figure 14-1). It is not effective when there are high rates of bleeding resulting from poor visualization and higher complication rates. It is

COLONOSCOPY

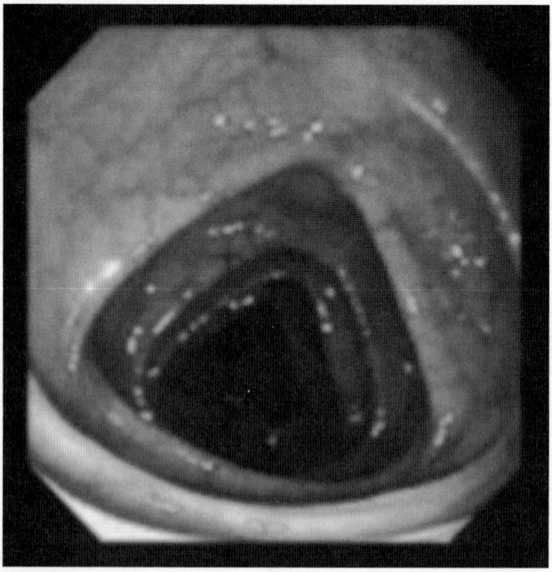

FIGURE 14-1
A View into a Normal Colon During Routine Colonoscopy

most useful in patients who have stopped bleeding or are bleeding at a slow rate. As well, there is limited efficacy in patients bleeding from diverticular disease, since there can be dozens to hundreds of diverticuli making the determination of the exact source of bleeding difficult.

Use **push endoscopy** in cases where no bleeding source is found in the upper tract or colon, and the suspicion is that bleeding is from the small bowel. The push endoscope is long and thin and can be "pushed" through the small bowel to inspect for lesions. Often, the scope is only effective for half to two thirds of the way through the small bowel. **Capsule endoscopy** is a new technology available in some centers, which uses a small capsule that is equipped with a camera and radiotransmitter. The patient swallows the capsule, and the radiotransmitter relays pictures from the camera as the capsule makes its way through the GI tract. The images are surprisingly clear, and the capsule is eventually released in the patient's stool.

■ DIAGNOSTIC PLAN

In all cases of blood per rectum, an **upper source** is first ruled out. Place a nasogastric tube and examine the effluent. Return of bilious fluid effectively eliminates an upper GI source. Obvious or occult blood will usually suggest an upper GI source and should be treated accordingly. In addition, a **rectal examination** and an **anoscopy** are performed on each patient to rule out bleeding that can easily be controlled with a local procedure.

Hemodynamically unstable patients first receive resuscitation with type-specific packed red cells and, if necessary, fresh frozen plasma and platelets. Consider the need for airway protection with endotracheal intubation in those patients in shock. Immediately assess the need to transfer the patient into a monitored bed, if that has not already been done.

Consider **radionucleotide** scan or **angiography** as the first diagnostic studies to find a bleeding source. Angiography has the ability to locate the precise source of the bleeding with active hemorrhage. Radionucleotide scan is more sensitive in picking up bleeding but is less specific in clearly identifying the exact location. Thus, these tests are not mutually exclusive and may be used together. Some centers have good success in using **colonoscopy** or **sigmoidoscopy** in patients with active bleeding. Colonoscopy is especially successful when a malignancy or AVM is suspected. Another advantage is that colonoscopy can be therapeutic but uses electrocautery attachments to coagulate AVMs or other identified sources of bleeding.

Hemodynamically stable patients with a single episode of hemorrhage or a positive guaiac study should be prepped and prepared for colonoscopy as the preferred study for evaluation. These patients can usually tolerate rapid intestinal lavage for colonoscopy preparation.

A small subset of patients with a lower GI bleed will have a negative upper and lower workup and indeed have a **small bowel source** of the bleeding. Making the diagnosis of small bowel bleeding is very difficult. Selective angiography of the superior mesenteric artery and celiac axis may show a source of extravasations. An option for treatment is **superselective embolization**, although this can lead to bowel ischemia. Another option is leaving the angiocatheter in place, performing an **exploratory laparotomy,** and resecting the bowel that is distal to the catheter.

After these investigations, patients will fall into two groups: those who have a source identified and those who do not have a definitive source identified.

Patients who have an exact source of bleeding have several options for treatment. In general, 80% of lower GI bleeds will halt spontaneously and the patient can be observed. If bleeding does not stop, treatment falls into two categories. The first are nonoperative treatments that include visceral **angiography** with possible embolization or colonoscopy with endoscopic coagulation or injection. Neither of these completely alleviates the possible need for surgery to the possibility of bowel wall necrosis post procedure. The last option is surgery including segmental colectomy or subtotal colectomy (Figure 14-2). A last option in a patient where severe bleeding continues with no source identifiable is a total abdominal colectomy with ileostomy.

■ DIFFERENTIAL DIAGNOSIS AND TREATMENT

Resuscitation

In all cases of hemodynamic instability, begin simultaneous resuscitation immediately while completing the initial workup. See **Chapter 13** for a full discussion of the resuscitation for a patient with a GI bleed.

Diverticulosis

Up to 50% of the general population has diverticulosis, and it is the most common cause of a lower GI hemorrhage. Fifteen percent of patients with diverticulosis will develop diverticular hemorrhage. This develops as inflammation in the wall erodes through the blood vessel in the neck of the diverticula in the colon (Chapter 10).

Although diverticular disease is most prevalent in the descending and sigmoid colon, the majority of diverticular bleeding (70%) arises in the right colon (Figure 14-3). The leading conjecture is that the wall of the right colon is thinner and, therefore, will bleed with less inflammation. The majority of diverticular bleeds are self-limiting (80%). When patients present, they will often be able to give a history of at least one previous episode of hematochezia or melanotic stools that resolved spontaneously. There are rarely any other findings in the history or physical examination to denote diverticular disease.

Make the diagnosis during significant hemorrhage by radionucleotide study or angiography. Localization by these maneuvers allows for a segmental colon resection if surgery is needed, although the majority of patients will not require surgical intervention (Figure 14-1). Surgery is required in approximately two

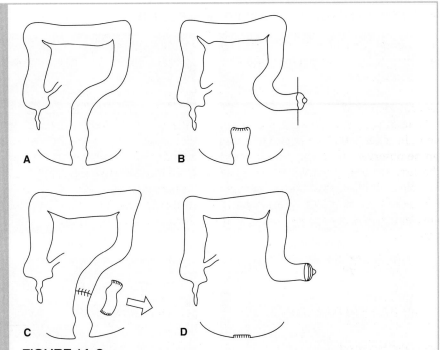

FIGURE 14-2
Types of Reconstruction after Colectomy Procedures, (A) Normal Anatomy, (B) the Hartman's Procedure, (c) Low Anterior Resection (LAR), and (D) Abdominal Perineal Resection (APR)

The patient is positioned in the modified lithotomy position to allow access to the rectum if needed. After a midline laparotomy, the colon is inspected throughout its course. The resection is then planned depending on the pathology and the indication for surgery. **Segmental resections** include the right, left, and transverse hemicolectomy (14-3). In these resections, the segment of colon to be removed is transected with a gastrointestinal anastomosis stapler, and the mesentery is ligated with clamps and ties. Anastomosis is performed by either a staple or a hand-sewn technique. For lesions in the distal colon, a **low anterior resection** removes the distal sigmoid and proximal rectum, with an anastomosis being created low in the pelvis. The **abdominal–perineal resection** is used for very low rectal lesions. Here the entire rectum and anus are resected, and the proximal colon is brought out as a permanent colostomy. In cases of perforated diverticulitis, rectal injuries, and sigmoid cancers, a Hartman's procedure may be done as a first-stage or permanent surgery. Here the sigmoid is resected, leaving a stump of rectum, while the proximal colon is brought out as anostomy. The Hartman's resection can be reanastomosed during a later surgery.

thirds of patients requiring >4 units PRBCs. These patients tend to be older than 65 years and have multiple comorbidities.

Angiodysplasia

Angiodysplasia can occur anywhere within the hollow viscus, but the colon is the most common site and, more specifically, the right colon (Figure 14-3).

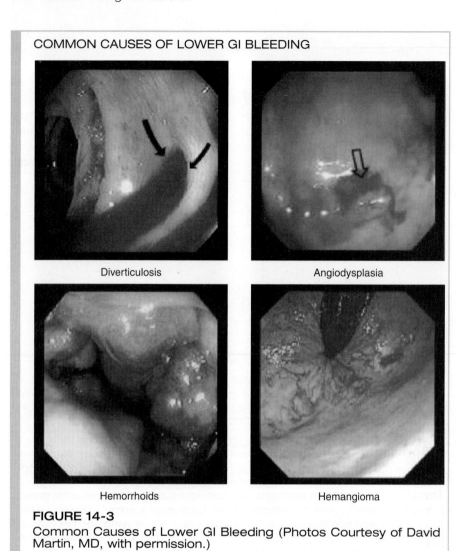

COMMON CAUSES OF LOWER GI BLEEDING

Diverticulosis

Angiodysplasia

Hemorrhoids

Hemangioma

FIGURE 14-3
Common Causes of Lower GI Bleeding (Photos Courtesy of David Martin, MD, with permission.)

The pathogenesis is a breakdown of the venules and capillaries, with congestion leading to formation of arteriovenous shunts. Diagnosis is by selective visceral angiography or colonoscopy. On angiography, it appears as a blush during the arterial phase followed by early venous drainage (Figure 14-3). Treatment is typically colonoscopic electrocauterization, with nonresponders requiring partial colectomy.

Colon Mass

Colonic neoplasms, most often adenocarcinoma, usually present as either in-testinal obstruction (see Chapter 10) or chronic occult hemorrhage in the form of melena. Occasionally, a colonic cancer can bleed acutely. Look for a history of weight loss, chronic anemia, and chronic constipation as signs of an occult malignancy. Make the diagnosis on either abdominal CT or colonoscopy. If CT is used, a complete colonoscopy is indicated to rule out synchronous lesions and to obtain tissue biopsy.

Colon adenocarcinoma can locally invade into the mesentery, local lymph nodes, and metastasis most often to the liver. Make the pathologic diagnosis by biopsy. Because the tumor becomes symptomatic only late in the disease, aggressive surveillance is recommended with fecal occult blood testing and routine sigmoidoscopies.

Ischemic Colitis

Bowel ischemia has many etiologies, including venous or arterial thrombosis, embolization, iatrogenic ligation after abdominal aortic aneurysm repair, thromboangiitis obliterans, and polyarteritis nodosa. Patients are usually older people and present complaining of low abdominal pain localizing to the left side with melena or hematochezia. Rectal examination is usually within normal limits. Diagnosis is made by inspecting the mucosa during colonoscopy. Although the mucosa may appear ischemic, it is difficult to determine if full-thickness necrosis is present in the bowel wall. Although some cases of partial necrosis can be treated conservatively with bowel rest and antibiotics, the majority of patients will need surgical exploration and partial colectomy.

Inflammatory Bowel Disease

Bloody diarrhea is a common symptom of Crohn's disease and ulcerative colitis. These patients are typically managed medically. A small number of patients (15%) with ulcerative colitis will present with greater than 20 bouts a day of fulminant bloody diarrhea. Diagnosis is by careful perianal examination and initial proctosigmoidoscopy. This may determine ulcerative colitis versus Crohn's disease, as the examination will reveal cobblestoning and linear ulceration in the Crohn's patient. If acute medical management fails, surgical intervention is recommended in cases of unrelenting hemorrhage (Figure 11-5).

Perirectal Disease

Hemorrhoids can be internal or external. Internal hemorrhoids are above the dentate line and covered with mucosa. Internal hemorrhoids do not cause pain, but they may bleed and prolapse. An **anal fissure** is a split in the anoderm. Ten percent occur anteriorly and 90% occur posteriorly. Symptoms can include tearing pain that lasts several hours with and after defecation. See **Chapter 19** for a full discussion of perirectal disease.

Selected Readings

Souba WW, ed. *ACS Surgery*. New York: WebMD. http://www.acssurgery.com/ visACS.htm (accessed 2-2008).

Cameron JL, ed. *Current Surgical Therapy*. 8th ed. New York, NY: Mosby; 2004.

15

Wounds and Wound Care

Jessica Brown, RN, MSN, ACNP-BC, CLNC ■ *Claudia E. Goettler, MD, FACS* ■ *Michael F. Rotondo, MD, FACS*

Key Points

■ Wound management is a large part of surgical practice and includes surgical incisions, burns, traumatic wounds, and infected tissue.

■ Good wound management requires regular reassessment to determine the best therapy and to assure adequate patient comfort.

■ Care of infected and necrotic wounds includes debridement of devitalized tissue by autolytic, enzymatic, mechanical, or surgical debridement.

■ Care of clean wounds includes adequate nutrition, allowing adequate wound coverage, regular wound care and assessment for surgical closure with flaps or skin grafts.

■ Burn wounds are challenging on account of the large surface area they may cover. Principles include frequent dressing changes, topical antibiotics, early surgical debridement and coverage with skin grafts or collagen-based biodressings.

■ Decubitus ulcers are best managed by prevention. When they do occur, debridement of necrotic tissue followed by aggressive wound care is the mainstay of treatment.

■ A soft-tissue abscess is usually a result of local infection and often requires surgical incision and drainage procedure with open packing.

■ GENERAL PRINCIPLES

Wounds and wound care is an inevitable part of surgical care. Wounds are formed by disease, injury, and intentionally by surgeons and practitioners to cure disease. Despite the wide variety of conditions that cause soft-tissue wounds, the management of them is similar. Most wounds, despite the cause, will heal naturally as long as they are kept free from infection and decessation. **Abnormal wound healing** occurs when one or more conditions interfere with normal wound healing. These conditions can be remembered by the mnemonic DIDN'T HEAL:

Diabetes: The long-term effects of diabetes impair wound healing by decreasing sensation and arterial inflow, diminishing cardiac output, causing poor peripheral perfusion, and impairing polymorphonuclear leukocyte phagocytosis.

Infection: Bacterial contamination is a necessary condition but is not sufficient for wound infection. A susceptible host and a wound environment are also required.

Drugs: Steroids and antimetabolites hinder proliferation of fibroblasts and collagen synthesis.

Nutritional problems: Malnutrition and deficiencies of vitamins A, C, and zinc impair normal wound-healing mechanisms.

Tissue necrosis: This condition results in local or systemic ischemia. Decreased blood supply may mark the onset of a long-term nonhealing ulcer.

Hypoxia: Inadequate tissue oxygenation as a result of local vasoconstriction may occur because of blood volume deficit, cardiac insufficiency, or severe anemia.

Excessive tension on wound edges: This leads to local tissue ischemia and necrosis.

Another wound: Competition between healing areas for the factors required for wound healing impairs healing at all sites.

Low temperature: A reduction of $1–1.5°C$ $(2–3°F)$ from normal core body temperature is responsible for slower healing.

■ INFECTED WOUNDS

Autolytic debridement uses the body's own enzymes and moisture to rehydrate, soften, and liquify hard eschar and slough. This can be accomplished with the use of occlusive or semiocclusive dressings that keep wound fluid in contact with necrotic tissue (Table 15-1).

TABLE 15-1.
Types of Autolytic Wound Debridement

	Characteristics	Indications	Contraindications	Technique	Advantages	Disadvantages	Types
Hydrocolloids	• Absorptive • Occlusive/semipermeable • Adhesive • Moisture retentive	• Light to moderately exudative wounds • Stage I–III ulcers	• Infected wounds • Exposed tendon/bone	• Change dressing every 3–5 days	• First-line dressing • Cost effective • Requires less care than other dressings • Sticks to wet/dry wounds • Conformable • Water resistant • Barrier against infection	• May become malodorous • Expensive (compared to saline) • Limits monitoring of wound	• Duoderm • Restore • Comfeel • Tegasorb
Hydrogels	• Semiocclusive dressing/filler • Moisture retentive • Adhesive/nonadhesive	• Light to moderately exudative wounds • Filler for deep/extensive wounds • Carrier for topical medicines • Stage II–III ulcers		• Change dressing every 5–7 days • Apply gel directly to wound/from syringe • Cover wound site with gauze/foam dressing • Secure in place with transparent film dressing	• Conformable • Filler for wound to keep moist healing environment • Cooling, soothing sensation/analgesia	• Needs moderate level of care • Requires dressing to hold in place • Expensive	• Nu-gel • Intrasite gel • Duoderm gel • Clearsite • Geliperm
Transparent film dressings	• Semipermeable, occlusive dressing • Allows gas and oxygen exchange • Retains exudates to create moist environment	• Nonexudative wounds • Stage I–III ulcers • Secure other wound dressings • Protects vulnerable areas from friction injury	• Wounds with sinus tracts/undermining • Infected wounds • Wounds with lots of exudate	• Change dressing every 3–7 days • Consider protecting skin edges from tearing • Check dressing daily	• Less care needed than gauze dressings • Conformable • Water resistant • Able to monitor wound without removal • Protects against infection	• Frequent dressing changes may cause skin damage • Expensive • Difficult to apply • No ability to absorb exudates	• Transparent adhesive dressing • Biocclu⁻ • Te⁻
Foam dressings	• Nonadherent • Semiocclusive dressing/filler	• Light to moderately exudative wounds • Combined with hydrogel dressing • Stage II–IV ulcers		• Change dressing every 7 days	• Insulate wound • Conformable	• Expensive	

TABLE 15-2.
Topical Ointments Used for Enzymatic Debridement

	Accuzyme	Panafil (Chlorophylline/) Papain/Urea) Gladase-C	Santyl (Collagenase)
Dose	830,000 units/g/10% ointment/spray	0.5%/521,700 units/g/10% ointment/spray	250 units/g
Frequency	Daily to BID	Daily to BID	Daily to BID
Available as	6 g tube	6 g tube	15 g tube
	30 g tube	30 g tube	30 g tube

Enzymatic debridement is the use of topical ointment to promote sloughing of necrotic tissue. Wound debridement is facilitated by enzymatic digestion. They are best used on wounds with a large amount of necrotic debris or eschar formation (Table 15-2). **Advantages** to enzymatic debridement include minimal or no damage to healthy tissues with proper applications. In addition, it may be used after surgical debridement and can be used in combination with autolytic and mechanical debridement. **Disadvantages** include inflammation or discomfort that may occur to healthy tissue. Logistically, it is expensive, requires a prescription, and often needs a skilled practitioner to apply to avoid damage to intact skin.

Mechanical debridement is the use of dressings to pull necrotic tissue off the wound. One application is a "**wet-to-dry**" dressing. When this wet dressing dries in the wound, it sticks to dead tissue, and, with manual removal of the dressing, nonselective debridement occurs. Since it works by sticking to the wound, wetting the dressing prior to removal is contraindicated. This type of debridement is best used in wounds with moderate amounts of necrotic debris (Table 15-3). **Hydrotherapy** is a type of mechanical debridement and involves

TABLE 15-3.
Solutions Used for Mechanical Debridement

	Sodium Chloride (NaCl)	Dakin's Solution (Sodium Hypochlorite)	Acetic Acid
Description	• Used when no germicidal agent required • Used as rinse to minimize fluid shifts • Decreases drying effect of other irritants	• Germicidal antiseptic wetting agent • Dissolves necrotic tissue/debris • Used as irrigant, cleanser, soak, or wet-to-dry dressing	• Effective against *Pseudomonas aeruginosa* • Can mask superinfections
Dose	0.9%	Full strength: 0.5% Half strength: 0.25%	0.5%
Frequency	Daily to PRN	Daily to TID	Daily

exposing the wound to a jet or a bath of water. It can be done at the bedside or in specialized facilities (whirlpool). The disadvantages are that it is nonselective and may traumatize healthy or healing tissue, prevent epithelialization, cause tissue maceration, and allow waterborne bacteria to contaminate wounds.

Surgical wound debridement is the fastest method of debridement. It is best used in wounds with large amounts of necrotic, infected tissues. Surgical debridement may be performed at the bedside if removing only necrotic tissue. This avoids excess loss of tissue. Without active infection, "less is more," as repeat debridement or wet-to-dry dressing can cause problems. **Advantages** to debridement are that it is fast and selective, extremely effective, and can be repeated often. **Disadvantages** are mostly related to pain and discomfort of patients. Care must always be given to providing adequate anesthetic or intravenous analgesia, if needed. It can also be costly, especially if an operating room is required. Lastly, it may not be possible on selected areas, such as close to bone or fascia, without worsening the wound.

Hyperbaric oxygen (HBO) therapy is an adjunct to wound care that involves forcing oxygen into a wound at high atmospheric pressure (Figure 15-1). It is a painless procedure in which a patient is placed in a clear, acrylic chamber under increased atmospheric pressure. The concept is that increasing the normal oxygen tension in the infected wounds causes a bactericidal effect, improving blood supply, and enhancing wound healing. HBO therapy is an **adjunct** and cannot replace physical debridement of infected or necrotic tissue. Optimal outcomes are achieved using a combination of therapies including antibiotics, surgery, and HBO, when available.

On account of the logistics of creating a high-pressure environment, there are significant **risks**. Limited personnel and equipment fit into the chambers; hence, "diving" is not appropriate for critical or unstable patients. The most common clinical side effect of the high pressure is perforated eardrums.

■ CLEAN WOUNDS

Once infection and necrosis have been eliminated, the goal is to facilitate wound healing. Wounds heal by forming **granulation** tissue, an immature, unstructured type of tissue that is very vascular and has the ability to fill in large spaces. Wounds also have the ability to **contract** over time, making the wound smaller. These lead to natural closure of even large wounds.

Standard wound care for a clean wound is keeping it moist and free from contamination. Often this includes using a "**wet-to-moist**" dressing. Unlike the wet-to-dry dressing, the goal is not debridement, but keeping the environment moist and not disturbing the frail granulation tissue when removing the dressing. Thus, the dressing is not allowed to dry out, wetting it if necessary between dressing changes.

The **negative pressure therapy** (NPT) dressing is a relatively new technology, which provides a clean, moist, negative pressure environment for wounds to heal. They can be homemade or commercially made devices. All have a dressing

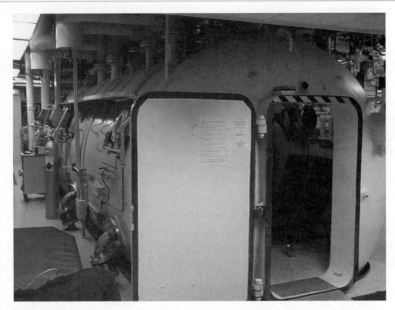

FIGURE 15-1.
A Typical Hyperbasic Oxygen Apparatus

A typical treatment protocol involves HBO, given aggressively after the first surgical debridement. Three treatment sessions, in a multiplace chamber with 100% oxygen for 90 minutes each, can be given in the first 24 hours. Appropriate air breaks are given as necessary. In a monoplace chamber, 100% oxygen is administered for 90 minutes per session. On the second day, twice-daily treatments can follow until granulation of the tissues is obtained to a total of 10–15 treatments.

There are several preparations to initiate prior to the procedure: Nicotine interferes with HBO and its effectiveness, so patients should not smoke during the treatment phase; to ensure safety, makeup, lotion, nail polish, hairspray, perfume, or deodorant containing petroleum or alcohol base cannot be worn due to flammability; and patients are asked to report symptoms of fever, cough, sore throat, or vomiting, as these illnesses may become worse with therapy.

In a monoplace chamber, the patient is placed on a padded table that slides into a long, cylindrical tube. A multiplace chamber can hold more than a dozen patients at a time.

The patient will be asked to change into 100% cotton clothing prior to the procedure. All metal, jewelry, contact lenses, and other prosthetic devices will be removed. In order to initiate the session, a technician gradually will increase the pressure in the chamber with 100% oxygen. With the increase in pressure, the patient may experience warmth or a "popping" sensation in the ears. When the chamber has reached the prescribed pressure, the patient may rest, sleep, watch television, or talk to the technician on a two-way intercom. The patient is monitored continuously throughout the procedure. At the end of the treatment, the pressure will gradually be decreased and the therapy session finished.

that contacts the wound, covered by an airtight plastic, and some form of suction device that is placed between the plastic and dressing.

There are several **advantages** to using negative pressure devices. Unlike wet-to-moist dressings, they only need to be changed every other or every third day, decreasing discomfort for the patient and saving resources. Formation of granulation tissue is encouraged by increased chemotaxins in the wound, whereas wound edema, swelling, and drainage are decreased. It is felt that wound contraction is accelerated due to the negative pressure, and the resulting granulation and contraction help to fill in "dents" with improved cosmetic outcome. Lastly, as the moist environment provides protection of underlying tissues, it is excellent over tissues that are at high risk of desiccation such as bone and tendon.

Disadvantages of NPT devices is the cost of the system, which is often offset by the shortened hospital stays and decreased resources needed to care for the wounds. Also, the devices create an anaerobic environment and thus can promote active infection if the wounds are not clean when the device is placed. Evidence of ongoing infection is a contraindication to this technology. It does not provide any debridement. The use over **enterocutaneous fistulae** to control drainage has been described; however, the research evidence of whether fistulae improve or worsen with negative pressure dressing therapy is not clear and thus caution should be used in these cases. Special considerations should be given when it is used over intestines to encourage granulation in an **open abdomen.** The bowel must be protected from abrasion that can cause fistulae. When using the commercial system, the soft white sponge or xeroform should be placed prior to the rough black sponge. With homemade systems, gauze should be separated from the bowel with xeroform.

■ BURN WOUNDS

Burns and abrasions functionally result in the same injury: variable loss of skin thickness. Abrasions seen in motor vehicle injuries are commonly known as "road rash" despite not being a rash at all. Burns are often from thermal injury but can also result from chemicals, radiation, or some medical conditions that cause the skin to slough off. Systemic **physiologic effects** occur with skin loss of more than 10–15% surface area. Estimate the size of the burn/abrasion using the "rule of nines," 1% of a patient's surface area is roughly the same size as the palm of the patient's hand. This is useful for measuring patchy areas of patients of all sizes. These rules can be used to determine the total affected surface area to allow calculation of fluid needs and communication with others.

Since the skin is a natural barrier, heat and fluid loss may be extensive; thus, it is important to keep the patient **warm** and **resuscitated.** Place a bladder catheter and use **urine output** as the best monitor of resuscitation. Provide tetanus prophylaxis in the form of a **tetanus booster**. In severely contaminated injuries, particularly involving farm machinery, **tetanus immune globulin** should be considered.

Adequate early **debridement** of devitalized skin is the keystone of burn care. All devitalized tissue should be removed, including blisters from burns and any necrotic flaps from abrasion injuries. Ground-in dirt must be removed, as it will result in permanent "tattooing" of the injuries. For significant burn injuries, this often necessitates general anesthesia and specialized equipment such as a shower and/or whirlpool tub. These are usually only available in burn centers.

Systemic antibiotics are *not* given. This practice results in selection of resistant wound organisms and will not decrease chance of burn-wound infection. If the patient develops a burn-wound infection, or cellulitis develops surrounding the burn wound, broad-spectrum antibiotics are then indicated. **Burn infections** appear as expanding dark or purple areas in the wound and require antibiotics and urgent debridement.

Depth determines healing. **Superficial** (first degree) wounds are red, tender, and without open areas—like sunburn. This will peel as skin heals underneath. Keeping it moist with lotion improves comfort and minimizes peeling and itching. **Superficial partial thickness** (second degree) wounds are pink, moist, blanching, painful, and blistered. Healing of these wounds is by epithelization. This will take several weeks for the basal cells to form new epithelia and new skin. The goal in care is to keep the wounds clean and moist to encourage epithelial migration. **Deep partial thickness** (second degree) is defined as red, nonblanching, and painful. In general, healing will take longer, on the order of 2 weeks, and often there will be some scar formation. The need for skin grafting is a clinical determination of whether skin graft will offer a functionally and cosmetically better outcome than waiting. **Full-thickness** (third degree) wounds are white or dark, leathery, exposed fat or muscle, and usually not painful as nerve endings are destroyed. If left alone, these wounds would heal by contraction over a long period of time. Unless very small, all third-degree wounds require excision and grafting to shorten healing time and improve function and cosmetic results.

Dressing choice for burns or large abrasions is variable (Table 15-4). A good dressing provides topical, antimicrobial control and a moist environment. Dressing changes should include gentle mechanical debridement with soap and water and a washcloth. **Occlusive** dressings prevent heat and moisture release but can make the wounds anaerobic and result in infection. Therefore, these should only be used on very clean wounds. **Enzymatic** debridement agents are used if an eschar is slow in lifting. This type of debridement is especially useful on areas where mechanical debridement is dangerous (fascia and tendon).

For deeper wounds, the standard of care is early **surgical debridement** of burn tissue and coverage with a biological covering. Split thickness skin-graft replacement with **autograft** (harvested from the patient) or placement of a temporary covering of **xenograft** (pigskin) is the most common covering. In addition, there are several commercially available **collagen-based dressings**.

Care of an autograft includes attention to the donor and recipient site. Split thickness skin-graft harvesting results in a superficial second-degree burn-type wound at the **donor site**. Coverage of this new wound is most often with **xeroform,** a nonadherent dressing impregnated with 3% bismuth tribromophenate.

TABLE 15-4.
Types of Burn/Abrasion Dressings

	Silvadene (Silver Sulfadiazine Topical)	Sulfamylon (Mafenide Topical)	Silver Impregnated Dressings	Bacitracin/Xeroform	Semiocclusive
Description	Inhibits dihydropteroate synthetase	Bacteriostatic for many organisms			
Characteristics	• Good penetration of eschar • Comfortable • Sulfa drug	• Excellent penetration of eschar • Painful • Used mostly for cartilage areas (ears)	• Causes black discoloration of wound	• Used on wounds without eschar due to poor penetration of antimicrobial protection • Comfortable • Use for face without additional covering • Excellent for epithelialization	• Very comfortable • Minimal dressings required • Only for very clean wounds without eschar • Requires systemic antibiotic coverage
Reactions	• Frequently reacts with wound fluids to produce yellowish, purulent-appearing material • Can cause dose-dependent neutropenia • Causes cataracts				
Dose	1% cream	8.5% cream or 5% solution			
How to apply	Apply thick (like cake icing) Daily to BID	Cream: apply thick (like cake icing) Daily to BID Solution: q6-8h & prn	Depending on dressing type, may be left in place for several days	Changed daily	May be left on for long periods (up to 2 weeks) as the wound heals underneath
Available as	1% 50 or 400 g jar 1% 20 or 85 g tube	Cream: 2 oz (56.7 g) tube, 4 oz (113.4 g) tube, and 16 oz (453.6 g) jar Solution: 50 g powder packet, when reconstituted with 1000 mL sterile water or saline = 5% sol			Biobrane Tegaderm

The xeroform dries onto the wound and acts as a scab. As the wound heals, the xeroform peels off.

Care of the skin-graft **recipient site** is also important. The skin graft must be immobilized until it has developed a blood supply. Typically, some type of bolster/pressure dressing is placed to prevent the graft from shifting. Depending on location, ambulation/activity may be limited to prevent shifting. The dressing is usually kept in place for 4–6 days at which time careful removal of the initial dressing is important to prevent lifting of the graft. After removal of the initial dressing, the area should be kept clean and moist to encourage epithelization of the open areas in the graft. This is usually done with daily xeroform and bacitracin. Graft that has successfully taken does not move and is pink, whereas a failed graft is gray and floats away.

■ DECUBITUS WOUNDS

Decubitus ulcers and pressure sores are often used synonymously and may commonly be referred to as a bed sore. A decubitus ulcer develops when pressure applied to the skin, soft tissue, muscle, and bone exceeds pressure for vascular flow. In gathering the patient's history, it is important to determine the medical cause for the ulcer. **Decubitus ulcers** form in individuals who are exposed to long episodes of continual pressure over body surfaces, causing ischemia and tissue anoxia. Permanent effects can occur in as little as 2 hours.

Several causes are responsible for the basic formation of decubitus ulcers. **Paralysis** and decreased sensation allow for skin breakdown by altering the body's response to pain. The skin is vulnerable to friction and shearing forces during movement. **Trauma** causing de-epithelization leads to transdermal water loss, creating maceration and adherence of skin to clothing and bedding. Patients who are sedated, restrained, demented, or neurologically impaired have **decreased mobility**. Less frequent position changes increase pressure over body prominences. **Contractures** and spasticity cause ulcers by exerting persistent pressure to tissues through flexion of a joint. A contracture keeps a joint in flexion, whereas spasticity applies friction and shearing forces to tissues.

Anemia and **vascular disease** decrease oxygen-rich blood from reaching the area of pressure sores and delay wound healing. **Malnutrition** and decreased protein intake are directly related to delayed wound healing. Other information that should be obtained during a history should include the onset, duration, other ulcers, wound care, and prior medical or surgical treatment. A patient's **social situation** can also impact treatment. Suitable support systems at home help to decrease the risk of recurrence.

Perform a **physical examination** documenting the specific location, size, and depth of the ulcer. Infection can be described by wound edge erythema, odor, drainage, and necrotic tissue or bone. On the basis of the depth of injury, ulcers can be classified into different stages (Table 15-5). It is a good practice to document the wound with a **digital photograph** that can be placed in the chart. This allows comparison over time and objective judgment of treatment effectiveness.

TABLE 15-5.
Staging of Pressure Ulcers

	Description	Signs/Symptoms	Interventions/ Dressing Type
Stage I	• Blanchable erythema over intact skin • Can resolve in 24 hours if direct pressure removed	• Warm, indurated area • Sensation of pain/itching • With continued pressure, erythematous area does not blanch and becomes white	• May require no dressing
Stage II	• Partial thickness skin loss • Damage or necrosis to epidermis, dermis, or both	• Superficial • Presents as abrasion, blister, or shallow crater	• Hydrocolloid occlusive dressing to provide a moist environment and aid in epithelialization
Stage III	• Full-thickness skin loss • Damage or necrosis to subcutaneous tissue • Does not extend through underlying fascia	• Presents as deep crater with or without undermining of adjacent tissues	• Wet-to-dry dressing • Isotonic sodium chloride solution • Dilute Dakin's solution • Hydrogel dressing • VAC dressing
Stage IV	• Full-thickness skin loss • Extensive destruction • Tissue necrosis • Damage to muscle, bone, tendon, or joint capsule	• Undermining and sinus tracts may be present	• Wet-to-dry dressing • Isotonic sodium chloride solution • Dilute Dakin's solution • Hydrogel dressing • VAC dressing • Daily whirlpool treatments • For contaminated, necrotic, or infected wounds, sharp surgical debridement is necessary

Order **laboratory** studies to help clarify the patient's overall condition. Determine the white blood cell (WBC) count on the **CBC** and look for abnormalities of electrolytes, glucose, BUN, and creatinine. Order an **erythrocyte sedimentation rate** (ESR). An ESR greater than 120 mm/h, in combination with a WBC count greater than 15,000/dL, can be indicative of osteomyelitis. Determining the **albumin** level helps to determine the patient's nutritional status. A value of at least 3.5 g/mL should be obtained before considering flap reconstruction to promote healing.

In wounds that have bone exposed, order **plain radiographs** to rule out the diagnosis of osteomyelitis. If nondiagnostic, a **bone scan** can also suggest the presence of osteomyelitis. A negative bone scan finding generally excludes osteomyelitis. However, it may be necessary to perform a bone biopsy to confirm positive bone scan findings.

The best treatment for decubitus wounds is **preventing** them from occurring in the first place. The mainstay for decubitus prevention is **frequent position changes**, at least every 2 hours, to alleviate direct pressure. Specialized mattresses have been developed with foam, air, and fluid to decrease pressure.

Wounds that have formed are treated aggressively to prevent worsening. The skin around the wound is kept clean and dry. Wound dressings for decubiti differ for each individual stage of the wound (Table 15-5). Ulcers that have not advanced beyond Stage II may heal by removing direct pressure. **Optimize nutrition**, particularly protein intake. Order supplements and/or tube feeds, if needed, along with weekly nutritional assessment including a pre-albumin level or 24-hour urine nitrogen.

■ ABSCESS WOUNDS

Abscesses are fluid-filled vesicles, usually caused by a bacterial infection, made up of both living and dead organisms as well as destroyed tissue from white blood cells. Abscesses are found in the soft tissue, such as the axilla, groin, or perineum, but may develop in any organ, breast, skin, or gums. Abscesses are found more commonly in men, elderly patients with serious medical conditions, the obese population, and patients with diabetes.

A **furuncle** is an abscess or a boil of walled off purulent material arising from a hair follicle. Furuncle lesions appear as an indurated, dull, red nodule with a central purulent core, usually beginning around a hair follicle or sebaceous gland. In a furuncle, a subcutaneous abscess can form and is associated with pain and a limited radius of surrounding cellulites. **Carbuncles** are clusters of small, shallow abscesses surrounding several hair follicles that connect under the skin. Carbuncles often result in extensive peeling of the skin, scar formation, and permanent hair loss.

Inflammation in the adjacent tissues causes pain and edema, including the subcutaneous fat, and is associated with systemic systems. Systemic indications typically include fever, fatigue, general malaise, and regional lymphadenopathy. **Sites** most often affected by carbuncles are the face, scalp, thighs, axilla, and inguinal area, and these can often occur in a pattern in areas that were previously shaved. A carbuncle on the back of the neck is found almost exclusively in diabetics.

Laboratory studies to consider are cultures, Gram stain, potassium hydroxide (KOH) prep and biopsy. **Cultures** help to determine accurate antibiotic therapy. **KOH** slides are obtained when a fungal infection is suspected. A significantly increased WBC count on the **CBC** can indicate systemic infection. Since many of these abscesses are commonly found in diabetics, evaluate the blood glucose for elevations.

Form a therapeutic treatment plan that is based upon history and physical examination findings. For uncomplicated lesions, use of **antibacterial soaps** and good hand-washing techniques are used. **Warm compresses** and cleansing represent the first line of treatment. **Heat** may accelerate healing, reduce inflammation, and alleviate pain. **Elevation** decreases edema and inflammation. Manipulation and surgical incision of small early lesions should be avoided because local or systemic infections can occur. For deep lesions, empiric treatment with topical and oral **antibiotics** that cover gram-positive organisms is indicated.

If the infection has spread as indicated by cellulitis or lymphatic streaking, or the abscess is located in the groin or face, **antibiotics** that target *Staphylococcus* are indicated to reduce further spreading. Recurrent furuncles are treated with oral antibiotics continuously for 1–2 months. Some carbuncles are complicated by significant cellulites and induration and will require a short course of IV antibiotics followed by oral antibiotics. Large abscesses, furuncles, and carbuncles may require an incision and drainage. If the wound is completely drained, antibiotics are not usually needed. Carbuncles are hard to eliminate because many small pus-filled pockets are difficult to find and drain, causing the need for antibiotics to often be continued for several months. A reduced-fat diet and weight loss program should be initiated, since carbuncles are more common in the obese.

Selected Readings

Bhumbra N, McCullough S. Skin and subcutaneous infections. *Prim Care Clin Office Pract.* 2003;30(1):1–24.

Brem H, Lyder C. Protocol for the successful treatment of pressure ulcers. *Am J Surg.* 2004;188(1):9S–17S.

Hartford C. Care of outpatient burns. In: Herndon D, ed. *Total Burn Care.* 2nd ed. Philadelphia: W.B. Saunders; 2001:71–80.

Kihiczak G, Schwartz R, Kapila R. Necrotizing fasciitis: A deadly infection. *J Eur Acad Dermatol Venerol.* 2006;20(4):365–369.

Lionelli G, Lawrence W. Wound dressings. *Surg Clin North Am.* 2003;83(3): 617–638.

Williams W, Phillips L. Pathophysiology of the burn wound. In: Herndon D, ed. *Total Burn Care.* 2nd ed. Philadelphia: W.B. Saunders; 2001:63–70.

16

Peripheral Vascular Insufficiency

Teresa Krosnick, PA-C ■ *G. Melville Williams, MD*

■ A careful history will differentiate acute versus chronic vascular insufficiency.

■ Document the strength and character of all pulses and describe all skin changes, both venous and arterial.

■ Advanced diagnostic techniques are utilized to obtain precise preoperative diagnoses. These include color flow, duplex imaging, computed tomography, magnetic resonance imaging three-dimensional CT(3-dCT) and the gold standard, angiography.

■ Claudication is pain with exertion of an extremity and signifies critical restriction of blood flow to the limb.

■ Rest pain is felt without limb exertion and signifies critical lack of blood flow to an extremity.

■ The judicious use of anticoagulants is critical in the surgical management of both arterial and venous disorders.

■ Significant aortoiliac or peripheral artery stenosis may be managed by angioplasty, stenting, endarterectomy or vascular bypass.

- Carefully selected therapeutic measures should be individualized for each specific clinical problem.

- Mesenteric ischemia caused by obstruction of the celiac and superior mesenteric artery can be chronic, or an acute, life threatening problem.

- A rare but limb threatening venous obstruction is Phlegmasia Cerulean Dolens.

- Thoracic outlet syndrome most often presents with neurologic symptoms or signs of acute venous obstruction of the upper limb.

■ HISTORY

Patients with peripheral vascular disease typically present with **chief complaints** such as extremity pain at rest, claudication, abdominal pain, limb swelling, or skin ulceration. Sudden onset of symptoms is often related to acute arterial ischemia, whereas long-standing problems, such as skin ulcers, are indicative of progressing arterial stenosis. Therefore, first define the chief complaint and events in the history of the present illness. This will allow the differential diagnosis to be refined and appropriate treatment to begin.

Determine if there is a history of acute pain, pallor, pulselessness, paresthesias, and paresis in the extremity suggestive of **acute arterial occlusion**. Acute occlusions are most often from emboli from the heart owing to atrial fibrillation, wall motion abnormality, cardiomegaly, ventricular wall aneurysm, acute MI, or valve disease. An embolism may also originate from an aortic aneurysm or ulcerated vascular plaque.

Ask the patient about any difficulty or pain with ambulating. This may be from **claudication** during exertion, especially walking, as a cramp or pain in the muscle group just distal to the area of disease. This is secondary to poor oxygen delivery and poor blood flow in a limb with significant arterial stenosis. It is reproducible and progressive and generally relieved within 1–5 minutes of rest. It is worse at a quick pace or when walking uphill. Symptoms can be stable or progressive, especially in patients who have symptoms with less and less activity.

Obtain any history of limb pain that occurs without exercise, or **rest pain**. Patients will describe this as a condition that awakens them at night, with the need to stand up or dangle the leg over the edge of the bed to get relief. Rest pain indicates critical stenosis and the need for urgent intervention.

If a patient presents with **skin necrosis** or breakdown of tissue or gangrene, clarify how long the skin changes have been present and how they have changed or been treated. Also, document any history of claudication and rest pain and how they may have changed at the time of tissue loss.

Infrequently, the presenting complaint is **abdominal pain**. Assess the type of pain, location, and duration of symptoms. Severe acute abdominal pain is worrisome for a ruptured aortic aneurysm or acute mesenteric occlusion, whereas chronic pain associated with eating can signal chronic mesenteric ischemia.

Perform a complete review of the **past medical history,** since most patients with peripheral vascular disease also suffer from a variety of chronic medical conditions that affect the diagnosis and treatment of the vascular problems. **Atherosclerosis** is a systemic disease associated with smoking, hypertension, renal disease, diabetes, coagulation defects, and dyslipidemia.

Peripheral vascular disease is highly associated with concomitant **coronary artery disease**. Investigate any previous history of myocardial infarction, congestive heart failure, dysrhythmias, or hypertension. **Cerebrovascular disease** is also prevalent in this patient population; thus enquire about previous strokes, neurologic symptoms, or previous carotid surgeries. Document all catheterizations, echocardiograms, stress tests, and halter-monitor testing and be as specific as possible about dates and subsequent surgeries. **Diabetes** is common in this patient population and can complicate treatment.

Since **smoking** is a primary risk factor for vascular disease, vascular patients frequently have advanced pulmonary disease. Document the smoking history as well as results from previous pulmonary function tests. Atherosclerosis may affect the renal vasculature and lead to chronic **renal insufficiency**. Finally, document any history of **autoimmune disease** such as systemic lupus erythematous, or vasculitis, both of which can cause significant, nonatherosclerotic vascular disease.

A history of **trauma**, either externally produced or iatrogenic (e.g., previous surgery or radiation), is important in the evaluation of dissections and aneurysms in patients without known atherosclerotic disease.

Obtain a **medication history**. Include dose, frequency, and time of dosing. Include when the patient began taking these medications and how the doses have been changed. All drug and other **allergies** must be documented, but specifically ask about allergens that will be involved in a vascular workup, including penicillin, sulfa, heparin, contrast dye, iodine, betadine, tape, latex, and seafood allergies.

■ PHYSICAL EXAMINATION

The physical examination of a vascular patient begins globally and then focuses on the current complaint. Evaluate the **pulse** strength and character at the superficial temporal, carotid, radial, femoral popliteal, posterior tibial, anterior tibial, and peroneal sites. Document any thrills or **pulsatile masses** that are appreciated on examination. Auscultate the carotid arteries while the patient holds their breath to assess for bruits indicating stenosis. Auscultate the heart listening for **murmurs**, which may reveal valvular disease or arrhythmias that can be the source of emboli. Auscultate the lungs for evidence of fluid overload or bronchospasm. Palpate and auscultate the abdomen for evidence of an **aneurysm**.

Note any body habitus features such as scoliosis, limb deformities, irregular gait, and obesity or cachetic habitus.

Patients should be examined wearing a gown for full examination. Look at both legs carefully and compare them with each other. Document pallor on elevation and rubor on dependency, atrophy, paralysis, and skin temperature.

Look for **trophic changes** such as thick nails, loss of hair. and shiny skin. Examine the feet looking at the heel and in between the toes. Look for signs of loss of tissue such as vascular insufficiency **ulcers** or gangrene. Ulcers or necrosis of the toes or fingers are often seen in embolization, whereas ulcers from venous stasis disease are found above the medial malleolus. **Dry gangrene** is desiccated and black and may be full thickness or superficial. **Wet gangrene** is foul smelling and moist.

If lower extremity stenosis is suspected, perform **ankle–brachial indexes (ABI)**. The ABI is a quick, noninvasive bedside measure of the adequacy of the blood flow to the distal lower extremity. A blood pressure cuff is placed on the calf, and a Doppler probe is placed on the posterior tibial artery until an audible signal is appreciated. The cuff is inflated until the signal is lost, indicating the systolic blood pressure. Concurrently, the brachial systolic pressure is recorded.

The ABI is defined as the lower extremity systolic pressure divided by the brachial systolic blood pressure. Thus the systolic pressure at the level of the posterior tibial artery is divided by the systolic pressure in the arm. An ABI of 0.9–1.2 is normal. Values between 0.9 and 0.3 indicate significant disease and are consistent with claudication. Rest pain and tissue loss generally occur with ABIs less than 0.3.

If the chief complaint is extremity swelling, examine the patient for other signs of **venous disease**. The leg should be surveyed for Brawny **edema**, hemosiderin deposits resulting in typical bluish-red discoloration, **dermatoliposclerosis** (hardening and toughening of the skin), loss of hair growth, pulse, or bruit. These signs are localized circumferentially, generally distal calf to the malleolus. While venous stasis ulceration can occur in several locations below the knee, they generally occur above or near the **medial maleolus**. They are generally wet wounds, which sometimes ooze copious quantities of serosanguinous fluid and may bleed profusely with mild trauma. In patients with suspected Deep vein thrombosis (DVT), feel for calf tenderness and attempt to elicit **Homan's sign,** pain with passive flexion of the foot.

In patients suspected of having a **thoracic outlet obstruction (TOS)** document pulse, deep tendon reflexes, strength, edema, pallor, rubor, ROM, and scalene tenderness. Palpate the supraclavicular area of the scalene muscle for tenderness, indicating a symptomatic cervical rib or entrapment. Perform the **elevated arm stress test (EAST)** examination in which the patient is asked to raise their arms over their head in a "stick em up" position and asked to open and close the fists over and over. Patients with TOS may develop claudication within 15 seconds or 2 minutes. Pallor is often observed in arterial TOS and rubor in venous TOS. Perform the **Adson's maneuver** by abducting and elevating the arm and finding a loss of pulse in the radial or ulnar artery, confirming arterial TOS.

■ LABORATORY STUDIES

If there is a suspicion of shock or acute blood loss from a ruptu... order a **CBC** to determine the need for transfusion and a **PT** and **PTT** to asses coagulation and need for reversal. In all patients, order an electrolyte panel to assess the **creatinine** and **BUN**, especially if contrast studies are being considered. Characterize the extent of **hyperlipidemia** by obtaining fasting lipid levels in all patients presenting with chronic problems.

In patients who present with acute occlusion, or symptomatic aneurysms, order a type and cross for possible **transfusion**. Consider obtaining cardiac enzymes to rule out acute coronary disease and myocardial infarction that may be associated or caused by the current peripheral vascular problem. Use the serum **beta naturetic peptide (BNP)** to gauge the amount of acute heart failure present on admission.

■ RADIOGRAPHIC STUDIES

Color flow duplex imaging is performed in the vascular laboratory. It can be used to study the flow of arteries, veins, bypass grafts, and hemodialysis grafts and to diagnose aneurysms, pseudoaneurysms, thrombus, fistulas, lymphoceles, hematomas, and abscesses. It can be used to study aortic, iliac, and lower extremity vessels. Two-dimensional imaging can provide measurements of the vessel. **pulse wave doppler** measures velocity at specific locations. Color is assigned based on the direction of the flow; brightness correlates to velocity.

Arteriography remains the diagnostic gold standard for peripheral vascular disease. Disease should be described as mild, moderate, or severe. The distribution and length of the disease are also characterized, as to whether it is focal or diffuse. Order an arteriogram to include the aorta and peripheral vascular runoff, allowing for diagnosis of inflow as well as outflow pathology. Since most patients will have concurrent renal disease, caution is used with administering IV contrast. **Hydrate** patients well prior to the injection of dye and consider **renal protection** strategies such as sodium bicarbonate, mannitol, or N-acestylcysteine prophylaxis. Patients with prior reactions to the contrast dye should be treated with a short course of **steroids** and premedicated with an antihistamine before the procedure.

Consider using **magnetic resonance angiogram (MRA)** as an alternative if the patient has a severe contrast allergy, renal failure, or a history of cholesterol embolization. It is also an alternative for patients with difficult access. It is 100% sensitive and 98% specific for occlusions. It allows differentiation of short- and long-segment stenosis. If it is timed correctly, it can capture reconstituted tibial runoff vessels distal to severe occlusive disease.

If available, consider **carbon dioxide angiography**, which may be the study of choice for diabetic patients with renal failure and/or severe reaction to contrast dye. It is more water soluble than oxygen and is rapidly eliminated by the lungs. It is safe for studies below the diaphragm but should not be used in the cerebral system, as it causes seizures. It may be used for diagnosis of renovascular hypertension and renal stenosis.

For unstable dissections and large vessel aneurysms, **three-dimensional CT (3-dCT)** is the study of choice. It will differentiate the true and false lumen and determine the origin of communicating branches. Order a 3-dCT to assess whether or not an aortic aneurysm may be treated using endovascular techniques. It will measure the lumen, the neck, the landing areas of the iliac vessel, and the degree of tortuosity of vessels with great accuracy. All of these variables must be assessed prior to ordering the endovascular grafts.

For patients suspected of having TOS, order an **ultrasound duplex** to measure waveforms in the subclavian artery or vein. Measurements are taken at rest and with the arms raised and positioned to see if the vessels are narrowed or occluded. **Cervical MRI** is used to characterize vessel entrapment and bone/soft-tissue anatomy in the area of the thoracic outlet. Consider **electromyography (EMG)** to detect diminished or flat waveforms suggestive of TOS. Also, consider obtaining a **nerve conduction study (NCS)** to diagnose cervical spine disease as well as carpal tunnel syndrome.

■ DIAGNOSTIC PLAN

Assessment of the information provided by the above history, physical examination, and subsequent testing is usually accomplished by a team including interventional radiologists, vascular surgeons, midlevel practitioners, and vascular technicians. The **history** and **physical examination** are used to characterize the clinical problem as arterial occlusion or aneurysm and venous occlusion/insufficiency. If surgical or interventional radiology techniques are required, order and review appropriate **laboratory studies** before proceeding.

Address suspected cardiac or pulmonary compromise by obtaining the necessary **subspecialty consults** with appropriate tests prior to surgery. When peripheral arterial bypass is anticipated, consider a **venous duplex** to survey the vein, as a potential graft should be completed prior to surgery.

Patients who present as hemodynamically unstable, with evidence of known or suspected **aortic aneurysm**, are considered for operative or endovascular intervention without further workup. Those with suspected **arterial occlusion** will have some type of imaging study to make an anatomic diagnosis.

Many medical institutions now combine **diagnostic arteriogram** using contrast dye with minimally invasive intervention including angioplasty, thrombectomy, and stent placement. Many of these interventional suites are fully functional operating rooms, and the patient can be converted quickly to an open procedure.

This spares the patient two anesthesia interventions and two operating times but requires foresight on behalf of the staff so that the patient is properly evaluated preoperatively.

If **venous stasis** or occlusion is suspected, order a **duplex Doppler** examination to diagnose a deep vein thrombosis. Consider a **chest CT** or a **ventilation-perfusion scan** in cases of suspected pulmonary embolism. If an extremity

examination shows severe swelling and cyanosis consistent v
sider performing a venogram with the capability of cathete·
sis. In cases of suspected TOS, start with a chest X-ray (CXR) to ·
ribs and then consider an MRI study to characterize the outlet anato·.

■ DIFFERENTIAL DIAGNOSIS AND TREATMENT

All patients need to be **NPO** and have **IV fluids** in anticipation of the need
for contrast studies and/or operative procedures. Diabetic patients should be
given **sliding scale insulin** with measured blood glucose every 6 hours. Patients
on coumadin who must be anticoagulated should be converted to heparin or
lovenox so that subsequent invasive procedures can be done safely. If lower
extremity cellulitis or infections are apparent or suspected, administer a broad-
spectrum intravenous antibiotic.

Patients with acute arterial occlusions are started immediately on **heparin,** if
not contraindicated. Heparin has a half-life of approximately 90 minutes and
can be reversed with **protamine**. Patients who have a history of **heparin-induced
thrombocytopenia (HIT)** should not be given heparin. HIT is defined as a 50% or
greater drop in baseline platelets with thrombus complications usually 5–10 days
after heparin exposure. These patients should have been tested for HIT antibod-
ies, as thrombocytopenia may be more profound with a subsequent exposure.
They should discontinue heparin and get a PTT. Consider **argatroban** as a substitute to heparin in this population.

Aortoiliac Occlusive Disease

Chronic and acute stenosis and occlusion of the aorta and iliac vessels present
as claudication, although rest pain can occur with acute occlusion. **Surgical procedures** to repair large artery occlusions causing inflow disease include thromboendarterectomy, percutaneous balloon angioplasty and stent placement, and
aortofemoral or bifemoral bypass (Figure 16-1). In cases where the occlusion is
not repairable (nonreconstructable), an axillary to the femoral artery (ax-fem)
bypass is considered. Aortoiliac **endarterectomy** and aortoiliac bypass have an
80% to 95% patency at 5 years. Aortoiliac **angioplasty** and stent placement have
an 80% patency at 5 years. An **ax-fem** procedure offers moderate hemodynamic
improvement and limited long-term patency.

Diet and exercise should be initiated and dyslipidemias treated appropriately.
Statins should be initiated to lower LDL, niacin, and fibrates to increase HDL and
genfibrozil and niacin to decrease triglycerides. Diabetic patients need to achieve
tight **glycemic control** and to be followed by a podiatrist. **Hypertension** should
be treated with appropriate agents, including beta blockers and angiotensin-
converting enzyme inhibitors, when appropriate.

These drugs are also beneficial perioperatively in reducing myocardial ischemia. **Exercise** is a key component in conservative therapy, as it improves
oxygen delivery to the extremities.

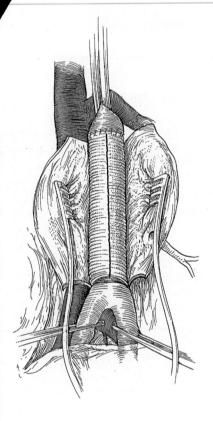

FIGURE 16-1

A Transabdominal Approach with an Interposition Graft to Repair an Abdominal Aortic Aneurysm

Patients undergoing thromboendarterectomy, aortic bypass, and aortofemoral or bifemoral bypass may undergo a retroperitoneal or transabdominal approach. The transabdominal approach is performed through a midline laparotomy and has the disadvantage of possible bowel injury and contamination during the surgery. The retroperitoneal approach is performed through a left flank incision, with patients being positioned on their right side, held by a beanbag. This approach involves dissection into the retroperitoneal space and keeps the intestines out of the surgical field. The left renal artery is the first landmark, and the aorta is dissected above and below the aneurysm.

A heparin dose is given, and 3 minutes later the aorta is clamped. Ideally, the clamp is placed just above the aneurysm, below the renal arteries. If this is not possible, the clamp may need to be above the renal vessels, a so-called suprarenal clamp. Suprarenal clamps will cause a period of renal ischemia, and, thus, patients are at a higher risk of perioperative renal dysfunction. Rarely, the clamp is placed even higher, above the celiac trunk (supraceliac clamp), which can cause a period of mesenteric ischemia. In all cases, the surgeon will record the time that these organs were not perfused as the "clamp time."

After clamping proximally and distally, the aorta is opened, the thrombus and plaque are removed, and small branches are oversewn with 3.0 prolene. A 16–20-mm Dacron graft is sewn end to end to the neck of the proximal aorta, and to the distal aorta with 4.0 or 5.0 prolene. The aneurysm sac is then closed around the graft, and the abdominal wall is closed usually in two layers closing fascia to fascia.

Cases of aortic, occlusive disease often involve the iliac arteries as well as the aorta. The techniques for exposing and clamping the aorta are similar. Typically, a bifurcated graft ("Y" shaped) will be sewn into the aorta proximally and to the iliac vessels distally or, if the iliacs are diseased, to the common femoral arteries.

Occasionally, there is a very short-segment stenosis in the distal aortal or common iliac artery. This may be treated with a thromboendarterectomy via surgical approaches and/or careful removal of the plaques and thrombus without placement of a graft. Alternatively, a short-segment focal stenosis may be treated with percutaneous balloon angioplasty and stent placement. Angioplasty or stent placement should not be used with dissection, occlusion, rupture, or embolization. Stents can be used in the setting of atherosclerotic disease, arteriovenous fistulas, and pseudoaneurysms and to access sites of remote arterial trauma. These are not appropriate for long-segment disease.

Peripheral Occlusive Disease

This includes stenosis and occlusion of limb vessels distal to the external iliac and axillary artery. **Procedures** to improve blood flow through theses areas include intravenous thrombolytic therapy, interventional procedures such as angioplasty, and open operative procedures.

Thrombolysis is an enzymatic dissolution of a clot in vessels too small to remove mechanically. Commonly used agents include tissue plasminogen activator (tPA) and urokinase. It is most frequently performed as a minimally invasive, percutaneous procedure, although it may also be performed during an open procedure. Absolute **contraindications** to thrombolysis include severe ischemia, which has already resulted in paresis or loss of muscle enervation. Other absolute contraindications include recent major trauma or surgery, especially involving the abdomen, chest or brain, pregnancy, or a stroke within the last 3 months. **Complications** of thrombolysis include bleeding and embolization of the partially lysed thrombus. This may be decreased by lysis of the last several centimeters of the thrombus.

Two common **interventional techniques** to clear occlusions and open stenosis are thrombectomy and angioplasty. Mechanical **thrombectomy** involves passing a balloon catheter through the thrombus and retrieving it out of the vessel. It may be performed as a percutaneous procedure or as an open operative procedure. Although effective for removing large quantities of clot from larger vessels, it may cause intimal damage. Percutaneous, transluminal **angioplasty** involves passing a balloon that actively dilates a segment of stenosis. It can be done alone, or in conjunction with placing a stent, to keep the stenosis patent. It is indicated for severe disabling claudication, ischemic rest pain, ulcers, and gangrene. It is contraindicated for embolic lesions, long segments of diffuse disease, or occlusions.

Open procedures to correct outflow disease include endarterectomy and open arterial bypass (Figure 16-2). A **bypass graft** may be combined with endarterectomy, thrombectomy, and angioplasty. The graft that is used for bypass can come from several sources, including greater **saphenous vein** from the ipsilateral or contralateral leg or a synthetic **Gortex** or **dacron** graft. The vein is reversed so that the venous valves do not hinder arterial flow. An anastomosis is the process of attaching a vein to an artery, artery to artery, vein to vein, or graft to vessel. Sutures are placed so that stitches are placed inside to outside on the vein and, then, outside to inside on the artery. Anastomoses are described based on whether these are sewn side to side or end to end.

In cases of failed bypass attempts, or in cases of progressive gangrene of an extremity, amputation becomes necessary. The level of amputation is determined by the extent of the ischemia and other anatomic considerations (Figure 16-3). Amputations for peripheral vascular disease carry a high morbidity and mortality rate related to the almost omnipresent associated cardiac disease in patients with such advanced peripheral vascular disease.

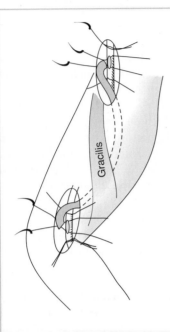

FIGURE 16-2

A Femoral to above Knee Popliteal (Fem-pop) Bypass

Both legs are prepped circumferentially if a vein graft is to be harvested. The feet are fully prepped and wrapped in sterile towels and clipped. Superficial femoral artery disease, which occurs between the femoral profunda junction and either above the knee or below the knee popliteal artery, is generally repaired with a bypass. A typical bypass begins with dissection in the groin and isolation of the femoral artery proximal to the obstruction. The distal target vessel is then dissected and isolated through a separate incision. Often the distal anastomosis is performed first. Intravenous heparin is given, and the vessel is clamped proximally and distally. A vertical arterotomy is made on the artery and the end of the graft is sewn into the side arterotomy made in the native vessel (end to side). The conduit is then tunneled under the skin so that the end is positioned next to the proximal artery site. The proximal artery is clamped, and the proximal anastomosis is performed. Before completing the anastomosis, the artery is flushed with heparinized saline and allowed to spray out, releasing any debris inside the artery. The clamps are all removed and the distal pulse is checked.

Bypass operations are characterized according to which vessels are connected. Common surgeries are the femoral–femoral and femoral–popliteal bypass. A femoral–distal bypass may travel from the femoral artery to a more distal target such as the posterior tibial, anterior tibial, or peroneal artery. Upper extremity bypasses are less common but include subclavian–brachial and brachial–radial bypass.

Mesenteric Ischemia

As vessels of the celiac trunk and superior and inferior mesenteric artery become diseased with atheroscerlosis, progressive stenosis occurs. The hallmark of chronic mesenteric ischemia is generalized **abdominal pain** that occurs after eating (see Chapter 11). Classically, these patients begin to avoid food on account of the pain it causes, so they lose weight and become cachexic.

Acute mesenteric occlusions can be life threatening on account of the subsequent bowel ischemia and necrosis (see Chapter 10). The physical examination reveals severe abdominal pain that is generalized and not worsened by palpation of the abdomen ("pain out of proportion to examination"). Acute ischemia can result from four distinct mechanisms. Mesenteric **thrombosis** occurs when an atherosclerotic plague finally becomes occluded, causing a full obstruction. Mesenteric **embolization** is often from clots in the heart or proximal aorta. Venous **ischemia** occurs with thrombosis of the superior or inferior mesenteric vein. Venous engorgement of the bowel causes sluggish flow and local bowel ischemia. Lastly, **nonocclusive mesenteric ischemia (NOMI)** is a diffuse spasm

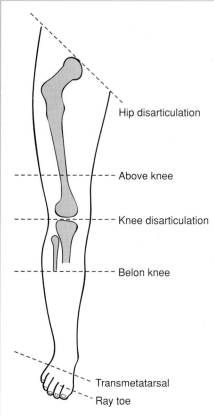

FIGURE 16-3
Various Levels for a Extremity Amputation

Amputation may be necessary to decrease infection, avoid sepsis, and relieve the patient from intense pain. The level of amputation is based on determining what incision is likely to heal, removing all ischemic tissue and decreasing surgical morbidity.

Amputations of the foot include digital amputation, ray, and transmetatarsal procedures. Primary amputation of **digits** 1–5 is dependent on lack of ischemia or cellulitis in the forefoot. Skin flaps may be necessary and may be cut as a circular flap along the base of the digit. The **ray amputation** is required when gangrene or ischemia extends into the metatarsophalangeal joint. Longitudinal incision is made to expose the distal metatarsophalangeal region, and the distal metatarsal is divided proximately. A **transmetatarsal** amputation is possible when gangrene, infection, or tissue loss extends into the forefoot but the plantar tissue is viable. All five mid-metatarsals are divided, and the plantar tissue is cut to allow for a posterior flap. All tendons are removed, and the plantar flap is closed primarily to the dorsal incision.

A **below-the-knee** or transtibial amputation **(BKA)** offers the most promise of rehabilitation and ambulation but may not be the best procedure if a femoral pulse is absent. The tibia is divided 10–15 cm below the knee joint, and the fibula is divided 2 cm proximal to the tibial section. A handsaw or gigli saw can be used to cut the bone, followed by a rongeur and file to even the bone. Several flaps are described, but the concept in all of them is adequate coverage of viable soft tissue over the bone stump. **Through-knee** amputations or disarticulation of the knee joint is a good choice when the patient has no chance of walking but can heal an amputation at this level. The disarticulated knee has a higher ability to bear weight.

Above-the-knee or transfemoral amputations are indicated in patients who are immobile and not expected to walk and when flexion contraction is significant at the level of the knee. The femur is usually divided at 12 cm above the knee or as close to that level as possible, as the longer the femur, the better the possibility of ambulation in patients who are able. An anterior–posterior flap is the most common. An inflow bypass procedure may be necessary prior to the amputation.

Finally, **hip disarticulation** may be necessary when an AKA does not heal or when sepsis or proximal gangrene is present. Incision is made from the anterior superior iliac spine to 2 cm below the pubic tubercle. This creates a flap that will be closed. The femoral head is exposed, and the capsule is incised. The obturator tendons are cut, and the femoral head is removed. Patients requiring this procedure have a poor prognosis.

of mesenteric arteries, which causes decreased blood supply to the bowel. It is associated with digitalis and dopamine use, or it can be idiosyncratic.

In all cases of suspected mesenteric occlusion, make the diagnosis as soon as possible to avoid ongoing bowel ischemia. **CT angiogram** or mesenteric **angiogram** will make the diagnosis. For acute thrombosis or embolization, treatment options include interventional **thrombectomy**/embolectomy with or without angioplasty, and open **mesenteric artery bypass**. For documented venous occlusion, start **heparin** infusion if not contraindicated. NOMI can be treated with intravascular injection of smooth muscle relaxants such as **papaverine**. In all cases, consult with a general surgeon and consider **exploratory laparotomy** as the gold-standard diagnosis for ischemic bowel and the possible need for bowel resection.

■ VENOUS DISEASE

In **venous disease**, deep vein thrombosis (DVT) **occurs in more than** 600,000 patients per year. Of those who are untreated, 50% will develop a pulmonary embolus (PE). PE accounts for 10%–15% of hospital mortality. **DVT** may be isolated or recurrent. Risk factors include previous DVT, period of immobility, extended general anesthesia, age greater than 70 years, adenocarcinoma, cardiac disease, fracture of the pelvis, hip, femur, tibia or fibula as well as soft-tissue injury of the limb, hip and knee replacements, coagulation defects, use of oral contraceptives or estrogen, pregnancy, or obesity. DVT should be suspected with new-onset leg pain, which may be accompanied by edema and erythema.

Patients with long-segment femoral or iliac DVTs are hospitalized and **heparinized**. Patients are treated with an initial heparin bolus, followed by a continuous infusion. The PTT is measured every 6 hours and heparin dose is adjusted until the PTT is >1.5 with the target range of 1.5–2.3. **Coumadin** is started with heparin in patients who are medically stable and who do not require surgical thrombectomy or vena cava insertion. All patients with a DVT should have **serial ultrasound** examinations to determine if proximal propagation of the clot is occurring. Support stockings should be ordered with instructions for moderate walking and daily elevation of the legs. **Vena Cava filters** may be necessary if there are contraindications to anticoagulants, or a PE occurs while anticoagulated. The Greenfield stainless steel or titanium filter or a Simon nitinol filter is inserted under fluoroscopic guidance.

Phlegmasia Cerulean Dolens

Severe ileofemoral venous thrombosis that may involve the vena cava or the calf is evidenced by massive edema, arterial compression, cyanosis, and ischemia. The majority of patients will have full capillary involvement and will develop irreversible venous gangrene involving skin and/or muscle. Physical examination also reveals a painful, **cyanotic leg** with the possibility of blebs and bullae on the skin. Plegmasia is a vascular emergency; thus, diagnosis and treatment must proceed quickly. Use duplex Doppler as a quick noninvasive bedside procedure, which can identify clot and track propagation. Consider a **magnetic resonance venogram (MRV)** or intravenous **venogram** to make the diagnosis.

Administer a **heparin** bolus followed by a continuous infusion. If heparin is contraindicated on account of a history of HIT, consider **danaparoid** or **lepirudin** infusions. If these conservative methods do not decrease the swelling, consider thrombolysis or thrombectomy. **Thrombolysis** is performed via a vein cut down in the foot or alternatively with an interventional procedure that inserts a catheter from the femoral vein into the clot distally. Percutaneous **thrombectomy** can decrease the significant clot burden of an ileofemoral clot and decrease the necessary thrombolysis. Surgical thrombectomy can be performed when a soft-tip venous Fogarty catheter is passed through the thrombus and pulled back to retrieve clot from the vein.

Venous Stasis Disease

Determine the primary contributing factor for the venous stasis. If the deep venous system is intact, and the superficial venous system is incompetent, **vein stripping** is considered after all venous wounds have been healed and do not recur for 6 months. Incompetent perforators or horizontal veins that communicate between the deep and superficial venous systems may be the cause of venous insufficiency ulcers. These can be diagnosed by ultrasound and treated by perforator ligation or venous stripping. History of DVT increases incidence of venous stasis changes, dermatoliposclerosis, and venous stasis ulcers.

Care of venous stasis ulcers follows the tenets of **general wound care** (see Chapter 15). Wash the wounds thoroughly with a clear antibiotic soap, as these patients may be afraid or unable to wash their own leg safely. Provide light debridement by washing the wound with mild-to-moderate pressure, using a surgical sponge or 4 × 4's. Consider the use of **Unna boots**, medicated kerlex materials that are wrapped with mild consistent pressure from the foot to just below the knee and covered with a dry kerlex and ace wrap. Conservative treatment of **support stockings**, elevation, and mild-to-moderate exercise to increase calf muscles and venous return are essential even if none of the venous stasis changes are apparent.

Thoracic Outlet Syndrome

TOS is an intermittent vascular occlusion caused by **compression** of the subclavian artery or vein. The thoracic outlet space is a triangle defined by the first rib at the base, the clavicle at the top, and the anterior and middle scalene muscle as the sides of the triangle. The subclavian vein, subclavian artery, and brachial plexus must pass through the thoracic outlet or over the first rib and under the clavicle to the arm. When any of these structures is compressed by this space either at rest or in provocative positions, TOS may occur. Sports injury, MVA, other trauma, repetitive motion, cervical rib (10%) scar tissue from a previous surgery, anatomically small space, connective tissue, or blood clotting disorder can all cause TOS.

Neurogenic TOS is the most common variant occurring most frequently in young women 20–40 years of age but is beyond the scope of this chapter. **Venous TOS** is the second most common and occurs more commonly in men. Several presentation variants have been described, including Paget–Schrotter syndrome, where there is a sudden swelling, pain, and rubor (red, blue, or purple skin color changes) in the hands or arms, or "effort thrombosis," which occurs during or after physical activity such as swimming or pitching ball. **Arterial TOS** occurs with compression of the subclavian artery and causes pain and weakness in the affected arm. There may be a decreased pulse at the wrist, and the hand may be cold. A supraclavicular pulsatile mass may be present. Overhead activities become very difficult.

For both arterial and venous TOS, obtain a **history of pain** including location and radiation, weakness, paresthesias, edema claudication, ischemia, and necrosis. Patients may be competitive athletes and musicians or may have jobs or hobbies requiring repetitive motions. Treatment is directed at relieving the anatomic obstruction, most often a **cervical rib** or an **impinging scalene muscle**. Surgical approach may be either transaxillary or supraclavicular. In both surgical procedures, the scalene muscle is sectioned and the first rib is removed. If there is a cervical rib present then that may be removed as well.

Takayasu's Arteritis

Takayasu's arteritis can lead to narrowing, **occlusion**, or **aneurysm** formation in the larger vessels such as the aortic arch and the larger branches of the aorta. The arteries to the arms and brain and viscera including the kidneys are most frequently affected, but this disease can also affect the arteries to the legs. Vasculitis is a systemic disease and may also cause a fever, anemia, and general malaise. On physical examination, the blood pressure in both arms may differ significantly, with a systolic difference greater than 30. Order an **MRI** or **CT** with contrast to define the level of disease. Treatment options include prednisone, cyclophosphamide, and methotrexate.

Raynaud's Disease

The hallmark of Raynaud's phenomenon is **vasospasm** of the arterial digits of the fingers and or toes. The digits develop pallor with the lack of blood flow and then turn blue secondary to a lack of oxygen. When the vessels relax, the blood returns, causing a red discoloration. This is usually accompanied by pain, throbbing, and numbness. These attacks may last from a few minutes to an hour. Secondary causes include **repetitive activity** such as playing the piano, rheumatoid arthritis, Sjogren's disease, thyroid disease, pulmonary hypertension, nicotine exposure, ergotamine, some OTC cold medications, oral contraceptives, and beta blockers, and previous trauma or frostbite treatment includes treating or changing the environment, stress or underlying disease, medications, and digital nerve blocks. Patients must avoid the cold, dress warmly, and move to a warm climate if symptoms are severe. **Analgesics** rarely help the pain. **Calcium channel blockers** such as nifedipine, amlodipine, or diltiazem may be prescribed. **Alpha blockers** such as prazosin or doxazosin may be effective. **Nitroglycerin** paste may be rubbed on the digits to vasodilate.

Buerger's Disease

Thromboangiitis obliterans is a small vessel disease associated with heavy smoking. The distal arterial vessels in the upper and lower extremities are affected. The proximal arteries in the extremities are usually normal. Lymphocytes are increased in number around the distal arteries, and a dense fibrous reaction occurs. The reaction is thought to be a localized response to the arsenic in smoke. This vascular disease in not amenable to bypass surgery and 20%–30% of patients will have an amputation of distal extremities within 10 years of diagnosis. Consider **calcium channel blockers** and pain control for treatment. In some cases, consider **lumbar sympathectomy** to decrease symptoms. Intra-arterial thrombolytic therapy may be helpful but is not widely used. These patients must be aggressively encouraged to quit smoking.

Selected Readings

Ernst CB, Stanley JC. *Current Therapy in Vascular Surgery*. St. Louis: Mosby; 1995.

Rutherford RB. *Atlas of Vascular Surgery*. Philadelphia: W.B. Saunders; 1993.

17

Neurologic Disturbances

Judy Nunes, PA-C ■ *Kenneth Vives, MD*

Key Points

■ Neurologic disturbances are distinguished from a mental status change in that they are focal neurologic deficits caused by a cerebral vascular event.

■ Stroke is the third most common cause of death in the United States and has a mortality rate of approximately 15%–30%.

■ Approximately 80% of all strokes are from a "low flow" state or thromboembolic event, 20% are hemorrhagic, including subarachnoid hemorrhage (SAH) and intraparenchymal hemorrhage.

■ There is a need for rapid diagnosis, determination of etiology, consideration of therapeutic options, and secondary prevention in the management of patients with stroke/transient ischemic attack (TIA).

■ Subarachnoid hemorrhage (SAH) without history of trauma causes approximately 5% of all strokes and affects 30,000 individuals per year in the United States. Approximately 80% of spontaneous SAH is due to a ruptured intracranial aneurysm.

■ Patients with a brain mass commonly present with headache, new-onset seizure, and behavioral changes.

■ The most common brain tumors in adults include meningioma, glioblastoma, and astrocytoma. Treatment includes a combined approach with surgery and radiotherapy.

■ HISTORY

Neurologic disturbances can be caused by either a cerebral vascular event or a brain mass. The most common presenting symptoms of **cerebral vascular events** are an acute onset of headache, unilateral weakness, or focal disturbances of speech and vision. Patients with a **brain mass** will complain of chronic headache, new-onset seizure, changes in behavior, or a progressive neurologic deficit. Headaches associated with increased intercerebral pressure from masses are typically generalized, worse in the morning, and associated with vomiting. Thus, the time, course, and severity of the initial symptoms are clues to the ultimate diagnosis.

Determine from the history of the present illness clues to the ultimate diagnosis. The symptoms of subarachnoid hemorrhage (SAH) usually have an abrupt onset and vary from headache to a comatose state. They are largely dependent on the extent, severity, and location of the hemorrhage. The typical headache is severe and of sudden onset, described as "worst headache of my life." This is thought to represent a sentinel hemorrhage and may improve before the patient seeks medical attention. Patients may also present in extremis with a history of becoming unresponsive after an initial complaint of severe headache and may even suffer sudden death as a result of massive SAH. Assess for associated symptoms such as nausea, emesis, photophobia, stiff neck, and loss of consciousness. Diplopia owing to cranial nerve deficits and low back pain owing to meningeal irritation may also occur. It is not uncommon that the onset of symptoms follows a period of strenuous activity, coughing, or straining.

A transient ischemic attack (TIA) is a sudden-onset neurologic deficit of less than 24 hours duration (usually minutes). Thought to be a "warning" of imminent stroke, the attacks often cause transient hemiplegia or speech changes. Crescendo TIAs are defined as more than two attacks within 24 hours and dictate emergent evaluation.

A **cerebrovascular accident** (CVA), or "stroke," is a syndrome characterized by the acute onset of a neurologic deficit that persists for at least 24 hours, reflects focal involvement of the CNS, and is a result of blood flow disturbance. Disruption in cerebral blood flow causes ischemia, which may be due to systemic hypotension (shock and MI), focal ischemia/infarct caused by thromboembolic phenomenon (cerebral vessels or cardiac in origin), intraparenchymal hemorrhage (long-standing hypertension, trauma, vasculitis, and amyloid angiopathy), and SAH.

Neurologic deficits depend on the vascular territories that the affected artery supplies. Thus, the clinical presentation can vary greatly, although the mechanism of blood flow disturbance is similar in most cases. **Amarosis fugax** is a phenomenon of transient monocular blindness owing to occlusion of central retinal artery (branch of ophthalmic and internal carotid artery). **Hemiplegia** and sensory loss are the most common presentation of a hemicerebral defect in the carotid distribution. **Aphasia** occurs if the speech center is involved. Cranial nerve deficit, cerebellar dysfunction, gait disturbance, dysarthria, and cortical blindness are all signs and symptoms of disturbances in the basilar or posterior circulation of the brain. Interview the family to obtain history of **odd behavior** or subtle changes in personalities that are often seen with the progression of brain tumors. Suspect a brain mass in any older patient who has a new-onset seizure.

Assess for risk factors for stroke, including a **family history** of stroke, diabetes mellitus, hypertension, tobacco smoking, hypercholesterolemia, atrial fibrillation, recent MI, hypercoagulable states, alcohol abuse, and use of oral contraceptives. Additional risks for hemorrhagic stroke include long-standing hypertension and amyloid angiopathy.

■ PHYSICAL EXAMINATION

The goal of the examination of a patient who presents with suspected cerebral ischemia is to gain information about the size, location, and etiology of the event. Focus is on a complete neurologic and cardiovascular examination. Cardiopulmonary status is quickly assessed to determine the adequacy of the airway, breathing, and circulation. A decreased mental status is not typical of isolated focal CVA and may indicate extensive hemisphere dysfunction, brainstem involvement of reticular activating system, or postictal state.

Neurologic evaluation includes a complete motor, sensory, coordination, reflex, cranial nerve, and mental status examination. Inspect the face for symmetry or presence of facial drop, slurred speech, or **dysarthria**. The pupil examination is revealing in certain instances of frontal ischemia or seizure activity. Expect a **frontal eye gaze** to the side of the lesion in a CVA or away from the focus of seizure activity. Include a fundoscopic examination to evaluate for **papilledema** or evidence of retinal artery occlusion. Unequal size and reactivity of the pupils may be evidence for a mass lesion compressing the third nerve such as in large intraparenchymal bleeding. **Subhyaloid hemorrhage** (ocular) is associated with SAH.

Acute stroke patients presenting with **hemiplegia** will exhibit weakness with or without sensory deficits. Although CVAs are an upper motor neuron disease, **tendon reflexes** are decreases in the acute phase, and patients will have down going toes on examination. Recall that right-sided cerebral lesions will result in left-sided weakness because of the crossing of motor fibers in the brainstem.

Nuchal rigidity is pathogenomic for SAH. Patients with SAH may demonstrate Kernig and Brudzinski signs. Typical focal neurologic deficits include **cranial nerve palsies** (oculomotor with resultant ptosis and anisocoria) and hemiparesis. Massive SAH may result in a comatose state, largely owing to intraparenchymal clot, hydrocephalus, ischemia, seizures, or elevated intracranial pressure.

■ LABORATORY STUDIES

Order a **CBC** to determine the white blood cell count to screen for possible infection and to rule on thrombocytopenia as a possible cause for cerebral bleeding. Hemorrhagic strokes, despite the severity, do not contain enough blood to decrease the red cell count appreciably. If anemia is present, other sources of blood loss must be sought. The **PT** is checked on all patients with a history of coumadin or heparin use and in patients with liver dysfunction.

CSF studies from lumbar puncture in patients with SAH often reveal an RBC count >100,000 with elevated protein, normal or decreased glucose, and xanthrochromia. A "traumatic tap" must be ruled out by comparing cell counts in tubes one and four to look for "clearing" of RBCs.

If a brain mass is suspected, consider obtaining **tumor markers**, including serum alpha-fetoprotein, human chorionic gonadotropin, and carcinoembryonic antigen, which can be elevated in neuroectodermal tumors. For suspected pituitary tumors, guide the neuroendocrine workup by the presenting symptoms, such as obtaining an ACTH level in patients presenting with Cushing's disease.

■ RADIOGRAPHIC STUIDIES

The immediate test of choice in patients with acute neurologic disturbances is a noncontrast **Head CT** (HCT). This will demonstrate an extra-axial bleed such as a subdural or epidural hemorrhage with great sensitivity. It will also diagnose SAH in >90% of cases. Patients with a negative HCT in whom there is a high clinical suspicion of SAH should undergo **lumbar puncture** to rule out the diagnosis.

In patients with CVA, the HCT is less sensitive acutely, since it may take up to 6 hours for ischemic changes to become evident on scan. In addition, HCT has limited visualization of posterior fossa and thus can miss some posterior strokes. In these cases, **magnetic resonance imaging** (MRI) of the brain with diffusion-weighted imaging (DWI) can be used to demonstrate early ischemic changes, evaluate the dural sinuses if concerned for thrombosis, and delineate critical lesions in the carotid, vertebral, and cerebral circulation.

In patients suspected to have a brain tumor, consider a head CT without and with IV contrast. The contrast study will highlight areas of swelling and possible ischemia associated with the mass. A MRI is also considered to differentiate types of tumor masses.

Consider an **EKG** in patients with SAH, since 50% of patients will have abnormal findings such as T-wave inversion, ST elevation or depression, and QT prolongation. A surge in catecholamine levels and sympathetic tone is the suspected mechanism for cardiac dysfunction. Cardiac enzymes are also frequently elevated.

■ DIAGNOSTIC PLAN

The **neurologic examination** is the first step in the diagnostic workup to establish etiology, and one should begin treatment aimed at maximizing recovery and preventing recurrence. **Cerebrovascular imaging** is used to confirm the diagnosis made on physical examination and determine the exact lesion causing the ischemia or hemorrhage. The most commonly used modalities are CT angiography, four-vessel conventional angiography, or magnetic resonance angiogram (MRA).

Both CT angiogram and conventional angiograms require IV contrast that is nephrotoxic. All patients undergoing these procedures need to have their renal function assessed with a serum creatinine and BUN. If elevated, consider mucomyst or sodium bicarbonate for renal protection. **CT angiogram** is often readily available and noninvasive and, thus, usually the first choice in determining vascular lesions such as aneurysms. **Conventional angiography** has the potential to be therapeutic as well as diagnostic, with the ability to deploy stents for large artery stenosis and embolization of bleeding sources such as aneurysms (Figure 17-1).

MRI/MRA with DWI can be used to evaluate for vascular lesions, define distribution of ischemia, and determine large artery stenosis such as in the carotid artery. The technology is not as readily available in all centers, and there is a small risk of nephrogenic systemic fibrosis with MR gadolinium (contrast).

To determine the site of embolization to the cerebral vessels, consider **duplex carotid ultrasonography** of the carotids to assess both physiologic (flow/velocity) and anatomic (plaque) characterizations. Ultrasound has a sensitivity and specificity of greater than 90%. Use cardiac **echocardiography** to assess valvular structures, aorta, and cardiac chambers for sources of emboli in thromboembolic stroke.

■ DIFFERENTIAL DIAGNOSIS AND TREATMENT

SAH from Ruptured Intracranial Aneurysm

A saccular or berry aneurysm is an out-pouching of an artery that is typically located at a branching point in the **circle of Willis** (Figure 17-1). Eighty-five percent of aneurysms occur in the anterior circulation and 15% in the posterior circulation. Major concerns of post-SAH are re-rupture of aneurysm (greatest risk within 24 hours of the hemorrhage), hydrocephalus (initially obstructive and later communicating), vasospasm with resulting neurologic deficit owing to ischemia and/or infarct, hyponatremia owing to cerebral salt wasting (brain natriuretic peptide release) or SIADH, and seizures (Figure 17-2).

Treatment goals are to stabilize the patient, exclude the aneurysm, and control complications. After providing basic life support for airway control and breathing support, treat hypertension with intravenous agents to control systolic blood pressure between 120 and 160. If continuous vasoactive medications are required, consider placing a radial arterial line for continuous blood pressure monitoring. Consider decompression of hydrocephalus caused by clotting of the third ventricle with **ventriculostomy**. Consider prophylaxis for seizures, vasospasm, and GI bleeding.

In the subacute phase, the main goal is to prevent rebleed by excluding aneurysm from circulation, while preserving parent vessel. The pertinent decision is whether the aneurysm will be secured by endovascular **coil embolization** or operative clipping. After the aneurysm is excluded, care involves providing the most favorable environment for maximal recovery. This includes recognizing and treating hyponatremia and vasospasm. Techniques for vasospasm control include head-up positioning and "**triple H**" **therapy**, hypertension, hemodilution,

CEREBRAL ANGIOGRAM AND EMBOLIZATION FOR ANEURYSMS

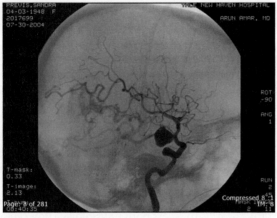

A

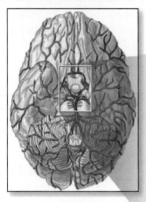

Bottom view of brain
and major arteries
of the brain

B

Berry aneurysm on the
anterior communicating
artery of the brain

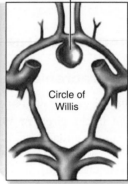

Circle of
Willis

FIGURE 17-1
A Cerebral Angiogram Showing an Aneurysm (A), and a View of the Circle of Willis from the Under Surface of the Brain

Using aseptic technique, and under fluoroscopic guidance, a femoral arterial puncture is performed using a 4 French catheter. A 6 French short sheath is inserted into the common femoral artery, and a 6 French guiding catheter is placed into the left internal carotid artery. A microcatheter is then advanced over a microwire. A continuous heparinized flush is used throughout the procedure in order to minimize thromboembolic events. Careful superselective angiography is performed to define the cerebral vascular anatomy of the intracranial circulation, and the aneurysm is identified (C). With the guiding catheter within the left internal carotid, a microcatheter is placed coaxially over a soft-tip wire in order to access the aneurysm. A GDC platinum coil is placed into the aneurysm forming the initial coil basket. Control angiography is performed, and the coil position is evaluated. If satisfactory, the coil is electrolytically detached. Additional platinum coil is placed into the initial coil basket, and control angiography is performed to assess patency. Once the aneurysm is occluded, angiography is again performed to ascertain obliteration and patency of parent vessels. The guiding catheter is withdrawn, and a 6 French angioseal device is used for hemostasis at the groin puncture site after inspection of the vasculature.

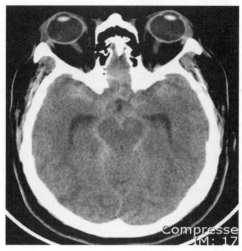

FIGURE 17-2
A Head CT Showing a Subarachnoid Hemorrhage

and hypervolemia. Patients with long-term CSF drainage need may be considered for permanent ventriculoperitoneal shunt.

SAH from Arteriovenous Malformation

Arteriovenous malformations (AVMs) account for less than 5% of all cases of SAH. They consist of a cluster of dilated abnormal blood vessels, which include artery–vein connections without an intervening capillary bed. Most common symptoms are caused by intracranial hemorrhage, although seizures and headache are also common presentations. The risk of rebleeding is thought to be 2%–4% per year. Risk factors for hemorrhage include deep venous drainage, small size, single draining vein, high-pressure feeding artery, male gender, and a diffuse nidus. Definitive **treatment** requires complete obliteration of the lesion by embolization, surgical resection, radiosurgery, or combination therapies.

Spontaneous SAH

SAH without identifiable lesion (negative neuroimaging studies—CT angiogram, conventional angiogram, and MR angiogram) accounts for approximately 10% of all cases of SAH. The typical pattern of hemorrhage is perimesencephalic in location and thought to be of venous origin. Treatment is similar to other forms of SAH.

Transient Ischemic Attack

TIAs are considered "prestroke" phenomena and thus prompt a full evaluation for a correctable cause. Patients should be evaluated for structural lesion with **imaging** such as carotid duplex ultrasound, MRA, or CTA. If significant carotid stenosis is identified, start **antiplatelet therapy** with aspirin (ASA) and consult a surgeon or interventionalist to consider carotid **endarterectomy** or stenting (Figure 17-3). If no lesion identified, consider antiplatelet therapy with ASA or ASA and Plavix. If the patient has underlying atrial fibrillation, dilated cardiomyopathy, or evidence of a mural thrombus, consider **anticoagulation** with heparin, with eventual conversion to coumadin. If the patient has a mechanical cardiac valve, anticoagulation is often maintained at a higher INR level.

Patients with **crescendo** TIAs are at higher risk of developing acute CVA. Consider admission and immediate anticoagulation with heparin after an HCT confirms no evidence of cerebral bleed.

Cerebrovascular Accident

The initial management of significant CVA includes admission to intensive care or specialized stroke unit. The first goal is to **optimize ventilation and oxygenation**. Consider continuous oxygen saturation, invasive blood pressure, and central venous pressure monitoring. Use caution with BP control, since 75% of patients with stroke will have transient rise in BP, which returns to normal within 72 hours; perform serial neurologic examinations; and watch for signs of elevated ICP (nausea, emesis, and worsening LOC) caused by worsening edema (peaks 3–5 days later). Consider serial CT scans, as clinical status dictates. If clinical situation deteriorates with signs of high intracerebral pressure, consider **decompressive craniectomy** with expansion duraplasty.

An **ischemic CVA** is also known as a "brain attack." Consider whether the patient is a candidate for **thrombolytic therapy**: (1) ischemic stroke symptom onset is within 3 hours and (2) there are no contraindications of such evidence of intracranial hemorrhage on CT, history of intracranial hemorrhage, uncontrolled hypertension SBP > 185, DBP > 110, known AVM, witnessed seizure at stroke onset, recent MI, GI bleed, or coagulopathy. Thrombolytic therapy with intravenous tissue plasminogen activator (tPA) may be considered in qualified stroke centers by trained personnel. If within 6 hours of symptom onset an acute occlusion is identified, consider intra-arterial thrombolytics (Figure 17-4).

If an ischemic stroke is identified, but there are contraindications to thrombolytics, consider **antiplatelet therapy** with ASA, ASA/dipyridamole, or ASA/Plavix. If an ischemic stroke is associated with chronic atrial fibrillation or valvular disease/prosthesis, then begin anticoagulation with heparin followed by coumadin. If carotid stenosis is identified on imaging studies, consult a surgeon or interventionalist for **carotid endarterectomy** or stenting in 5–8 weeks once neurologic examination has stabilized (Figure 17-3). In all cases of ischemic stroke, manage modifiable risk factors as a means of secondary prevention. This includes managing hypertension, smoking cessation, lipid management (LDL

CAROTID ENDARTERECTOMY

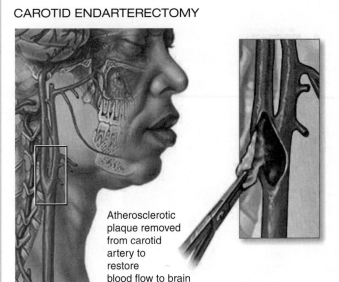

Atherosclerotic plaque removed from carotid artery to restore blood flow to brain

FIGURE 17-3
The Location and Procedure for Performing a Carotid Endarterectomy

Patient is placed supine with head turned 15–20 degrees to the opposite side. An incision is made at the anterior border of the sternocleidomastoid muscle (~8 cm). The platysma is divided, and the dissection continued until the carotid sheath is identified. The sheath is entered proximal to the bifurcation with care, not to manipulate the bifurcation. The internal jugular vein is identified; any other veins (such as facial) are taken to allow adequate mobilization of the internal jugular. The common carotid artery is dissected with careful attention, not to injure the recurrent laryngeal and vagus nerves. Local infiltrate using 1% lidocaine is used in the region of the carotid sinus nerve in order to prevent bradycardia and hypotension. The external carotid artery is isolated, and proximal branches are temporarily occluded. Silastic loops are placed around the common and internal carotids (in the event that a shunt should be necessary). Hypertension is induced by anesthesia, and an IV bolus of 5000 units of heparin is given. The internal (ICA), external (ECA), and the common carotid arteries (CCA) are clamped. An arteriotomy is made using a scalpel and extended (Potts scissors) into the internal carotid to a point beyond the plaque. If EEG is reduced to 50% of the baseline, the SBP is increased to 200. If the EEG does not improve, a silastic shunt is inserted from the common carotid into the internal carotid. Back bleeding is controlled, and blunt dissection is used to separate the plaque from the media. Prolene tacking sutures are placed across the cuff of the intima of the ICA. The field is copiously irrigated with heparinized saline. The arteriotomy closure is performed with Prolene (5-6.0) via a primary closure. The distal portion is closed with a running suture beginning at the proximal end of the incision. The running sutures are tightened, and the proximal and distal sutures are tied together. The shunt, if used, is removed, and the clip is removed from the ECA and CCA, allowing any debris and air to be flushed into the external system. The clip is removed from the ICA, and suture line is inspected. A drain is placed through an inferiorly placed stab wound, and the platysma is reapproximated with 3.0 vicryl sutures. The subcutaneous tissues are closed with vicryl suture, and the skin is closed with staples or Steri-Strips.

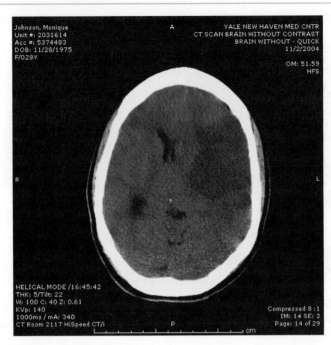

FIGURE 17-4
A Head CT Showing an Ischemic Stroke

target < 100 and HDL > 40) with statin, weight loss, physical exercise, and encouraging moderation in alcohol consumption.

Hemorrhagic CVA is treated in the same manner during the acute period with the increased concern for intracerebral hypertension caused by mass effect (Figure 17-5). Thrombolytics are contraindicated. Consult a neurosurgeon early to consider intracerebral pressure monitoring and possible craniotomy for clot evacuation (Figure 17-6). Serial HCTs will help to determine expansion or secondary bleeding. A hemorrhagic stroke needs to be differentiated from an acute subdural hematoma (Figure 17-7), epidural hematoma (Figure 17-8), and intraparenchymal hematoma (Figure 17-9), all of which are more common in patients with significant trauma.

Fibromuscular Dysplasia

Fibromuscular dysplasia (FMD) selectively affects the carotid and vertebral arteries and is a common cause of extra-cranial carotid stenosis. FMD has been implicated in some carotid dissections and increases one's risk of intracranial aneurysm formation. It is best diagnosed with conventional angiography and treated with antiplatelet therapy (ASA). The location of the lesion (near skull

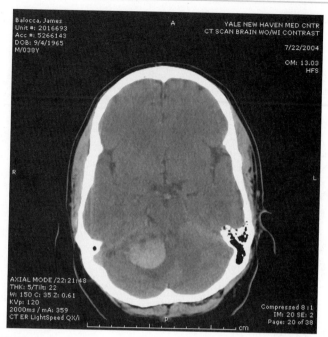

FIGURE 17-5
A Head CT Showing a Hemorrhagic Stroke

base) and pathophysiology (vessels tend to be "friable") present technical challenges for surgical therapy.

Carotid Dissection

Carotid dissection with compromised flow or embolization may occur spontaneously or following blunt trauma. Traumatic lesions usually involve vascular disruption at the level of the second vertebral body. This may result in occlusion, near occlusion, or thromboembolus. Most lesions are treated with full anticoagulation with heparin. If there is a contraindication to heparin, such as with an associated traumatic injury, consider ASA or Plavix-only therapy. Surgery is rarely indicated; however, endovascular stenting is a newer technology and may be considered in some cases.

Brain Tumor

A brain mass is distinguished from intercerebral bleeding and hydrocephalus as a solid lesion within the parenchyma of the brain matter. Make the diagnosis by HCT or MRI. Narrow the differential diagnosis by noting the location and

CRANIOTOMY

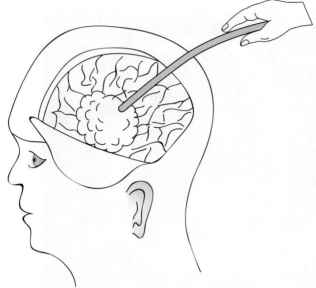

FIGURE 17-6
A View into a Left Temporal Craniotomy During Clot Evacuation

The patient is placed in a supine position on the operating room table; IV access and monitoring equipment including a radial arterial line are placed. The patient is intubated, paralyzed, and maintained under general anesthesia. The patient's head is turned to allow for minimal brain retraction and optimal exposure, and skull fixation is applied. The operative region is shaved in a strip fashion, prepped, drapped, and a curvilinear incision is made. Hemostasis of the scalp is obtained with the use of Raney clips, and the flap (galea, temporalis fascia, and muscle) is reflected anteriorly and secured in place. Multiple burr holes are made in the bone with a power drill, and a bone flap is raised and removed. Hemostasis of the bone is obtained with the use of bone wax, and epidural tacking sutures are placed. The dura is sharply incised in a curvilinear fashion and reflected. The surgical cavity is copiously irrigated, and any bleeding points are coagulated with bipolar cautery. Once hemostasis is certain, papaverine is applied to the region and closing begins with placement of a dural graft. The bone flap is replaced and secured using a mini-plating system. The incision is closed in layers with the temporalis muscle and fascia closed with interrupted vicryl sutures. The galea is closed with interrupted sutures and the skin with staples.

character of the mass on imaging studies. **Glioblastoma multiforme**, which comprises 23% of all brain tumors in adults, are found in the cerebral cortex and often present with signs of increased intracranial pressure on account of their rapid growth. **Meningiomas** account for another 26% of all tumors. They are found adjacent to the dura and can be seen in patients who have had prior radiation therapy for other diseases. **Astrocytomas** are common (13%) slow-growing tumors arising from the cerebral cortex in young adults. Various **neuroendocrine**

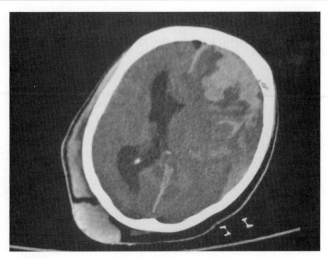

FIGURE 17-7
A Head CT Showing a Subdural Hematoma

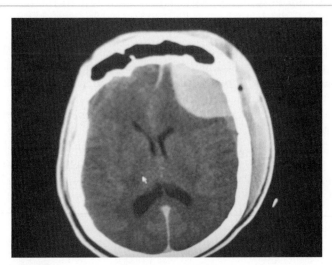

FIGURE 17-8
A Head CT Showing an Epidural Hematoma

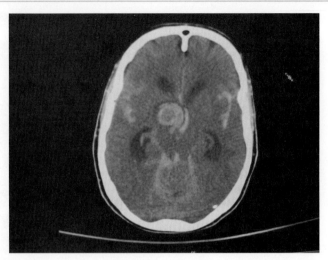

FIGURE 17-9
A Head CT Showing an Intraparanchymal Hematoma

tumors can arise from the pituitary gland, causing a myriad of symptoms depending on the tumor function. A classic pattern of metastatic tumor to the brain is the finding of multiple, widespread lesions, most often found at the gray–white interface.

Direct the medical care toward correcting abnormalities in electrolyte balance and endocrine pathology. Consider steroid therapy in patients with signs of acute increase in intracerebral pressure. In patients with new-onset seizures, begin antiepileptic therapy immediately.

Surgical intervention is considered to accomplish one or more clearly defined goals: biopsy for definitive diagnosis, excision for debulking or cure, excision to relieve symptoms owing to increased ICP, or excision for relief of symptoms related to compression from the mass. Consider **radiation therapy** as an adjunct to surgery for a majority of tumors. **Guided radiation** (radiosurgery) is a newer technique that delivers much localized radiation to involved tissue while sparing radiation to normal brain. Specific technologies include the linear accelerator, gamma knife, and proton beam therapy.

Selected Readings

Mayberg MR, Batjer HH, Dacey R, et al. Guidelines for the management of SAH: A statement for healthcare professionals from Stroke Council of the AHA. *Circulation.* 1994;90:2592–2605.

Greenberg MS, ed.*Handbook of Neurosurgery.* 5th ed. New York: Thieme; 2001.

Molyneux AJ, Kerr RS, Yu LM, et al. International Subarachnoid Aneurysm Trial (ISAT) of neurosurgical clipping versus endovascular coiling in 2143 patients with ruptured intracranial aneurysms: A randomised comparison of effects on survival, dependency, seizures, rebleeding, subgroups, and aneurysm occlusion.*Lancet.* 2005;366:809–817.

Molyneux A, Kerr R, Stratton I, et al. International Subarachnoid Aneurysm Trial (ISAT) of neurosurgical clipping versus endovascular coiling in 2143 patients with ruptured intracranial aneurysms: A randomised trial. *Lancet.* 2002;360:1267–1274.

Ropper AH, Brown RH. *Adams and Victors' Principles of Neurology.* 8th ed. Chapter 34: Cerebrovascular Diseases. McGraw-Hill; 2005.

Samuels MA. *Manual of Neurologic Therapeutics.* 7th ed. Lippincott, Williams and Wilkins; 2004.

18

Masses

Jenna Gates, PA-C, MHS ■ *Jeffrey A. Drebin, MD, PhD*

Key Points

■ Asymptomatic masses are discovered on self-examination, examination by clinicians, and radiographic imaging. A mass can cause symptoms by compression, obstruction, or release of physiologic substances.

■ Radiographic studies, especially ultrasound, computed tomography (CT), and magnetic resonance imaging (MRI), lead to a narrow differential diagnosis in most cases.

■ Fine needle aspiration (FNA) and incisional and excisional biopsies are the most common techniques used to provide a definitive diagnosis of a mass.

■ Brain lesions cause symptoms by increasing intracranial pressure. The most common brain tumor is a meningioma.

■ Thyroid cancer most often presents as a single, painless thyroid nodule that does not take up iodine-131 on scintigraphy.

■ The most prevalent thyroid cancer is papillary type. Papillary cancer has an ability to spread first to local lymph nodes and then widely.

■ Squamous cell carcinomas (SCCs) of the neck most often originate from the oral cavity or salivary glands. SCC that has spread to the neck nodes is treated with primary cancer excision and modified radical neck dissection.

■ The diagnosis of a breast mass is made by FNA, core biopsy, or open biopsy, depending on the clinical situation and location of the mass.

- Women with breast cancer have the option of lumpectomy with axillary node sampling or modified radical mastectomy with similar outcomes. Radiation, chemotherapy, and hormonal therapy are frequently used as adjuncts.

- Pancreatic tumors vary by cell type and malignancy potential. Adenocarcinoma of the pancreas is treated with pancreatic resection.

- All gastric ulcers are to be considered a malignancy until proven otherwise. Definitive diagnosis is made on biopsy.

- Metastatic cancer to the liver is more common than the development of a primary hepatic tumor.

■ MEDICAL HISTORY

The discovery of a mass either on physical examination or during a radiographic study will provoke a search for a definitive diagnosis and often lead to surgical biopsy or excision. If the patient discovers a mass on self-examination, this is often the chief complaint. In others, the **chief complaint** can be varied: hoarseness with neck masses, recurrent pneumonia in lung masses, or abdominal pain with gastrointestinal masses. If a mass is found on examination, first determine when it was noted, changes in size and the time course of that change, and associated symptoms. For masses found on radiographic study, determine the reason for the study, the chief complaint that prompted the study, and the recent history that brought the patient to medical attention.

The character, location, and radiation of abdominal and pelvic pain owing to a mass are highly variable. Pancreatic masses or expanding (or rupturing) aneurysms characteristically cause epigastric pain that radiates to the back. Upper abdominal masses that cause irritation to the diaphragm characteristically cause radiation to the ipsilateral shoulder. Severe, acute abdominal pain may represent peritonitis caused by intraperitoneal hemorrhage from rupture of an ovarian mass. Many masses of the intestines are asymptomatic until they cause obstruction or perforation.

Guide the history of the **present illness** by the location of the mass. For a neck mass, determine the time course of swelling, noting any oral infections or previous thyroid disease. Patients with a breast mass are asked how it was discovered, how frequently self-breast examinations are performed, and whether there is abnormal nipple discharge. In all cases, determine if there has been an associated **weight loss**, anorexia, or constitutional symptoms suggestive of a malignant neoplasm.

Patients with a **family history** of cancer may have an increased risk of developing a malignant mass. In patients with colon or pancreatic cancer, there is the need for earlier and more frequent screening as well as the need for possible genetic testing and counseling. Conduct a history of recent **travel**, especially in regard to travel outside of the United States or those who have recently emigrated from other regions of the world. Many diseases that cause infection masses, especially involving the lymph nodes, can be contracted outside the United States.

Review the **social history**, as it relates to smoking, alcohol, and drug use. It is thought that smoking may be a risk factor for developing many types of cancer. Patients with a history of heavy alcohol use are at risk of gastric, esophageal, and liver malignancies. A thorough **medication history** including use of anticoagulants is important for safely scheduling biopsies or surgical procedures that will decrease the risk of bleeding risk as well as spontaneous hemorrhage with hematoma forming a mass. In women, ask about the **menstrual history** and determine if there are abnormal bleeding patterns as seen with some ovarian tumors.

■ PHYSICAL EXAMINATION

Perform both a **generalized examination** and a **directed examination** pertaining to the region that contains the mass. If the mass is palpable, determine its relative **size and position**. Mobile masses are often located in superficial tissues, whereas fixed, immobile masses are often affixed to deep structures. The finding of a **fluctuance** suggests a fluid-filled mass, whereas hard masses are often solid. Observe the overlying area for **skin changes**. Erythema and warmth suggest an infection, whereas skin retraction, such as peau d'orange on the breast, suggests invasive cancer.

Auscultate and percuss the **chest** in cases of a pulmonary mass to determine if there is consolidated lung or the presence of an effusion. Palpate the **abdomen** for characteristics of the mass including size, texture (hard, pulsatile, fluctuant, soft, etc.), region of the abdomen involved, tenderness, and fixation to underlying structures. Palpable, pulsatile mass above or around the umbilicus is of concern for an abdominal aneurysm. An enlarged, palpable, nontender liver mass may represent hepatocellular carcinoma (HCC). Epigastric or right upper quadrant tenderness or fullness may be the result of cystic or solid lesions in the pancreas or liver. Native or incisional **hernias** may present as abdominal wall masses and differentiated by their location and sudden onset of symptoms.

Ascites is present in patients with liver mass such as metastases or primary HCC, as well as in some women with gynecological malignancies. In patients with pelvic pain or with a suspicion of a pelvic mass, perform a **gynecologic examination** with a bimanual examination to feel for masses of the uterus and adnexa. Obtain cultures that may lead to the diagnosis of PID or tubo-ovarian abscess.

On the general examination, palpate all areas for evidence of lymphadenopathy. Generalized lymph node enlargement is seen with systemic diseases such as HIV and tuberculosis, whereas localized lymphadenopathy suggests an active infection. Palpate for **Virchow's** node (left supraclavicular node) or **Sister Mary**

Joseph's node (umbilical node), indicating metastatic disease from pancreatic or other gastrointestinal cancer.

■ LABORATORY STUDIES

Order a **complete blood count** (CBC) with differential. Abscesses are generally, but not always, associated with leukocytosis. Anemia may be found in patients with gastrointestinal malignancies or acutely in patients with ruptured aneurysms or retroperitoneal hemorrhage. Consider **liver function tests** (LFTs) in patients with a suspected abdominal mass. Elevated transaminases are seen in patients with liver abscesses, perihepatic inflammatory processes such as acute cholecystitis, and primary or metastatic liver tumors. Elevated alkaline phosphatase is helpful in determining cause or in monitoring cholestasis. It can be elevated in liver disease that obstructs the biliary system (tumor or stone). Elevated serum bilirubin is useful in diagnosing hepatobiliary or pancreatic diseases that cause jaundice.

Obtain **coagulation studies** (PT/PTT/INR) prior to surgical biopsies or operative procedures. Correction with vitamin K or fresh frozen plasma (FFP) may be needed in patients taking anticoagulants or those with previous liver disease.

Elevated serum **amylase** and **lipase** occurs when there is obstruction of the pancreatic duct from stones or tumors, biliary tract disease, or complications from pancreatitis (pseudocyst or abscess). Fluid amylase and lipase are generally high in cystic fluid analysis from FNA of pancreatic pseudocysts and low in cystic tumors.

Consider hormonal assays where indicated. **Alpha-fetoprotein** (AFP) is increased in primary HCC, metastatic cancer of the liver, and germ-cell tumors of the testes or ovaries or may also be slightly elevated in chronic hepatitis. **B-human chorionic gonadotropin** (BHCG) may be elevated in neuroendocrine tumors, trophoblastic tumors, and testicular malignancies. **Carbohydrate antigen** (CA 19-9) is a tumor marker of pancreatic adenocarcinoma and cholangiocarcinoma. The **carcinoembryonic antigen** (CEA) is primarily used to monitor metastatic or recurrent adenocarcinoma of the colon as well as prognosis. The **CA-125** is elevated in some ovarian cancers.

Order **thyroid function tests** (TFT) in patients with a neck mass. Of all the thyroid tests, the thyroid-stimulating hormone level is the most sensitive for distinguishing a hyperfunctioning thyroid gland (TSH suppressed) from a hypofunctioning one (TSH elevated).

■ RADIOGRAPHIC STUDIES

Review a **chest X-ray** (CXR) as a useful screening modality for detecting pulmonary masses and malignant pleural effusions resulting from neoplasms. Consider obtaining a plain **abdominal film** (KUB) to confirm the presence of free air from a perforated gastric, duodenal, or colonic mass. Obtain an **ultrasound** to evaluate solid and fluid-filled abdominal organs and masses. Because the presence of air/gas does not facilitate transmission of ultrasound signal, it is less helpful in evaluating hollow intestinal organs (stomach and bowel) or structures lying behind hollow organs. Vascular invasion of tumor thrombus can be detected on duplex ultrasound.

Order an **abdominal CT** as the most sensitive and specific imaging study in detection of benign or malignant masses in the head, neck, chest, abdomen, and soft tissue. Consider an **MRI** as an alternate to contrast-enhanced CT for detection of masses and to provide special investigations such as MR cholangiopancreatography (MRCP), a noninvasive imaging study, to evaluate the biliary tract or MR angiogram to evaluate vascular involvement by tumors. Consider a **positron emission tomography** (PET) scan to assess spread of malignancy from primary tumor.

Consider other radiographic techniques as needed. **Endoscopic retrograde cholangiography (ERCP)** may be diagnostic and/or therapeutic. Brushings and biopsies of periampullar lesions can be obtained for diagnosis as well as ductal stenting to relieve obstruction. **Endoscopic ultrasound (EUS)** with fine-needle aspiration is used for patients with pancreatic and periampullary masses in assessing tumor character and size as well as vascular involvement. **Upper GI contrast** studies are used to evaluate esophageal and gastric masses, and **lower GI contrast** studies are considered in patients with a suspected colon mass. Although **mammography** is still the standard of care for the evaluation of breast lesions, consider **MRI** of the breast as an alternative.

■ DIAGNOSTIC PLAN

Once a mass is discovered, the two goals of the investigation are to define the anatomy of the mass and to make a pathologic diagnosis. Three-dimensional imaging makes the **anatomic localization** possible for the great majority of masses. MRI is often more sensitive to determine invasion vs. approximation of tumor into surrounding structures.

Once the anatomy is determined, obtain tissue to make a definitive **pathologic diagnosis**. For cystic breast masses, thyroid masses, and some GI tumors, use **FNA** to obtain cells for examination. The FNA is a specialized skill, and therefore only credentialed clinicians should perform the procedure. FNA has the advantage of being a quick, outpatient procedure, which can provide a diagnosis in the majority of samples if the sample is obtained and fixed correctly.

Obtain an **incisional biopsy** to sample tissue in large masses or those in which treatment depends heavily on the pathologic diagnosis. Consider an incisional or percutaneous biopsy in masses of the brain, lung, abdominal cavity, or soft tissue. Masses that involve the breast, soft tissue, and ovary are amendable to **excisional biopsy**, where the entire mass is removed with surrounding tissue. At the time of surgery, consider a **frozen section** where a pathologist immediately examines the specimen to determine that the tumor is contained in the specimen and that the margins are free of tumor.

With the anatomy and pathologic diagnosis completed, determine if a **metastatic disease** workup is indicated. This may require additional imaging and possibly additional biopsies to determine if there is evidence of metastatic spread of malignant tumors. Use the evidence for metastatic disease to help plan the treatment of the primary tumor.

■ DIFFERENTIAL DIAGNOSIS AND TREATMENT

Brain

Masses within the cranial cavity are often found on head CT after complaints of headache or nonspecific neurologic disturbances such as changes in personality and behavior. Occasionally these are noted on scans performed for other reasons, such as after a trauma. The most common tumors include meningioma, glioblastoma, and astrocytoma. Other conditions that can cause a mass are bleeding (contusions and hemorrhagic infarcts) and hydrocephalus. See **Chapter 17** for a full discussion of brain tumors.

Neck

Determine the **location** and the **duration of symptoms** to narrow the diagnosis of a neck mass. Acute onset of a tender mass in the neck is indicative of an infectious or inflammatory process, often involving the lymph nodes or salivary glands. A chronic, enlarging midline mass is seen in thyroid cancer and noncancerous goiter disease. Perform a comprehensive head and neck evaluation including an oral examination. Consider consultation with a head and neck service to perform a **direct laryngoscopy** to examine the pharynx, larynx, and epiglottis if indicated.

Infection
If the history and examination are consistent with an infection, start antibiotic therapy and admit the patient for observation if **airway patency** is a concern. Obtain a **neck CT scan** to identify an abscess that will require surgical drainage. If surgical drainage is performed, direct the antibiotic therapy by culture results. In patients who are not cultured, choose antibiotics that have coverage for anaerobic and mixed flora.

Thyroid Mass
Use the history of the present illness and physical examination to distinguish between a thyroid goiter and a possible thyroid tumor, although this is not always possible. If there is any doubt, all thyroid masses are to be considered tumors until proven otherwise. The most common cause of a goiter worldwide is iodine deficiency, although rarely seen in the United States. The most common cause of goiter in the United States is **Hashimoto's thyroiditis**, an autoimmune disease seen in women. The diagnosis is made by FNA, and treatment includes thyroid hormone replacement.

For a suspicious thyroid mass, obtain an **ultrasound** to define the anatomy. If ultrasound confirms that the mass is in the thyroid, characterize the lesion as solid or cystic. Along with ultrasound, consider using **nuclear scintigraphy** (iodine 131) to determine if the tumor mass takes up tracer ("hot") or does not ("cold"). Multiple "hot" nodules are indicative of goiter, whereas a single "cold" nodule is highly suspicious for cancer.

To make a definitive diagnosis, obtain an **FNA** of the mass. Performing an FNA is a skill and requires specific equipment and technique. Treatment is then guided by the pathologic diagnosis and clinical situation. The most common type of thyroid cancer, **papillary** (85%), is treated with either partial or total thyroidectomy, depending on the size and involvement of lymph nodes (Figure 18-1). Papillary cancer can spread to the nodes and become metastatic; thus, a lymph node dissection is often included in the primary surgery. **Follicular**-type thyroid cancer is often difficult to distinguish from a benign adenoma that is similar histologically on FNA. Thus, often the final diagnosis is not possible until the mass has been removed and examined in permanent section. **Anaplastic** and **medullary** tumors are less common but more aggressive cancers that often invade surrounding tissue. Treatment is complete resection with lymph node dissection and sometimes with a radical neck dissection.

Neck Masses

Neck masses not involving the thyroid include cancers of the salivary glands and oral cavity, lymphoma, metastatic lymph node disease, and a host of congenital cystic structures. The history of a slow-growing, single mass is the most suspicious for a primary neck cancer. Obtain a **neck CT** or MRI to help localize the mass and determine involved structures. Perform an **FNA** for definitive diagnosis. If the FNA shows a malignancy, determine the primary site if possible. This often requires an **examination under anesthesia** (EUA) where a full oral, pharyngeal, esophageal, and tracheal examination can be performed. If a primary cancer is discovered, obtain a biopsy and use three-dimensional images to plan a resection.

If a primary **SCC** is identified, total excision is performed, if possible. If metastatic disease to lymph nodes in the neck are found or suspected, consider a **modified radical neck dissection** (Figure 18-2). Occasionally, a single lymph node with SCC will be found without evidence for a primary lesion on EUA and radiographic workup. In these cases, consider resection of the lymph node with an associated neck dissection. **Radiation therapy** is considered and an adjunct to surgery.

Chest

Masses in the lung or esophagus are the two most common lesions found in the chest. Have a concern for a lung cancer in patients who present with chest pain, cough, or hemoptysis, especially if there is a past history of weight loss and smoking. The most common chief complaint in patients with esophageal masses is difficulty or pain with swallowing, or chronic symptoms of GERD. See **Chapter 12** for a full discussion of lung and esophageal tumors.

THYROID RESECTION

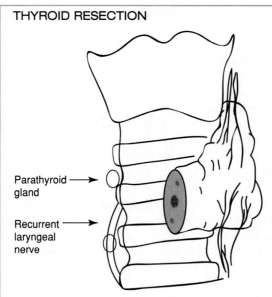

Parathyroid gland

Recurrent laryngeal nerve

FIGURE 18-1
View of the anterior neck with the right thyroid lobe removed

The patient is positioned with a roll or inflatable device behind the upper back to extend the neck. After drape and prep of the neck, a collar-type incision is made along a skin crease of the lower neck. Skin flaps are advanced superiorly and inferiorly to expose the middle neck. The strap muscles are divided in the midline and retracted, exposing the thyroid gland.

The dissection of the thyroid is dependent on identifying, and avoiding injury to, the recurrent laryngeal nerve. The thyroid arteries and veins are found laterally and ligated. The thyroid is reflected away from the recurrent laryngeal nerve, and the parathyroid glands are identified. A partial thyroidectomy involves the removal of half (hemithyroidectomy) of nearly all (subtotal) thyroid tissue. A total thyroidectomy removes all thyroid tissue from both sides. If a partial thyroidectomy is performed, the tissue is removed without an extensive search for all parathyroid glands. During total and subtotal resections, care is taken to leave at least one parathyroid gland in place to allow for normal parathyroid function.

Minimizing complications of thyroid surgery involve avoidance of recurrent laryngeal nerve injury and inadvertent total parathyroid resection. The recurrent laryngeal nerve acts to abduct the vocal cords and thus is important in speech and protecting the airway from aspiration. Recurrent nerve injury results in hoarse voice and difficulty with secretions. Most injuries are not full transactions, but nerve contusions from retraction, and will resolve spontaneously. Subtotal thyroidectomy is often performed over total resection because a small rim of tissue is left on one side to protect the parathyroid glands. Inadvertent total parathyroid resection leads to profound and intractable hypocalcemia.

RADICAL NECK DISSECTION

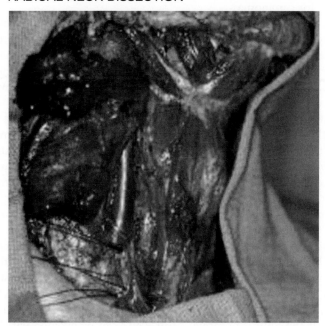

FIGURE 18-2
A view into the right neck during a radical neck dissection

The patient is positioned with the head extended and turned away from the operative field. A curvilinear incision is made from the sternal notch up toward the mastoid process and back toward the lateral clavicle posteriorly. The operative goal is to resect all tissue at or above the level of the sternocleidomastoid muscle (SCM), along with the internal jugular vein and all associated lymphatic tissue. The dissection begins by dissecting the spinal accessory nerve from the insertion of the SCM and transecting the muscle at its insertion. Inferiorly the omohyoid muscle is transected, along with all of the branches of the external jugular vein. As the internal jugular vein and SCM are retracted superiorly, all small vessel and nerve fibers are transected. The lymphatic tissue laterally is kept with the specimen. The resection is complete when the specimen is freed from underneath the spinal accessory nerve. The wound is then closed over Jackson–Pratt drains.

Breast

Most women will present with a breast mass found either on **self-examination** or by routine examination by a clinician. Breast cancer in men is often discovered as a mass near the nipple, which may be associated with nipple discharge. Investigate the **present history** of when the mass was discovered and what routine breast examinations were done in the past. **Pain** is not often associated with a finding of a breast mass but, if present, determines the duration and whether the patient had any previous episodes of pain. Intermittent, painful masses are consistent with fibrocystic disease, while the finding of a first-time, painless mass is more concerning for carcinoma.

Consider radiographic testing to characterize the mass and aid in planning for eventual biopsy. Order an **ultrasound** to see if the lesion is cystic or solid. A cystic lesion is more amendable to using an **FNA** to rule out malignancy than a solid lesion. Order a **mammogram** if not already done to rule out metachronous lesions in the ipsilateral or contralateral breast. Alternatively, consider an **MRI** to provide the same type of information.

For single breast mass, the diagnostic gold standard is **excisional biopsy**. If the mass is deep or otherwise difficult to palpate, needle localization is performed before surgery. Alternatively, consider a **core needle biopsy** where localization and wide biopsy with a large core needle are performed at the same time under radiographic guidance. Breast cancer is staged by **histological type**, size, lymph node involvement, and presence of metastasis. The most common forms are infiltrating ductal carcinoma (75%), followed by invasive lobular (8%) and non-invasive cancer (6%).

Once a diagnosis is made, involve a surgeon who has extensive experience in breast surgery to help with the complex decision making in forming a treatment plan. In most cases, offer **breast-conserving surgery**, which consist of lumpectomy with axillary node dissection (AND). An alternate to a full AND is the **sentinel node biopsy** (SNB), where only a single node is examined for cancer infiltration. If the SNB is negative, a full AND can be avoided with the same local recurrence rate and overall survival. In all cases, radiation therapy is recommended and is the leading reason why some women do not opt for breast-conserving therapy.

In patients who do not qualify, or refuse breast-conserving surgery, offer **modified radical mastectomy** (MRM) (Figure 18-3) for surgical resection. Since MRM removes the entire breast, it can be combined with immediate or subsequent breast reconstruction. For patients who receive either breast-conserving surgery or MRM, consider a course of adjuvant chemotherapy to decrease the recurrence rate. Consider hormonal therapy as another adjunct that is used in advanced disease for some types of tumors.

Abdomen

Pancreatic Mass

Cystic lesions of the pancreas include pseudocysts and cystic neoplasms. **Pancreatic pseudocysts** are lined with inflammatory tissue, communicate with the pancreatic duct, and develop secondary to acute or chronic pancreatitis or, in some cases, blunt abdominal trauma. Pseudocysts form after disruption of the pancreatic duct, causing leakage of pancreatic enzymes forming a fluid collection. Start by offering nonoperative management for uncomplicated, small, asymptomatic pseudocysts. If the patient is symptomatic or the pseudocyst is enlarging, consider one of several drainage procedures. **Percutaneous drainage** can be used in patients who are symptomatic or at high risk and may not be able to tolerate a surgical procedure. **Endoscopic drainage** entails forming a connection between the stomach and cyst via an EGD. **Surgical drainage** may include excision of

MODIFIED RADICAL MASTECTOMY

Sitrone breast tissue

Sitrone

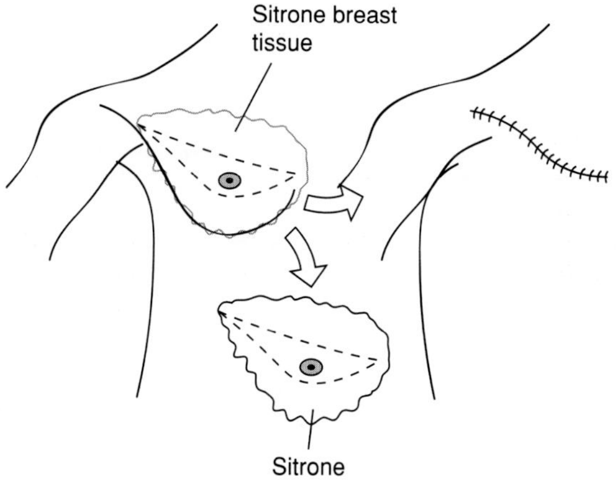

FIGURE 18-3
The extent of breast tissue removal during a modified radical mastectomy

The patient is positioned with the arm extended outward to expose the axilla on the side of surgery. An incision is made, which runs from the axilla, around the nipple to the medial breast margin. Skin flaps are then raised superiorly and inferiorly toward the extent of breast tissue in all areas. The breast tissue is then dissected off the pectoralis fascia en bloc. The dissection is carried into the axilla with resection of all axillary lymph nodes up to the axillary vein. The skin is then reapproximated over Jackson–Pratt drains, and a compression dressing is applied to decrease the collection of serum under the skin incision.

pseudocyst or internal drainage, such as **cystgastrostomy**, which involves opening the cyst and anastomosing the wall to a gastrotomy incision. Biopsy of the cyst wall should always be obtained to rule out malignancy.

Cystic neoplasms can be difficult to distinguish from pseudocysts on imaging. **Serous cystadenomas** are usually benign with low malignant potential, arise from acinar cells, and more often occur in the pancreatic head. **Mucinous cystadenomas** are usually located in the pancreatic body or tail but can be located in the head, are filled with mucin, arise from ductular cells, and can be premalignant or malignant. The treatment of choice is surgical resection and histology because of the potential of malignant mucinous cystadenomas.

Solid pancreatic masses include adenocarcinoma and neuroendocrine tumors. **Adenocarcinoma** of the exocrine pancreas is usually ductal in origin and most often located in the pancreatic head. Patients may present with symptoms of abdominal pain, weight loss, and, often, obstructive jaundice. Adenocarcinoma of the pancreas is an aggressive tumor that often causes symptoms after the disease has advanced to the liver and lymph nodes. Elevated serum tumor markers, especially CA19-9, increase the suspicion for pancreatic cancer. Make the anatomic diagnosis on **imaging studies** such as CT scan and MRI. Consult a gastroenterologist to perform **ERCP** with brushings, or **EUS** with **FNA** to make the pathologic

THE WHIPPLE PROCEDURE

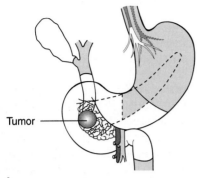
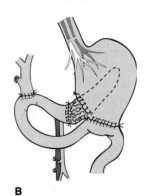

Tumor

A

B

FIGURE 18-4
The extent of excision (A) and final reconstruction (B) during a Whipple procedure

The classic pancreaticoduodenectomy, also referred to as the Whipple procedure, is most often performed for periampullar carcinoma of the pancreas, duodenum, or bile duct. The patient is positioned supine, and either a midline or bilateral subcostal incision is used to access the abdominal cavity. The first part of the operation entails a definitive exploration to determine resectability. Evidence of metastatic disease not seen on preoperative imaging, or invasion of the tumor into structures such as the portal vein, often declares the tumor nonresectable. In these cases, a palliative "double bypass" procedure is considered, which entails a gastroenterostomy and a bile duct diversion. This allows the patient to become free of obstructive symptoms related to the mass.

If a full resection is possible, the surgery proceeds as follows. The duodenum is mobilized, and the common bile duct is transected. Either the distal stomach is transected (classic Whipple) or the duodenum is transected after the pylorus (pyloric sparing). The body of the pancreas is then dissected from the mesenteric vessels just behind, and transected sharply with a knife. The specimen, which now contains the duodenal sweep and pancreatic head, is removed. The structures are then reconnected in one of several ways. One common reconstruction is anastomosing a Rou-en-y limb of jejunum to the pancreatic head, then to the bile duct, and then to the duodenal or gastric stump.

Complications from this procedure include leaks from one or more of the sites of anastomosis. Of all the connections, the one between the jejunum and the pancreatic body is the most prone to leaks and pancreatic fistula. Most cases of pancreatic leak and fistula will resolve spontaneously and rarely need reoperation.

diagnosis. Treatment for pancreatic adenocarcinoma varies, depending on location and stage of disease. Patients who have a mass in the pancreatic head or periampullary region without evidence of metastatic disease are offered pancreaticoduodenectomy for possible cure (Figure 18-4). Patients with unresectable disease may undergo a palliative bypass, which includes a gastrojejunostomy and hepaticojejunostomy to prevent or relieve gastric outlet and biliary obstruction. Total pancreatectomy is sometimes necessary if the tumor continues to be present in cut edge of pancreas and free margins cannot be obtained.

Neuroendocrine tumors of the endocrine pancreas include **insulinomas** and **gastrinomas**. Nonfunctioning neuroendocrine tumors are more common than functioning tumors. Since they are slow-growing tumors and rarely invasive, offer local excision as the best surgical option.

Hepatic Mass

A liver mass is most often found on physical examination or discovered by CT, MRI, or ultrasound. **Hemangiomas, focal nodular hyperplasia**, and **hepatic adenomas** are the most common benign neoplasms of the liver. **Simple cysts** are usually solitary, benign, slow growing, and asymptomatic. **Polycystic liver disease** is congenital and is associated with numerous cysts, small and large in size, scattered throughout both lobes of the liver. Two types of **liver abscesses** are pyogenic and amebic. They can be single, multiple, parasitic, bacterial, or fungal. **Pyogenic abscesses** form secondary to abdominal infections, usually resulting from biliary tract disease (acute cholecystitis or cholangitis) or infections at sites drained by the portal vein (appendicitis, diverticulitis, bowel perforation, or IBD). Include systemic broad-spectrum antibiotic coverage in the treatment because 20%–50% of the abscesses are polymicrobial. Also, include appropriate drainage of the abscess cavity. **Amebic abscesses** are caused by *Entamoeba histolytica*. Obtain a history of travel through, or emigration from, areas affected with endemic amebic disease. Treatment is systemic metronidazole for up to 2 weeks.

Expect **liver metastases** to be more common than primary hepatic carcinoma as a cause of malignant hepatic mass. The most common malignancies to metastasize to the liver are colon, stomach, pancreas, breast, and lung, but other sites of neoplasms should be considered when searching for primary site. Treatment of liver metastases can include surgical resection by either wedge resection or formal **hepatectomy** (Figure 18-5), intraoperative radio frequency ablation, and/or adjuvant chemotherapy. **Primary HCC** is the most common malignant neoplasm originating in the liver. Once diagnosis is made, evaluation for surgical resection should be considered. The extent of hepatectomy, segmental vs. lobectomy, is decided by the size and the location of the mass as well as the presence of increased vascularity or vessel involvement (Figure 18-5). **Cholangiocarcinoma** arises from cells in the bile duct epithelium and has a poor prognosis. Risk factors for malignant bile duct tumors include history of primary sclerosing cholangitis, choledochal cysts, ulcerative colitis, and parasitic infestations such as liver flukes.

Gastric Mass

On account of the distendability of the stomach wall, gastric masses often do not become symptomatic until they become large or have a secondary complication such as bleeding or perforation. The mass is, therefore, often found during CT scan imaging for abdominal pain or during EGD for the suspicion of peptic ulcer disease. A **gastric ulcer** can form a mass that is seen on imaging or during endoscopy (see Chapter 11). Always consider the possibility of

LIVER RESECTION

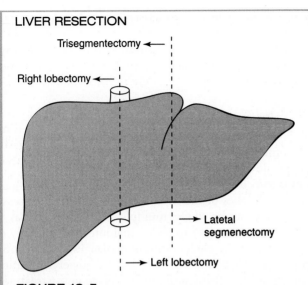

FIGURE 18-5
The lines of resection for different types of liver surgery

In the supine position, the abdomen is entered via a right subcostal incision. The first goal is dissection and control of the structures of the porta hepatitus, including the portal vein, hepatic artery, and common bile duct. Intraoperative ultrasound is used to localize the mass, look for additional masses missed on previous imaging, and delineate the hepatic anatomy in regard to major branch points of the main vessels within the liver parenchyma.

There are several types of hepatic resection, based on the complex internal anatomy of the liver. A **right lobectomy** involves the removal of all tissue supplied by the right hepatic artery and right portal vein. The external dissection is along the Cantlie's line, the anatomic plane between the gallbladder and vena cava. Likewise, resection of hepatic tissue to the left of Cantlie's line constitutes a left **hepatic lobectomy**. If the mass is found at the confluence of the right and left vascular distributions, a **trisegmentectomy** can be performed, which involves the resection of all tissue lateral to the falciform ligament. A **lateral segmentectomy** involves the removal of all tissue to the left of the falciform ligament.

The principles for each resection are similar. Arterial, venous, and bile drainage to the segment to be removed is first ligated, followed by slow and deliberate resection of parenchymal tissue with a bouvie or harmonic scalpel. Care is taken to formally ligate larger vessels. The hepatic drainage from the liver is by way of three hepatic veins, which sit precariously behind the liver, a short distance from the vena cava. Identification and ligation of these veins represent the time of most risk of bleeding, since these vessels can tear easily and are hard to control if damaged.

gastric cancer in any patient found to have a gastric ulcer anywhere in the stomach.

Although several types of **gastric cancer** are described, by far the most prevalent is adenocarcinoma. Find a history of smoking, heavy alcohol use, or previous *H. pylori* infection. In rare cases, a palpable mass is noted on physical examination. Look for chronic anemia and an elevated CEA on laboratory studies. Although ulcers and masses are both seen on upper gastrointestinal **contrast studies** and **abdominal CT**, they are often only distinguishable by histological examination and thus require a biopsy. Make the definitive diagnosis by performing a full-thickness **biopsy** of the mucosa and submucosa during **EGD** or surgery.

Offer surgical resection as the only treatment for cure. Consider a distal **gastrectomy** for smaller lesions without evidence of lymph node metastasis. Tumors in the proximal stomach are resected by performing a proximal or total gastrectomy. Overall prognosis for patients with gastric cancer is poor; thus, attempt to make a diagnosis by early EGD and biopsy in any patient with a history or symptoms associated with the disease.

Colon Mass

Colon cancer may be asymptomatic until the mass causes bleeding, obstruction, or perforation. Colon cancer that presents in one of these ways has a poor prognosis; thus, early detection programs, such as occult blood examination and surveillance colonoscopy, are warranted to detect cancer early. See **Chapter 14** for a full discussion of colon cancer.

Pelvic Mass

This is often of endometrial or ovarian origin. The most common acquired pelvic mass is pregnancy, which is most often suggested by the history and physical examination. Make the diagnosis using pelvic ultrasound and CT scan. The treatment for most ovarian masses is oopherectomy. Masses within the uterus, such as lieomyoma, are treated with either partial resection or total hysterectomy. See **Chapter 21** for a full discussion of pelvic masses.

Extremity

Soft-tissue masses are most often discovered on self-examination or during a clinician's examination. Masses found in the location of lymph nodes are characterized as to whether there is a soft-tissue mass or lymphadenopathy. Care is taken to biopsy soft-tissue masses correctly so as to allow for definitive resection if the biopsy reveals sarcoma. See **Chapter 26** for a full discussion of extremity masses.

Selected Readings

Sitzmann JV. Malignant liver tumors. In: Cameron JL, ed. *Current Surgical Therapy.* 6th ed. New York: Mosby; 1998.

Patino Jose F. Gastric cancer. In: Cameron JL, ed. *Current Surgical Therapy*. 6th ed. New York: Mosby; 1998.

Yeo CJ. Periampular cancer In: Cameron JL, ed. *Current Surgical Therapy*. 6th ed. New York: Mosby; 1998.

Weber T, Schilling T, Buchler MK. Thyroid carcinoma [review]. *Curr Opin Oncol.* 2006;18:30–35.

Kademani D. Oral cancer [review]. *Mayo Clin Proc.* 2007;82:878–887.

19

Anal Pain

Michael David Fejka III, PA-C ∎ *Najjia N. Mahmoud, MD*

Key Points

- Thrombosed external hemorrhoids are a major cause of severe anal pain and discomfort, whereas internal hemorrhoids (above the dentate line) usually cause painless bleeding and may prolapse with defecation.

- Anal fissure is a common cause of anal pain and is diagnosed by bight red blood and knife-like anal pain associated with bowel movements. Inspection of the anal verge with gentle retraction of the gluteal cleft can secure the diagnosis of an anal fissure.

- Fifty percent of anorectal abscesses develop into anorectal fistulas. Fistulas are chronic and associated with irritation and drainage, but abscesses are acute and should be incised and drained. Antibiotics are not typically required to treat abscesses and should not be used as a substitute for proper drainage.

- Pilonidal cysts are more common in men and usually occur between puberty and 40 years of age. Their location high in the gluteal cleft and association with small midline pits or pores differentiate them from anorectal abscesses.

∎ HISTORY

Anal pain can be characterized by a series of pertinent questions directed specifically at the symptoms of the patient. Allow the patient to describe the problem in his or her own words. Questions are asked tactfully in order to build trust while discussing a sensitive and private area of the body. A **chief complaint** of anal pain is differentiated and identified by location (anal or perianal), character (sharp or dull), and duration (constant or intermittent), in addition to exacerbating and relieving factors. It is important to determine if the discomfort is associated with defecation. Symptoms such as **rectal bleeding** or **mucus discharge** are classified by color (bright red or dark), amount, and timing (in reference to defecation) and whether it is associated with pain.

A review of the patient's **bowel habits** enquiring about frequency, consistency, and recent changes is included for completeness. A review of **family history** of colon cancer is an essential component of the patient's medical profile. Although rectal cancers rarely cause pain, low rectal adenocarcinomas and anal canal and margin squamous cell cancers may. These tumors may be confused by the patient and the practitioner alike for more common hemorrhoidal complaints. A careful history and physical examination will clarify the diagnosis. To complete the history, enquire whether the patient has had a flexible sigmoidoscopic or colonoscopic examination and record the results. Many anorectal problems can be diagnosed by history alone and confirmed with a gentle physical examination.

■ PHYSICAL EXAMINATION

The key components to a thorough **anorectal examination** of the perineal region consist of patient positioning, inspection, and digital palpation. Initial findings during this inspection may warrant anoscopy or proctoscopy. To enhance exposure, a movable procedure table allows the examiner to place the patient in the prone **jackknife position**. However, the position involves kneeling and placing head and shoulders in a dependent position and may not be the optimal position for some elderly arthritic or cardiac patients.

The left lateral decubitus or **Sims position** is ideal for patients who are unable to tolerate the prone position or when a movable table is unavailable. To preserve modesty, provide adequate draping and have a chaperone for members of the opposite sex during physical inspection.

Begin **inspection** with careful examination of buttocks and then move to the sacrococcygeal regions. Identify all scars, **skin lesions**, and sinus tracts that could confirm a history of anorectal abscess or pilonidal disease. Note any **skin changes**, excoriations, or painful lumps at the anal verge that can lead to diagnoses such as pruritus ani, thrombosed external hemorrhoids, or abscesses. Continue with gentle retraction of the buttocks to investigate the **perianal skin** for swelling, erythema, soilage, or possible tears in the anoderm at the anal verge (fissure). In many cases, sentinel skin tags or hypertrophied anal papilla can be found adjacent to the anal verge or at the proximal edge of the fissure. Often, white fibers of the internal sphincter are visualized at the base of the fissure, which confirms the diagnosis of chronic anal fissure. Ninety percent of all **anal fissures** are located at the posterior midline. Only 10% of fissures (mostly in women) are located at the anterior midline. An "atypical" fissure is one that is located off the midline and should raise suspicion for Crohn's disease.

Clinical features of **anorectal abscess** are best described by the four cardinal signs of inflammation: rubor, calor, dolor, and tumor (swelling). Many anorectal abscesses do not present with swelling initially because the perirectal fat in the ischiorectal fossa is easily distensible and may hide signs of infection. Induration and/or intense pain around the perianal or perirectal space may lead to a diagnosis of anorectal abscess. Patients may complain of pain with minimal external signs or symptoms. Gentle palpation of the area usually elicits pain in the area of the abscess. Swelling and fluctuance are considered late signs of anorectal abscess, and the drainage of pus usually coincides with a decrease in pain. It is possible to diagnose the cause of anal pain from close inspection and palpation of the perineum. A **digital rectal examination** is then performed to assess for mass lesions and sphincter tone. However, severe complaints of anal pain may preclude inspection, digital rectal examination, or both. In this case, an **examination under anesthesia** (EUA) is mandatory.

Thrombosed external hemorrhoids are often described by patients as "painful," "hard," "grape," or "marble-like" swelling on the anal verge. On physical examination, they are very firm, painful, and typically nonfluctuant and nonerythematous. There may be a small opening or area of necrosis on the overlying skin with clot or bright red blood coming from within.

■ LABORATORY STUDIES

There are few blood or laboratory tests that can aid in the diagnosis of anal pain; however, an elevated white blood cell count may strengthen the suspicion of an underlying anorectal abscess. Anal fissures and thrombosed external hemorrhoids are not associated with any laboratory deviation.

Order a **CBC** in patients with anal pain associated with bleeding to evaluate the hemoglobin and red cell indices. Evidence of chronic anemia should prompt a workup for a gastrointestinal neoplasm after the anal pain is addressed. A **colonoscopy** would be indicated for patients who have not had one recently.

■ RADIOGRAPHIC STUDIES

The diagnosis of anal pain is primarily a clinical diagnosis, and physical examination is by far the most accurate and useful modality. In cases where physical examination either is not helpful or does not adequately account for the patient's symptoms, order a **computed tomography** (CT) to aid in the diagnosis of deep perirectal abscesses or associated abdominal processes such as diverticulitis.

MRI and **endoanal ultrasound** have a role in the evaluation of recurrent or atypical anal fistulas. The evaluation of the course of the tract from the internal to the external opening may help in operative planning. However, there is no indication for these studies in the evaluation of acute perianal or perirectal abscesses.

SURGERY FOR HEMORRHOID DISEASE

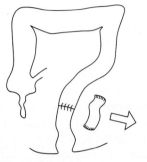

FIGURE 19-1
Internal Hemorrhoids as Viewed During Colonoscopy

All anorectal procedures should be done by practitioners with experience and training. The proximity of the anal sphincter mechanism increases the potential for harm to this structure, resulting in fecal incontinence. While it may be appropriate in many instances to do some of these procedures in the emergency department or office setting, several general requirements must be met. A clean, well-lighted area with access to sterile surgical instruments is essential. Effective pain management may be achieved with local, monitored sedation; regional block; or general anesthesia. If either the facility or the pain management is inadequate, the procedure should be done in the operating room where both these issues are routinely addressed; good sedation and good exposure of the area are ensured; and unexpected situations and findings can be safely managed.

In regard to **thrombosed hemorrhoids,** the benefit of excising or expressing the clot from a thrombosed hemorrhoid is limited to the first 48 hours after presentation. After this time, the clot becomes organized and very difficult to express. With the patient in the left lateral Sims or prone jackknife position, expose the area by taping the buttocks apart and clean the area with an antiseptic solution. Instill 1% lidocaine with epinephrine (approximately 5–7 cc) slowly, directly underneath the thrombosed hemorrhoid. With a sharp, curved scissors or scalpel either excise the hemorrhoid completely or incise over the hemorrhoid and express the clot. Stop bleeding with electrocautery or chemical cautery. There is typically no need to close the defect with sutures unless significant bleeding occurs. Then only absorbable sutures (chromic or vicryl) should be used.

Sigmoidoscopy and colonoscopy may be useful procedures to exclude a neoplasm or Crohn-related diagnosis. In these cases, the ability to biopsy to obtain a tissue diagnosis is important.

■ DIAGNOSTIC PLAN

Careful history taking and physical examination are of paramount importance. There is a limited role for CT scan. If the patient is complaining of anal pain and the office or emergency department physical examination is limited by pain, the patient should be scheduled for an EUA as soon as possible. It is possible that an intersphincteric abscess or abscess in the deep postanal space is present and yet not visible. These are more easily appreciated in the operating room under general or spinal anesthesia and may be incised and drained simultaneously.

■ DIFFERENTIAL DIAGNOSIS AND TREATMENT

Hemorrhoids

Engorged perirectal veins may occur as a result of prolonged immobility, straining with defecation, and certain medical conditions such as liver failure. Hemorrhoids may enlarge from either prolonged straining during defecation or diarrhea and are commonly perceived as enlarged and swollen or more protuberant during late pregnancy, when venous return is impeded by the large gravid uterus. Patients often characterize all anal pain as "hemorrhoids," thus making this problem the most commonly reported condition causing anal pain. However, in reality, hemorrhoidal disease is a far less common cause of pain than a fissure or abscess and cause significant pain only when thrombosed.

The dentate line, located approximately 1.5 cm above the anal verge, separates internal and external hemorrhoids. Increased pressure (chronic obstructive pulmonary disease, late pregnancy, and constipation) and prolonged trauma (diarrhea and hard stools) can cause bright red blood to appear during defecation or between stools secondary to ulceration of the mucosa overlying the hemorrhoidal arteriovenous complexes (see Chapter 14).

Internal Hemorrhoids

These will usually **not cause pain** and can be seen in the right anterolateral, posterolateral, and left lateral positions of the anal canal. They may, as mentioned, prolapse through the anal canal and create hygiene issues. Patients may notice blood on the toilet paper or blood dripping in the water. Chronic bleeding can result in **anemia**. In most cases, the bleeding hemorrhoid will eventually clot without significant hemodynamic consequences but may make hygiene difficult. Internal hemorrhoids are classified by degree of prolapse through the anus and whether or not the hemorrhoid reduces spontaneously or manually (Table 19-1).

Management of **first-degree hemorrhoids** includes altering the diet to bulk and soften the stools, thereby alleviating straining or diarrhea and reducing trauma to the anal canal. Although it is very uncommon for internal first-degree hemorrhoids to be symptomatic, the management of bleeding in these rare cases consists of insoluble fiber therapy (bran, psyllium, etc.) along with plenty of noncaffeinated fluids. There are several treatment options for bleeding **second-degree hemorrhoids** (prolapse with spontaneous reduction), including rubber band ligation, infrared coagulation, and dietary modifications, as outlined. The treatment for **third- and fourth-degree hemorrhoids** include the above treatments and/or surgical hemorrhoidectomy.

TABLE 19-1.
Grading and Management of Internal Hemorrhoids

Grade	Prolapse	Symptoms	Treatment
1	None	Bleeding	High-fiber diet/ constipation management
2	Occurs with BM but reduces spontaneously	Bleeding, mild discomfort	Rubber band ligation High-fiber diet
3	Occurs with BM or exertion but requires manual reduction	Bleeding, discomfort, soiling, pruritus	Rubber band Hemorrhoidectomy
4	Not reducible	Pain, bleeding, thrombosis, massive swelling, discharge	Pain control, bed rest, stool softners

External Hemorrhoids

These present with an acute **painful** lump or swelling at the anal verge and are often associated with pregnancy or intense physical exertion. Thrombosed hemorrhoids may be surgically excised or lanced with expression of the clot with local anesthesia within 48 hours of presentation; however, most cases completely resolve within 2 weeks without any interventions. The nonsurgical treatment involves oral pain medication, stool softeners, sitz baths, and a high-fiber diet.

Anorectal Fissure

A fissure is a small painful tear or defect in the anal mucosa usually in the **posterior midline** but sometimes located anteriorly. Trauma to the area is felt to cause tears that fail to heal because of relatively reduced blood flow to the anal midline. Many patients report that symptoms coincide with large bulky stools or have a history of **constipation**. Chronic diarrhea may also cause traumatic injury to the anal verge. Anal fissures are either acute (less than 6 months in duration) or chronic (present for more than 6 months). Acute fissures often spontaneously heal. These respond quite well to conservative, nonsurgical therapy, as outlined below. Chronic fissures should also be given a trial of medical therapy, but the response rate is significantly worse than that seen with acute fissures. Up to 80% of patients with acute fissures heal with **fiber therapy** alone. One to two tablespoons of insoluble fiber in one to two cups of water daily usually achieve results in approximately 6–8 weeks. Since inadequate hydration is a significant cause of constipation, emphasize increasing water and juice intake along with the fiber.

For fissures that fail to respond to fiber alone, **nitroglycerin ointment** applied to the anal verge twice per day may increase the rate of healing. Patients should be warned, however, that up to 50% of those treated develop a severe, although short-lived, headache. Although the headache responds to acetaminophen and often only occurs for the first 2 weeks of treatment, those prone to migraines may elect to forego this option. Topical **nifedipine** reduces internal sphincter pressure and correlates with decreased pain scores and healing. Nifedipine is an alternative to nitroglycerin and does not cause headache. **Botox** (botulinum) injection is a treatment for chronic fissure that involves an injection of botulinum toxin into the internal sphincter. The toxin causes a temporary paralysis of the internal sphincter that lowers sphincter pressures and lasts approximately 3 months. Although it is generally believed to be quite safe and can be applied in the office setting, it must be very accurately injected into the internal sphincter. This can be difficult and painful, and there are reported cases of temporary incontinence from this treatment. It is also the most costly option.

For those who fail conservative medical management, a **lateral internal sphincterotomy** is associated with a 95% rate of healing with resolution of symptoms in approximately 1–2 weeks (Figure 19-2). The procedure involves careful localization of the internal sphincter followed by division of one-quarter to one-third of the fibers on the lateral aspect of the anal verge. This results in a reduction of resting tone that permits better perfusion and subsequent healing. The procedure should be done by a surgeon in the operating room under local, spinal, or general anesthesia.

■ PERIRECTAL ABSCESS

Perianal abscesses presents with anorectal pain, swelling, and possibly fever. Overlying erythema may signal concomitant cellulites. Perianal abscesses are located at the anal verge. **Ischiorectal abscesses** produce a discrete area of fluctuance, swelling, and tenderness in the gluteal region (Figure 19-3). Patients with **intersphincteric abscess** complain of dull anal pain with a sense of fullness in the rectum and may have purulent discharge with defecation. Many patients have no physical signs during rectal examination other than exquisite pain and need to be examined under anesthesia. **Supralevator abscesses** are rare and result from an upward spread toward the puborectalis muscle or downward from diverticulitis or pelvic inflammatory disease. Symptoms are similar to those of intersphincteric or ischiorectal fossa abscesses, and diagnosis is difficult. The underlying diagnosis may be suspected if the patient has a concomitant-related problem resulting in pelvic sepsis. CT imaging or MRI is needed to clarify the course of the fistula and diagnose any other preexisting problems. In all cases the treatment is abscess drainage (Figure 19-4). The procedure is best performed under general anesthesia so that a good exam of the anal canal and full abscess drainage can be performed.

Anorectal Fistula

Abscesses are acute events causing gradual onset of severe perianal pain. **Fistulas** are chronic conditions that arise from abscesses. Although fistulas drain, close, open again, cause local irritation, and become reinfected, they typically

LATERAL INTERNAL SPHINCTEROTOMY

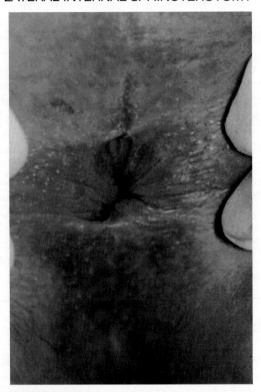

FIGURE 19-2
A Anal Fissure

The theory behind the lateral internal sphincterotomy (LIS) is that fissures set up a cycle of pain where the mucosa is torn by local trauma; the pain this causes makes the internal sphincter spasm, which leads to constipation and the eventually traumatic bowel movements that make the fissure worse. The concept is that relieving the spasm of the internal sphincter by cutting it will break allow easier bowel movements and break the cycle of pain.

This operation is elective and should be done by a general or colorectal surgeon with special training in this procedure. This procedure can be done under local, monitored sedation; regional block; or general anesthesia. The patient is positioned in the prone jackknife position, with the buttocks taped apart and the perineum cleaned with a sterile solution. Examination of the anus is performed to determine location of the fissure. A retractor is used to expose the lateral aspect of the anal canal and feel for the intersphincteric groove—the space between the external and internal anal sphincter. During the "open technique," direct visualization of the internal sphincter and subsequent division of approximately one-quarter to one third of this structure are performed. The "closed technique" refers to the use of a thin scalpel placed submucosally either in the anal canal or intersphincteric groove to divide blindly one-quarter to one third of the internal sphincter. The anal fissure itself is left in situ. Excision or debridement of the fissure may leave a larger, more difficult nonhealing wound and is contraindicated.

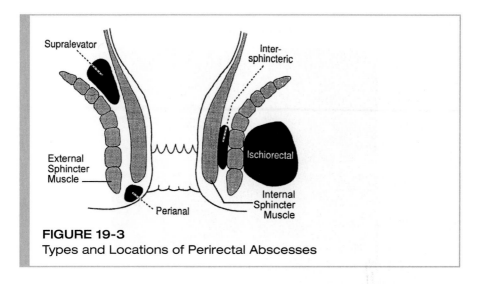

FIGURE 19-3
Types and Locations of Perirectal Abscesses

do not cause pain. Perirectal abscesses are cryptoglandular in origin and begin in the anal glands that empty into the anal crypts. Anal crypts are located at the dentate line, and infection tends to occur in several typical locations. Perianal and intersphincteric abscesses account for the majority of cases, followed by the far less common intersphincteric and supralevator abscesses. Patients who are **immunocompromised** by **diabetes** or chemotherapy are particularly vulnerable to progression and extension of the infection into the surrounding perineal tissues. **Fournier's gangrene** is a life-threatening illness, which usually begins with perirectal suppuration and describes the necrotizing fasciitis and sepsis that follows. Immediate operative drainage of perirectal abscesses in the operating room is essential in these patients to avoid this complication. A "trial" of oral antibiotics has no role in the treatment of perianal abscess in any patient and results in delay of treatment. This maneuver could be life-threatening in the diabetic or immunocompromised.

Pilonidal Cyst

Pilonidal disease involves subcutaneous infection of small midline "pits" or pores in the upper gluteal cleft. Migration of loose body hairs into the pores introduces bacteria that cause abscess formation and pain. The term pilonidal cyst is derived from Latin meaning "nest of hair" and most frequently affects young adults. Pilonidal disease is diagnosed clinically with an acutely inflamed mass overlying the coccyx, which can present as an acute abscess with fluctuance and erythema or develop into a chronic recurrent draining sinus or sinuses.

Acute abscess formation causes a gradual (2–3 days) onset of severe pain, swelling, and induration without a visible sinus tract. A simple incision and drainage are the preferred treatment for any first occurrence. The wound is left open, and covered, but typically not packed. Complete drainage of the infected

PERIRECTAL ABSCESS DRAINAGE

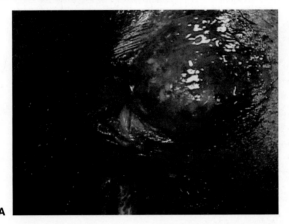

A

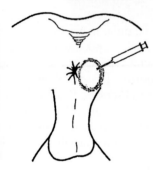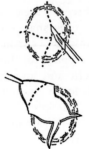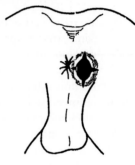

B

FIGURE 19-4

A Perirectal Abscess and Illustration of the Abscess Drainage Procedure

A small easily palpable perianal or ischiorectal fossa abscess in a healthy patient may be drained under local anesthesia in the emergency department or office setting (A). A diabetic or immunocompromised patient, a large complicated abscess, or unexplained anal pain with no external findings needs to be evaluated under anesthesia in the operating room by a surgeon with the appropriate training. Recurrence and continued or progressive sepsis occur most commonly owing to inadequate drainage. The patient is positioned in the lateral Sims or prone jackknife position, with buttocks taped apart if required. After injection with local lidocaine, an incision is made over the area that is most fluctuant until pus is expressed. Open the area with the scalpel adequately enough to allow the passage of a small hemostat clamp. With the clamp gently spread in the cavity, all loculated collections are broken apart. a small tab or plug of tissue from the edge of the incision is carefully excised so that the opening stays open to drain (B). A clean dressing is placed over the area after obtaining hemostasis. There is no need to pack the cavity after drainage or while it heals.

cyst obviates the need for antibiotics. Unfortunately, without excision of the underlying cyst, recurrent disease occurs in approximately 70% of cases.

Recurrent infection or the development of a chronic draining sinus or sinuses merit surgical treatment. **Definitive excision** should be done when the sinus is draining, but not fluctuant or erythematous. Recurrent abscess is treated with repeat incision and drainage. When the incision is healed, a local excision of the cyst with overlying sinus is done electively and can be closed primarily. This procedure should be done in an operating room by an experienced surgeon.

Neglected advanced pilonidal disease or disease that recurs following local excision may require **complex excision** with **advancement flap** or other surgical techniques. A surgical team consisting of a general or colorectal surgeon and a plastic surgeon is sometimes required. Pilonidal disease typically does not require antibiotics except if extensive cellulitis is noted before intervention. There are often high recurrence rates and slow-healing wounds, particularly if the wound is left open following wide local excision.

Selected Readings

Beck DE. *Handbook of Colorectal Surgery*. 2nd ed. New York: Marcel Dekker, 2003.

Fazio VW, Church JM, Delancey CP. *Current Therapy in Colon and Rectal Surgery*. 2nd ed. St. Louis: Mosby, Inc., 2007.

Townsend C. *Sabiston Textbook of Surgery*. 17th ed.

20

Abnormal Uterine Bleeding

Abigail Tripp Berman, AB ■ *Virgen Milagros Figueroa, BS, RPA-C* ■ *Donovan Dixon, MD*

Key Points

- Abnormal uterine bleeding (AUB) includes any disorder in which there is too much or too little bleeding in either a regular or an irregular pattern.

- Dysfunctional uterine bleeding (DUB) is a diagnosis of exclusion, usually secondary to anovulation.

- The most common causes of postmenopausal vaginal bleeding are vaginal/endometrial atrophy and exogenous estrogen use.

- Evaluation of AUB includes a thorough history and physical examination, pregnancy test, CBC, thyroid-stimulating hormone (TSH), prolactin, and follicle-stimulating hormone (FSH), as well as pelvic ultrasound potentially followed by endometrial biopsy.

- In any patient older than 35 years, an endometrial biopsy must be performed to rule out endometrial hyperplasia and cancer, even if another cause of the bleeding has been identified.

- The treatment of DUB is hormonal therapy. In acute hemorrhage in DUB, intravenous estrogen can be used to stop the bleeding.

- AUB treatment is designed for the specific cause and utilizes a mixture of medical and surgical approaches.

■ HISTORY

AUB refers to any departure from the norm in the menstrual cycle. This may be defined as uterine bleeding occurring at unexpected times or of abnormal duration, frequency, or amount. The etiology of AUB can be divided into "known causes" and "dysfunctional causes" of uterine bleeding. AUB must always be differentiated from bleeding originating in the urinary or gastrointestinal tracts.

Ascertain the specific **chief complaint** since patterns of AUB are associated with specific pathologies. The patient's **menstrual history** should include the timing of bleeding, including number of days of flow, the quantity of bleeding with the number of pads/tampons used daily, as well as the impact on daily living. The normal menstrual cycle averages 28 days in length, with a duration average of 4 days and an average blood loss of 40 mL. **Menorrhagia** (prolonged >7 days) or excessive (>80 mL) uterine bleeding occurring at regular intervals is associated with uterine fibroids, adenomyosis, endometrial hyperplasia or polyps, and endometrial or cervical cancer. **Metrorrhagia** is characterized by bleeding that occurs between regular menstrual periods, usually less than or equal to menses, and **menometrorrhagia** is defined as prolonged or excessive bleeding at irregular intervals. Both of these patterns are associated with cervical lesions, endometrial polyps, and carcinoma. In addition, uterine fibroids and adenomyositis (endometrial tissue in the myometrium of the uterus) tend to cause menometrorrhagia but not metrorrhagia. **Polymenorrhea**, which can often be confused with metrorrhagia, is defined as regular periods that occur less than 21 days apart, as seen in cases of anovulation.

Evaluate the history for evidence of a **bleeding disorder**—including a family history as well as asking about any unusual bleeding from gums, easy bruising, and prolonged bleeding from minor cuts. Also probe the history for evidence of a possible **endocrine disorder**. Ask about symptoms of hypothyroidism: weight gain, constipation, hair loss, fatigue, and edema. Also ask about possible symptoms of **hyperprolactinemia** including **galactorrhea**. Lastly, take a full **sexual history** including any methods of contraception. Intrauterine devices (IUD), oral contraceptive pills (OCP), vaginal rings, and topical patches can all be classified as iatrogenic causes of vaginal bleeding.

■ PHYSICAL EXAMINATION

Perform a full **gynecologic examination** to see if there is any gross bleeding. In addition, a **bimanual examination** is performed to palpate any uterine or adnexal masses—although it would not be possible to discriminate among fibroids, adenomyosis, pregnancy, or cancer. Obtain a **pap smear** and **cervical cultures** to rule out cervical cancer and infection, respectively. The urethra is inspected to reveal overt lesions. Perform a digital **rectal examination** or anoscopy with occult blood testing to rule out a gastrointestinal or rectal cause of bleeding.

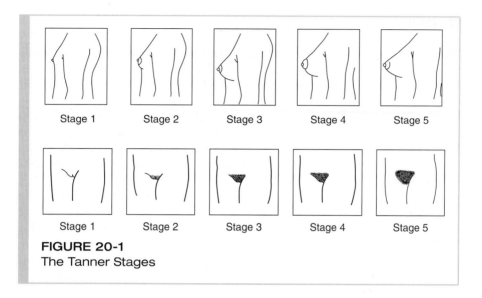

Stage 1   Stage 2   Stage 3   Stage 4   Stage 5

Stage 1   Stage 2   Stage 3   Stage 4   Stage 5

FIGURE 20-1
The Tanner Stages

Determine the **Tanner stage** to note the patient's level of puberty (Figure 20-1). If the patient fails to have a Tanner stage appropriate for age, consider a primary amenorrhea such as Turner's syndrome.

■ LABORATORY STUDIES

Obtain a **pregnancy test** (urine or serum beta-HCG), since the most common cause of AUB during the reproductive years are pregnancy-related disorders, such as abortions, ectopic pregnancies, and trophoblastic disease. In addition, obtain a **CBC** to rule out chronic anemia, which can be seen with recurrent bleeding in an excess of 80 mL/cycle. Consider a **TSH** and **prolactin** level to rule out hypothyroidism or hyperprolactinemia associated with a pituitary prolactinoma. If menopause or premature ovarian failure (PMOF) is suspected, a **serum FSH** is obtained. In addition, if a bleeding disorder is suspected, review **coagulation studies**, such as the platelet count, PT and PTT, and fibrinogen levels.

■ RADIOGRAPHIC STUDIES

Order a **pelvic ultrasound** as the radiographic study of choice. This can confirm the presence of fibroids, polyps, hyperplasia, or masses. If abnormalities are detected, consider **hysterosalpingogram** to further define structural abnormalities. Occasionally, consider an **MRI** to characterize anatomic structures, especially in patients in early pregnancy. If a patient is anovulatory and has menorrhagia, the patient must be evaluated for the presence of uterine lesions by ultrasound, hysterosalpingogram, or **hysteroscopy**.

■ DIAGNOSTIC PLAN

Perform a thorough history and a detailed menstrual history as the most important aspects of making a diagnosis. Direct laboratory studies to rule in or rule out specific conditions that are suggested by the history and physical examination. Ordering a battery of endocrine profiles in every patient is not warranted.

Use the **pelvic ultrasound**, performed with both a transabdominal and a transvaginal approach, to provide quick and accurate anatomic information about structural problems. Once an anatomic abnormality is found, such as an endometrial mass, consider **hysterosalpingogram**, **hysteroscopy**, or abdominal **laparoscopy** to definitively diagnose the anatomy and to obtain biopsies.

Lastly, several procedures can be performed to further aid in diagnosis. An **endometrial biopsy** should be performed in any woman aged 35 years or older to look for endometrial hyperplasia or cancer *even* if another source of bleeding has been identified. In addition, a biopsy should be performed on younger women if they are obese and have oligomenorrhea. Hysteroscopy can also be performed for direct visualization of intrauterine pathology, and this can be combined with dilation and curettage (D&C), which provides tissue.

■ DIFFERENTIAL DIAGNOSIS AND TREATMENT

Endometrial Abnormalities

Symptomatic fibroids (leiomyomas), polyps, hyperplasia, and adenomyosis are the most common causes of AUB. Endometrial **fibroids** can be associated with intermittent lower abdominal pain and larger masses may be palpated on examination. The diagnosis is made on pelvic ultrasound. Consider a course of **OCP** as first-line therapy. Several surgical options can also be considered. **Myomectomy** involves an operative procedure to remove the fibroid from the uterus, leaving the endometrium intact.

Endometrial **hyperplasia** is treated with progestin, which stops endometrial growth and supports and organizes the endometrium so that sloughing is more uniform. If refractory, endometrial hyperplasia can be treated with dilation and curettage (D&C), where the endometrium is scrapped away, or hysterectomy. **Adenomyosis** is an abnormal in-growth of the endometrial layer into the smooth muscle layers of the endometrium. Elicit a history of hypermenorrhea, polymenorrhea, or intermenstrual bleeding in middle-aged women. Consider medical management with progestin or gonadotropin-releasing hormone analogs.

Surgery is considered for endometrial bleeding, which does not respond to medical treatment, for bleeding resulting in hemodynamic instability or for patients who do not desire future fertility and/or have concomitant pelvic disease that is surgically correctible. **Endometrial ablation** destroys the basalis layer of the endometrium using a variety of techniques including laser, cryoablation, hydrothermal ablation, or bipolar mesh ablation. A **hysterectomy** is a curative operation for atypical hyperplasia, endometrial cancer, or bleeding that does not

TOTAL ABDOMINAL HYSTERECTOMY

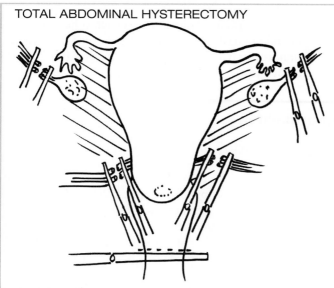

FIGURE 20-2
The hysterectomy procedure showing division of the true ovarian ligament, uterine vessels and vaginal cuff.

With the patient in the supine position, the legs are supported in a modified lithotomy position to allow access to the vagina. The most common incision is the Pfannenstiel where the skin incision is made horizontally along a skin crease below the belt line. Skin flaps are mobilized superiorly and inferiorly and then the fascia is opened vertically in the midline.

The dissection begins with division of the broad ligament and ligation of the uterine arteries and veins. Care is taken during this stage not to injure the ureters, which lie just below the uterine vessels. Dissection continues around the outside of the cervix until the superior portion of the vagina is free on all sides. At this point, if an oopherectomy is to be included in the resection, the ovarian vessels are ligated in the true ovarian ligament. If the ovaries are to be spared, the fallopian tubes on both sides are dissected free from the ovaries.

With the uterus and ovaries being free, the vagina is transected just below the cervix and the specimen is removed. The vaginal cuff is then closed by sutures or a stapling device. The fascia is closed in the midline, and the skin is closed with subcutaneous suture.

respond to less invasive uterus-sparing surgeries (Figure 20-2). Transcervical resection of the endometrium is a new minimally invasive technique, which is sometimes an alternative to hysterectomy.

Endometrial Cancer

Suspect endometrial cancer in any postmenopausal woman who develops vaginal bleeding. Although the peak incidence is in the fifth and sixth decades, the disease is occasionally seen in younger women. The disease progresses from endometrial hyperplasia to atypical hyperplasia to frank cancer; thus, surveillance and diagnosis are possible by performing **endometrial biopsy**.

The treatment of cervical and endometrial cancers requires complex management, including various surgical options, radiation, and chemotherapy. Usually, the surgical treatment for endometrial cancer is a total abdominal hysterectomy and bilateral salpingo-oophorectomy (Figure 20-2). The prognosis is 70%–90% at 5 years for cancers caught early.

Endocrine Abnormalities

Suspect abnormal bleeding secondary to **hypothyroidism** by the history, confirmed by hormone studies. Treatment is with thyroid hormone replacement and long-term regulation of thyroid function. In patients with a known or suspected pituitary **prolactinoma**, offer dopamine agonists such as bromocriptine or surgical removal. **Anovulatory** DUB is treated with hormonal therapy—OCP or cyclic progestin if estrogen is contraindicated. If there is severe, acute bleeding, intravenous estrogen can be given. In patients with significant but not life-threatening bleeding, a high-dose oral estrogen or OCP taper regimen can be started.

Medical management of postmenopausal vaginal and **endometrial atrophy** should be treated with estrogen (oral or cream/ring), which causes rapid growth of endometrium over a denuded or raw epithelial surface.

Postmenopausal Bleeding

Bleeding for more than 12 months after menopause or at irregular intervals while on hormone replacement therapy requires a special consideration. Menopause can be confirmed by measuring the **FSH** with a level more than 30 mIU/mL being diagnostic. The most common cause of postmenopausal bleeding is endometrial and/or vaginal atrophy and exogenous estrogens (accounting for about 30% each). In all cases, have a suspicion for endometrial cancer as well as ovarian cancer, which can secrete estrogen and thus produce endometrial bleeding. Common nongynecologic causes of bleeding in postmenopausal women include GI bleeding from a tumor or rectal bleeding from hemorrhoids, an anal fissure, or a rectal prolapse.

Dysfunctional Uterine Bleeding

DUB is a diagnosis of exclusion when no pathological cause of AUB is identified. The most common mechanism of bleeding in this case is **anovulation**. The ovary has continuous estradiol production without formation of the corpus luteum. This produces progesterone, which leads to a continuously proliferating endometrium that may outgrow the blood supply and necrose. Thus, sloughing of the endometrium occurs in an irregular fashion. Anovulation is common during several periods of a woman's life, such as adolescence, perimenopause, lactation, and pregnancy. Therefore, DUB can occur during these times. There are also pathologic conditions that lead to anovulation and thus DUB. These include hypothyroidism, hyperprolactinemia, hyperandrogenism, and PMOF.

In ovulatory women with dysfunctional bleeding, consider treatment with nonsteroidal anti-inflammatory agents, which inhibit prostaglandin release, which in turn decreases vasodilatation, thus causing less menstrual bleeding.

Selected Readings

Munro MG. Endometrial ablation: Where have we been? Where are we going? [review]. *Clin Obstet Gynecol.* 2006;49(4):736–766.

Osei J, Critchley H. Menorrhagia, mechanisms, and targeted therapies [review]. *Curr Opin Obstet Gynecol.* 2005;17(4):411–418.

Pitkin J. Dysfunctional uterine bleeding [review]. *BMJ.* 2007;334(7603): 1110–1111.

21

Pelvic Pain

Abigail Tripp Berman, AB ■ *Virgen Milagros Figueroa, BS, PA-C* ■ *Donovan D. Dixon, MD*

Key Points

- Primary dysmenorrhea begins shortly after menarche, whereas secondary dysmenorrhea occurs with other pelvic pathology.

- Mittelschmertz represents pain during ovulation, although the exact mechanism is unclear.

- Pelvic inflammatory disease (PID), most often gonorrheal or chlamydial, is suspected in every woman with acute or chronic pelvic pain. The physical examination is only 60% sensitive in making the diagnosis.

- Endometriosis is a common cause of chronic pelvic pain that becomes worse during menstruation. Many patients respond to treatment with danazol or oral contraceptive pills (OCPs).

- Ectopic pregnancy is uncommon but can be life threatening. Pelvic ultrasound may be insensitive to detecting a tubal pregnancy before 5 weeks gestation.

- The most common types of pelvic masses that cause pain are ovarian cysts, ovarian cancer, and uterine fibroids. Pelvic ultrasound is used to distinguish ovarian from uterine masses.

■ HISTORY

Characterize the **chief complaint** as pelvic pain, dysmenorrhea (pain during menstruation), or dyspareunia (painful intercourse). Determine the quality and location of pain, along with associated findings of constitutional symptoms such as nausea and vomiting. Determine the relation to menstruation as well as exacerbating/remitting factors.

Pelvic pain can be characterized as chronic or acute. Chronic pelvic pain is defined as nonspecific pelvic pain for more than 6 months, which may or may not be relieved by analgesics (narcotics and nonsteroidal anti-inflammatory agents [NSAIDs]). In pelvic pain, often the patient is unclear of when symptoms began. In contrast, acute pelvic pain is short in duration (<6 months) and is generally associated with tissue damage appropriate to the degree of symptoms.

The pain of primary **dysmenorrhea** tends to start on the first or second day of menstruation, whereas menstruation actually relieves the pain in endometriosis. In secondary dysmenorrhea, look for a history of scarring or congenital abnormalities of the cervical os that might indicate that the patient has a cervical stenosis. Pelvic pain associated with **dyspareunia** may indicate an infectious or inflammatory condition, such as PID or pelvic adhesions.

Obtain a complete **sexual history**, with attention to determining previous sexually transmitted diseases, number of partners, and any prior sexual abuse. Elicit a social history including work conditions, leisure activities, stressors, marital status, children, and substance abuse problems. In patients with chronic pelvic pain, consider a history of past abdominal surgeries, endometriosis, adenomyosis, or polycystic ovarian disease as risk factors for the development of pelvic adhesions.

Pain associated with **pregnancy** has a unique differential diagnosis. Acute pelvic pain with vaginal bleeding can result from an ectopic pregnancy, miscarriage, placental abruption, or placenta accrete. In women who are newly postpartum, consider endometritis, septic thrombophlebitis, retained products of conception, or pelvic abscess. Determine the last menstrual period (LMP), estimated date of conception (EDC), and therefore the estimated gestational age (EGA) to guide the diagnosis of pregnancy-related conditions.

■ LABORATORY STUDIES

In all reproductive-age women, obtain a urine **beta-HCG** to determine if the patient is pregnant. If an ectopic pregnancy or spontaneous abortion is suspected, obtain serial serum HCG measurements to determine the rate of rise or fall of values. If PID is suspected, obtain a **CBC** for leukocytosis and consider ordering an **erythrocyte sedimentation rate** (ESR) and **C-reactive protein** level to help establish the diagnosis of pelvic infection. During pelvic examination, obtain gonorrhea and chlamydial cultures to confirm the diagnosis. An elevated CA-125 level consistent with an ovarian malignancy.

■ RADIOGRAPHIC STUDIES

Order a **pelvic ultrasound** as a quick, bedside test to examine pelvic structures. The transvaginal approach, although a more uncomfortable test, will provide a greater resolution for adnexal structures and detection of embryonic implantation during ectopic pregnancy. In patients with abdominal pain radiating to the pelvis, order a **CT scan** as the most sensitive and specific study for abdominal anatomy. Alternatively, consider an **MRI** to characterize anatomic structures, especially in patients in early pregnancy. If a patient is anovulatory and has menorrhagia associated with pain, evaluate for the presence of uterine lesions by ultrasound, **hysterosalpingogram**, or **hysteroscopy**.

■ PHYSICAL EXAMINATION

Patients with pelvic pain warrant a full **general physical** examination before attention is placed on the pelvic examination. Perform a detailed abdominal examination with auscultation, percussion, and palpation to determine if there is generalized peritonitis or other evidence of an intra-abdominal catastrophe. The most common causes of frank peritonitis from a pelvic source are PID, ruptured ovarian cyst, ovarian torsion, and ectopic pregnancy.

Perform a full **gynecologic examination** including a **bimanual examination** to palpate any uterine or adnexal masses. Obtain a **pap smear** and **cervical cultures** to rule out cervical cancer and infection, respectively. The urethra is inspected to reveal overt lesions.

■ DIFFERENTIAL DIAGNOSIS AND TREATMENT

Dysmenorrhea

Elicit a history of painful cramping sensations in the lower abdomen just before or during menses. The pain is often accompanied by other symptoms, such as sweating, tachycardia, headaches, nausea, vomiting, diarrhea, and tremulousness. The severity ranges from mild to severe and bedridden. Approximately half of menstruating women experience some form of dysmenorrhea. **Primary dysmenorrhea** begins at or shortly after menarche and is usually not accompanied by pelvic pathology. **Secondary dysmenorrhea** is associated with other pelvic conditions, including endometriosis, fibroids, adenomyosis, PID, and cervical stenosis (see Chapter 20).

Offer **NSAIDs** as treatment for primary dysmenorrhea. NSAIDs have been shown to block the production of the likely destructive prostaglandins. Commonly used NSAIDs include aspirin, ibuprofen, and naproxen; all these agents should be taken 1 day before the anticipated pain. Consider treatment with **OCPs** in primary dysmenorrhea to inhibit ovulation, decreasing endometrial proliferation and prostaglandin production. Often, if patients have been treated long term with OCP, their symptoms will remain quiescent even if the OCP is discontinued.

Recommend **supportive adjuncts** such as massage, heating pads, exercise, acupuncture, and nerve stimulation. Counsel patients that primary dysmenorrhea will decrease in their thirties as well as with pregnancy. **Surgical treatments** including cervical dilation, presacral neurectomy, and hysterectomy are mentioned for historical purposes but are no longer offered as treatment options.

Mittelschmertz

Physiologic causes of pelvic pain include pain associated with ovulation as well as premenstrual or menstrual pain. Mittelschmertz is technically defined as abnormal pain midway between menstrual periods, often related to ovulation. The actual mechanism is not clear, although it may come from peritoneal irritation by the follicular fluid. Typically, it is described as an aching, dull pain at midcycle in one lower quadrant of moderate severity.

The **diagnosis** of Mittelschmertz is suggested by the onset at midcycle, moderate severity, and short duration. The diagnosis of primary dysmenorrheal is one of exclusion, where no organic cause can be identified (it is often mistaken for endometriosis).

Pelvic Infections and Inflammations

PID is a disorder that includes acute infections of the uterus, fallopian tubes, and ovaries, with subsequent scar and adhesion formation that can lead to chronic pain and infertility. Seek a **history** of prior sexually transmitted disease, intrauterine device (IUD) for contraception, or recent unprotected sexual intercourse as known predisposing factors for a new infection. Suspect active PID infection with **cervical motion tenderness** during bimanual examination, although the physical examination is only 60% sensitive in detecting the disease. Make the definitive diagnosis by observing pus from the cervical os during **pelvic examination** or pus in the pelvic cavity during **laparoscopy**.

The most common organisms causing acute PID infection are *Neisseria gonorrhoeae* and *Chlamydia trachomatis*. Consider **antibiotic treatment** in patients with documented or suspected infection. Treatment schemes differ depending on culture results and reliability of the patient to take the appropriate medication.

Previous pelvic surgery, PID, and endometriosis are common causes of **pelvic adhesions**. If pelvic adhesions are found to be the cause of the pain, the definitive treatment is diagnostic laparoscopy (Figure 21-1) with lysis of adhesions.

Endometriosis

Endometriosis is defined by the presence of functioning endometrial tissue in location other than the uterus. The most common sites of involvement are the ovaries, tissue around the uterus, and the peritoneal cavity. Pain is caused when the tissue enlarges in reaction to the normal hormonal regulation of the ovulatory cycle. Over time, adhesions can form in areas of active disease, causing further pain or **infertility.**

Consider the diagnosis in patients who have pelvic pain that is exacerbated during menstruation. Make the definitive diagnosis by **diagnostic laparoscopy** (Figure 21-1). Medical treatment will control symptoms but will not eliminate the condition. Several **hormonal agents** are available to attenuate the ovulatory cycle, such as danazol, progestins, and OCPs. Offer surgical treatment

DIAGNOSTIC LAPAROSCOPY

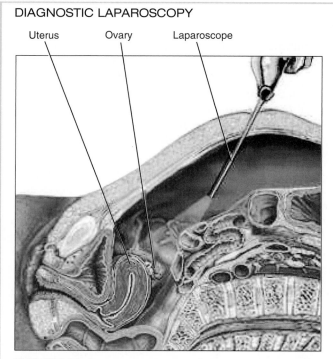

Uterus   Ovary   Laparoscope

FIGURE 21-1
A view into the peritoneum during diagnostic laparoscopy

Patients with cryptic pelvic pain or a newly diagnosed pelvic mass often undergo diagnostic laparoscopy for diagnosis and possible treatment of common pelvic conditions that cause pain. The patient is positioned supine, and the operation begins with an incision around the umbilicus and placement of a large laparoscopic port into the abdominal cavity. The peritoneal is inflated with CO_2, and a camera is placed through the port. Under direct vision, two additional ports are placed in the lower abdomen so that instruments can be introduced into the operative field. The contents of the pelvis and entire abdominal cavity are the inspected. Laparoscopy provides excellent visualization of pelvic structures.

Several therapeutic maneuvers can be performed during laparoscopy. Adhesions causing pain or infertility can be lysed, endometriosis can be cauterized, and tubal abscess can be drained. When the procedure is finished, the ports are taken out under direct vision to assure that there is no bleeding. The periumbilical port is then closed formally with sutures at the fascia, and the skin over each port site is closed.

for patients who have failed medical management of those who have fertility difficulties secondary to the disease. The goal of conservative surgery is to obliterate ectopic endometrial tissue and free adhesions. This can be done typically with laparoscopic surgery. In patients who have failed conservative management, consider total abdominal **hysterectomy** with bilateral salpingo-oopherectomy (see Chapter 20, Figure 20-2). This surgery removes both the most common sites of implants and the hormonal drive that exacerbates disease in the peritoneum or elsewhere.

Ectopic Pregnancy

The vast majority of abnormal implantations of a fertilized egg, leading to an ectopic pregnancy, occur in the **fallopian tube**. With embryonic growth, the tube is stretched, causing pain. Undiagnosed, tubal rupture with life-threatening bleeding may occur. On account of this, have a high index of suspicion for a possible ectopic pregnancy in all premenopausal women with abdominal pain. Order a **beta-HCG** to determine if there is a pregnancy. Obtain a **pelvic ultrasound** as the definitive study to confirm the location of the implantation as in the uterus, or in an ectopic location.

In patients with a very early pregnancy, less than 5 weeks, the diagnosis of ectopic pregnancy is difficult because of the small size of the embryo. In these cases, consider obtaining **serial beta-HCG** levels. In general, the beta-HCG will increase by 66% every 48 hours in an intrauterine pregnancy, but not in an ectopic pregnancy. Patients with a confirmed ectopic pregnancy are offered **surgery** as the definitive treatment to remove the embryo. Other options include the administration of **methotrexate** to induce embryo demise.

Infrequently, patients will present with acute abdominal pain and shock, indicating a **rupture** and free bleeding. Begin resuscitation with fluid and blood products as indicated and arrange for immediate exploratory laparotomy. Often, the only surgical option after tubal rupture is unilateral **salphingectomy**.

Pelvic Mass

Although tumors can form from any structure in the pelvis, in women pelvic masses are most likely ovarian or uterine in nature. The most common benign causes of mass in the pelvis include ovarian cysts (follicular and luteal) uterine fibroids and pregnancy. All masses noted on physical examination or imaging are to be considered a malignancy until proven otherwise. The most common cancer in the pelvis is ovarian carcinoma.

Ovarian Cancer
It can develop from one of the many types of tissue present in the ovary. Obtain a history of pelvic pain and abnormal vaginal bleeding, especially in postmenopausal women. Make the diagnosis of an ovarian mass by **transvaginal ultrasound** or by **abdominal CT**. Definitive diagnosis is made at the time of surgery. If an ovarian mass is found at operation that is suspicious for cancer,

biopsy is not recommended on account of the risk for malignant cell spread into the peritoneal cavity. The decision to perform oopherectomy versus a total abdominal hysterectomy with bilateral salpingo-oopherectomy is made on consideration of tumor size, local spread, and whether the patient desires a subsequent pregnancy. The 5-year survival depends on the stage of disease, ranging from 85% for stage I to 20–35% for stages III and IV disease.

Endometrial Mass

The most common uterine mass is leiomyoma or **uterine fibroid**. Fibroids are benign masses caused by the overproliferation of uterine smooth muscle cells. Patients often have a chief complaint of pelvic pressure, vague and ill defined. Often the masses are discovered on routine examination. Acute hemorrhage into a fibroid can occasionally cause acute lower abdominal pain. Make the diagnosis by pelvic ultrasound. Although there is a possibility of **uterine sarcoma**, a malignant version of the simple fibroid, the risk is extremely low. Thus, surgery is offered only for patients who are symptomatic with pain, abnormal vaginal bleeding, or infertility concerns. Surgery can include a partial resection of the fibroid or hysterectomy.

Selected Readings

CDC, Workowski KA, Berman SM. Sexually transmitted diseases treatment guidelines, 2006. *MMWR Recomm Rep.* 2006;55(RR-11):1–94.

ACOG Committee on Practice Bulletins. Medical management of endometriosis. Number 11, December 1999 (replaces Technical Bulletin Number 184, September 1993). Clinical management guidelines for obstetrician-gynecologists. *Int J Gynaecol Obstet.* 2000;71(2):183–196.

American Society for Reproductive Medicine. Revised American Society for Reproductive Medicine classification of endometriosis: 1996. *Fertil Steril.* 1997;67(5):817–821.

Yao M, Tulandi T. Current status of surgical and nonsurgical management of ectopic pregnancy. *Fertil Steril.* 1997;67(3):421–433.

Goff BA, Mandel LS, Melancon CH, Muntz HG. Frequency of symptoms of ovarian cancer in women presenting to primary care clinics. *JAMA.* 2004;291(22):2705–2712.

22

Neck and Back Pain

John N. Awad, MD ■ *Robert V. Dawe, MD*

Key Points

■ The history and physical examination are paramount in limiting the differential diagnosis in patients with neck and back pain.

■ "Red flags" in the history indicate potential for a serious pathology and include trauma, cancer, constitutional symptoms, night pain, associated infection, or associated neurologic deficits.

■ Plain radiographs are still considered as the first radiographic diagnostic tool.

■ Computerized tomography (CT) scan is used to characterize fractures and bony abnormalities.

■ Magnetic resonance imaging (MRI) is utilized to examine ligamentous and disc structures.

■ Patients without "red flags" in the history can be observed for a period of 6 weeks, since most neck and back pain will resolve spontaneously. Those with "red flags" will have further radiographic testing.

■ Common causes of neck and back pain include musculoligamentous strain, herniated nucleolus pulposus (HNP), and osteoporotic fractures.

■ The vast majority of patients with common neck and back pain syndromes are treated with medication and physical therapy. Surgery is considered in patients who fail first-line therapy or have acute, significant neurologic deficits.

■ HISTORY

Mechanical neck and low back pain (N&LBP) are one of the most common complaints necessitating medical care. Nearly 80%–90% of adults aged 50 years or less will experience some form of neck and or back pain. Unfortunately, it is difficult to identify the exact pathologic pain generator in most cases; therefore, the medical history is an integral portion of the workup that is commonly overlooked.

First delineate **pain symptoms** to rule out serious conditions. Look for elements in the present illness commonly called "**red flags**," that may indicate a serious pathoanatomic condition that may warrant an urgent workup. These include a history of trauma, cancer, constitutional symptoms, night pain, immunosuppression, recent infection, bladder/bowel dysfunction, bilateral neurologic deficits, saddle anesthesia, progressive neurologic deficit, and progressive or unremitting pain. If a patient demonstrates any of these symptoms or signs then further workup is warranted on an urgent basis.

The urgency of diagnosis and treatment is determined by the **history of the present illness**. Acute urinary or bowel retention/incontinence, significant motor loss, saddle anesthesia, or a progressive unremitting pain may indicate a surgical emergency, while chronic N&LBP with no neurologic deficits may not require emergent imaging or workup. Significant trauma should alert the practitioner to frank or subtle fractures or instability. A history of previous neoplasm, constitutional symptoms, immunosuppression, or night pain may signal tumor or infection as the etiology of the pain.

Determine the **time course** of the symptoms. An acute symptom associated with any "red flag" requires further workup and a high index of suspicion. Chronic pain with no neurologic symptoms and no change in character can be approached in a less aggressive manner. If available, obtain previous medical records that may help with the diagnosis.

Characterize the symptoms to whether it is associated with **arm or leg pain**. Differentiate this type of pain from a less well-defined deep aching pain that is confined to the sclerotomes of the spine, commonly known as referred pain. Neck pain associated with extremity pain may indicate a disc herniation.

Determine the **quality** of the pain. A "burning" quality stereotypically indicates a neurogenic cause, whereas pain midline or more in the paraspinal region indicates a muscular origin. **Night pain** should increase the practitioner's awareness for an underlying pathologic cause.

Age can be important in narrowing the differential diagnosis. **Younger** patients are more susceptible to acute disc herniations, discogenic axial back pain, and primary bone tumors, whereas **older** patients are more susceptible to compression fractures, stenosis, or metastatic disease. Some processes are age independent such as osteomyelitis. N&LBP is an uncommon complaint in very young children.

Determine if there are any aggravating or alleviating factors. Pain that is aggravated by movement or prolonged sitting or standing indicates a mechanical compression mechanism. Elicit any precipitating events that may have contributed to the current symptoms. Even simple things like a bump during a car ride or sneeze can be important. These are often associated with compression fractures.

Review **past medical history**, which may contribute to the current symptomatology. Musculoskeletal syndromes such as myofascial pain syndromes and **fibromyalgia** can present as acute neck and back pain. These patients require a thorough and judicious workup to rule out any other cause before the symptoms are attributed to their known syndrome. Systemic **arthropathies** such as rheumatoid and psoriatic arthritis are associated with spinal involvement that can predispose the patient to significant instability, especially in the cervical spine.

Psychosocial and **economic** factors can be quite illustrative in the examination of a patient with N&LBP. A factor of **secondary gain** can be a component of the patient's symptoms. It is important to determine if the patient has a pending litigation or may receive some form of compensation for the injury. Also enquire about the patients' job situation: whether they are satisfied with their job, since depression or significant stressors may be contributing to the symptom complex.

■ PHYSICAL EXAMINATION

Although several similarities exist between examining a patient with neck or back pain, a few important differences exist to warrant separation of the two examinations.

Back Examination

The back examination includes determining the range of motion (flexion, extension, lateral bending, and rotation) of the back, hips, and knees. Complaints of hip and knee pain can often be secondary to spinal etiology and vice versa; back pain can be secondary to hip pathology. Many patients describe hip pain as a lateral buttock or thigh pain, usually secondary to spine pathology, whereas groin pain typically indicates a hip problem or a high disc herniation.

Perform the **Waddell signs** to determine if the pain is nonneurogenic. If the pain is neurogenic in character, the **straight leg raise** (SLR) performed while the patient is seated should elicit the same response of pain as if lying down. Have the patient then perform a total body rotation; this should not elicit pain, since the spine is kept in line during the maneuver.

Palpate the back and abdomen. Pain elicited in the sacroiliac region may indicate a sacroilitis rather than a true spinal disorder, whereas midline point tenderness may be indicative of a fracture. Also many **intra-abdominal** processes can mimic back pain. Appendicitis, bowel perforation, abdominal aortic aneurysm, perirectal abscess, pancreatitis, cholelcystitis, pelvic inflammatory disease, prostatitis, urinary tract infection, and kidney stones can all present initially as low back pain.

The **neurologic examination** is critical and is performed serially in any patient with a detected neurologic deficit, although there are considerable variation and cross over. Specific muscle groups and sensory nerves receive the majority of their innervation by a specific nerve root (Table 22-1). **Motor testing** is performed on all myotomes and given a grade of 0–5 (Table 22-2). This is important to document accurately, since this will help determine if the weakness is progressive or static. A progressive neurologic deficit indicates that urgent treatment may be necessary. A static deficit that is not acute may be observed depending on the clinical situation.

Sensory testing is critical and should correspond to any motor findings if present. This is tested to light touch such as a cotton applicator as well as to sharp objects. If myelopathy is suspected, perform position and vibration testing. As with motor testing, each nerve root acts as an individual sensory dermatome on the skin (Figure 22-1).

Examine the **Reflexes** to discern upper vs. lower motor neuron pathologies, as well as involvement of specific nerve roots. Superficial reflexes include the abdominal, cremasteric, and anal reflexes. They are elicited by skin stimulation. Abnormalities indicate an upper motor neuron lesion (cortex or spinal cord). Pathologic reflexes, such as the Hoffman, Babinski, and Oppenheim tests, are mediated by the central nervous system and indicate a central lesion. Deep tendon reflexes are normal reflexes in which the lower motor neuron tract is stimulated. There absence may be indicative of a postganglionic nerve root injury. If the patient is hyperreflexic, have a concern for an upper motor neuron lesion. Perform a **rectal examination** to document sensation and rectal tone.

Provocative tests help to elicit for a disc herniation. The classic test for L5 nerve root irritation is the **SLR** with ankle dorsiflexion. A variation of this is the **crossed straight leg raise** test (CSLR). To confirm the finding the **bowstring test** can be performed, which involves flexing the knee while the hip is flexed 90 degrees. This should relieve the pain by releasing the tension on the sciatic nerve. The reversed SLR, or more commonly known as the **femoral stretch test**, places L2–4 nerve roots on stretch and is diagnostic of compression of these roots. In order to confirm the SLR, the tripod or **flip test** can be performed. In this maneuver, the patient is sitting upright, the hip is flexed to 90 degrees, and the knee is fully extended. This places the nerve root on tension. If the patients truly have irritation of the nerve, they will try to lean back in order to reduce the tension. Other tests include the **Hoover test** or **Waddell's signs**, which test to see if the patient is malingering or the pain is nonorganic in nature.

TABLE 22-1.
The Motor and Sensory Examination for Spinal Levels

Nerve Root	Motor Distribution (Myotome)	Sensory Distribution (Dermatome)	Reflex
C5	• Deltoid (shoulder abduction) • Biceps (elbow flexion and supination)	• Lateral shoulder and arm	• Biceps
C6	• Biceps • Wrist extension: extensor carpi radialis longus and brevis	• Lateral forearm, thumb, and radial half of index finger	• Biceps • Brachioradialis
C7	• Triceps (elbow extension) • Wrist flexion: flexor carpi radialis and ulnaris	• Middle finger	• Triceps
C8	• Finger abduction/adduction (finger interossei) • Finger flexors (grip) (flexor digitorum superficialis and profundus)	• Ulnar forearm • Small and ring finger	• None
T1	• Finger abduction/adduction	• Medial half of arm	• None
T12 and L1–3	• Hip flexion (iliopsoas)	• L1: oblique band on the upper anterior portion of the thigh immediately below the inguinal ligament • L2: between L1 and L3 • L3: oblique band on anterior thigh immediately above patella	• None
L2–4	• Knee extension (quadriceps) (femoral nerve) • Hip adduction (obturator nerve)		• Patellar (mainly L4)
L4	• Knee extension (quadriceps) • Foot dorsiflexion/inversion (tibialis anterior)	• Medial leg and medial malleolus	• Patellar
L5	• Large toe extension (extensor hallicus longus) • Foot dorsiflexors • Hip abductors (gluteus maximus)	• Dorsum of foot and lateral half of large toe	• None
S1	• Foot plantarflexion (gastrocnemius) • Foot eversion (peroneus longus)	• Lateral malleolus, lateral foot, and plantar surface	• Achilles
S2–5	• Bladder control • Intrinsic foot muscles	• Concentric rings around anus (S2 outermost and S5 innermost) • Perineum (penis and vulva)	

273

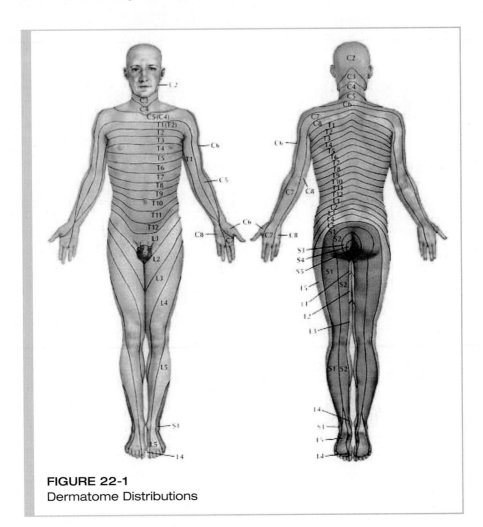

FIGURE 22-1
Dermatome Distributions

Although rare, meningeal irritation from intradural neoplasms and intradural inflammatory conditions needs to be ruled out if there is a suspicion. Maneuvers such as **Kerning's** and **Milgram** tests, along with the Valsalva maneuver, all may be indicative of an intradural process. Sacroiliac joint injuries can be difficult to diagnose, but certain classic provocative tests can help to elicit the pain. These include the **Fabere** and **pelvic rock tests** and **Gaenslen's sign**.

Cervical Spine

The same principles as the lumbar spine apply to the cervical spine with a few considerations, since the spinal cord exists at this level. Subtle injury and instability can manifest itself several weeks after the initial injury, especially if it is ligamentous in origin. There it is important to be vigilant and to perform repeated examinations and radiographs.

TABLE 22-2.
Grading System for the Motor Examination

0: No muscle activity
1: Muscle twitch
2: Full range of motion with gravity removed
3: Full range of motion against gravity
4: Full range of motion against gravity and can offer some resistance to testing. This is the only grade that is subjective in nature and can further be quantified with a "+" or "−"
5: Full range of motion and can fully resist the examiner

Upper motor neuron injury is more likely to occur at this level, since the spinal cord exists rather than individual nerve rootlets. Document the reflexes and other provocative tests as mentioned in the lumbar section. Patients with cervical cord pathology will present with hyperreflexia, wide-based shuffling gate, pathologic reflexes such as Babinski and Hoffmans' reflexes, sustained clonus, and difficulty with fine motor skills.

Care is taken to do a full neurologic examination in every patient. Some cervical pathologies, such as central cord syndrome, can present with isolated arm weakness with a normal lower extremity examination.

■ LABORATORY STUDIES

The purpose of laboratories in the workup of spinal is limited. They are of value if an infection, an autoimmune disease, or a neoplasm is suspected. For a suspicion of infection, order a **CBC** to look for elevations in the white blood cell count, **eosinophil sedimentation rate** (ESR), and **C-reactive protein** level. In patients suspected of having an **autoimmune disease**, consider ordering antinuclear antibody (ANA), RF, or a Lyme titer if in an indigenous area. In cases of compression fractures, suspect multiple myeloma and order serum protein electrophoresis.

■ RADIOGRAPHIC STUDUIES

As opposed to laboratory studies, imaging plays a key role in the workup of N&LBP. Radiographs remain the mainstay of diagnosis and imaging. These should not be ignored for newer modalities, since they provide valuable information that other modalities cannot easily offer.

Unless a "red flag" exists and the patient is younger than 15 years or older than 60 years, **plain radiographs** are obtained if the pain persists for more than 6 weeks. Traditional anterior–posterior or lateral radiographs centered on the area of interest is usually adequate. If the patient is young, then oblique views are included to visualize the pars intra-articularis to see if there are any defects. If instability is suspected or if there was significant trauma, then order flexion/extension views to document any occult instability.

Order an **MRI** as a superior modality in visualizing soft-tissue elements such as nerves, tendons, ligaments, muscle, and intervertebral discs. An MRI should be ordered if the patient presents with a neurologic deficit (sensory or motor), if tumor or infection are suspected, or if an occult compression fracture is suspected that is not well visualized on plain radiographs. In general, T1-weighted images highlight fat and therefore are preferred in viewing anatomy, whereas T2-weighted images highlight water and therefore assist in visualizing pathology. STIR images help identify ligamentous injury or fracture when trauma is suspected.

Use **CT** in cases where osseous anatomy needs to be better visualized. This modality is very useful in cases of trauma to better characterize the fracture patterns or in congenital deformities of the spine. CT combined with a myelogram, in which a dye is injected into the subarachnoid space, is considered to visualize the central and lateral recesses and nerve sheaths. Although MRI has largely replaced this modality, CT myelogram is helpful in cases where metallic implants have been used, obscuring MRI images.

Bone scan/SPECT scan is a modality that tries to quantify metabolic activity of the bone tissue. It is a sensitive diagnostic tool used to detect stress fractures, spondylolysis, infection, and tumors. It is typically used as a screening test if the whole spine needs to be imaged, since the exact location cannot be identified. It will help direct the practitioner where to order more specific, higher-resolution tests such as MRI or CT scan. It is very useful in cases of metastatic tumors, since the whole body can be imaged at once. It has greater sensitivity to detect tumors or infection much earlier than plain radiographs.

Consider **electromyelography** (EMG) and **nerve conduction** test (NCT) to evaluate the status of muscle innervations and axonal conduction integrity, respectively. They are useful in cases of radiculopathy where it is unclear whether the compression is secondary to an individual nerve root being compromised (e.g., herniated disc) versus a peripheral compression syndrome (e.g., carpal tunnel).

■ DIAGNOSTIC PLAN

Most often the medical **history** and **physical examination** will lead to a short differential diagnosis list. Laboratories and radiographic studies are usually only needed to confirm the diagnosis and help direct treatment. Too often clinicians over rely on radiographic imaging to make a diagnosis. This can lead to erroneous tests and unnecessary treatments. This is especially true in case of isolated neck or back pain with no neurologic findings.

If a "red flag" is not present or if the patient is not at the two ends of the age spectrum (younger than 15 or older than 60 years), then 6 weeks of **observation** is appropriate. Most N&LBP will significantly improve within this time interval.

If a "**red flag**" is present, or if the patient is younger than 15 or older than 60 years, or if it has been longer than 6 weeks since the symptoms starts, then further diagnostic workup is warranted. Start with **plain radiographs**. These should be centered over the area of interest. AP and lateral radiographs are usually sufficient. If instability is suspected, or in cases of trauma, flexion and extension can help visualize any abnormal movement of the vertebrae. If the patient is young and a spondylolysis is suspected, then oblique radiographs should be included.

If X-rays are not conclusive then further imaging is considered. Order an **MRI** as the next test. This is especially helpful if the patient presents with a radiculopathy or if X-rays reveal a pathologic process. It is also useful if an occult compression fracture is suspected. Order a **CT scan** in cases where a fracture has been diagnosed, but detailed anatomic picture of the fracture in three planes is needed. Consider bone/SPECT scans in cases of metastasis, spondylolysis if X-ray is negative, or occult fractures where the exact position is difficult to pinpoint. It is a highly sensitive test but not very specific; thus, it is typically used to identify a general area of a pathologic process.

Based on the history, physical examination, and appropriate imaging modalities, **laboratory studies** may be ordered. If a tumor is suspected, order the appropriate tumor markers.

■ DIFFERENTIAL DIAGNOSIS AND TREATMENT

Musculoligamentous Strain

This is a very common finding in patients with acute back pain. The true etiology is unclear, but trauma to the multiple ligamentous and tendonous attachments is thought to be the underlying pathology. In general, the majority of these patients improve within 6–12 weeks. Typically, supportive care with **nonsteroidal anti-inflammatory** agents (NSAIDs), **physical therapy**, and **time** are sufficient in the majority of patients. If the patient does not significantly improve within 6 weeks, then a formal workup with imaging studies (X-rays and MRI) and possibly laboratory work are performed.

Herniated Nucleolus Pulposus

This is one of the most common causes of acute neck or low back pain with or without radiculopathy. The fragmentation of the nucleus pulposus and inner annulus is largely asymptomatic, secondary to the lack of innervations. Pain results when the outer annulus, which contains the nervous structure for the intervertebral disc, is compromised. The mechanism is most likely multifactorial but involves stimulation of the nerve endings in the outer annulus, direct nerve root, and the chemical inflammatory cascade induced by the exposed nucleus pulposus. HNP is thought to be part of the natural history of a degenerated intervertebral disc. If associated with a radiculopathy, the HNP typically impinges on the traversing nerve root (e.g., an L4–5 HNP causes an L5 radiculopathy). The posterior paracentral part of the annulus is the weakest part of the annulus; thus, it is hypothesized that this is the cause for this area being the most common location of an HNP.

Treatment initially is nonoperative. The majority will improve in 6–12 weeks. In cases with or without radiculopathy, consider a short course of **oral steroids** (commonly known as a medrol dose pack), if not contraindicated, to help relieve the back and/or leg pain. Combine this with **physical therapy** and traditional **NSAIDs**. If these do not give significant symptomatic relief then consider **epidural steroid injections**. In cases where radiculopathy continues despite these treatment attempts, offer surgical decompression. Surgical treatment for discogenic back pain without radiculopathy is controversial and should be thoroughly discussed with the patient.

There are a few cases of HNP that warrant emergent surgical decompression. If there is acute and progressive arm or leg weakness, rapidly progressive cervical myelopathy, or cauda equina syndrome (see below), the patient should undergo surgical decompression emergently (Figure 22-2). If the above conditions have been preexistent or nonprogressive then there is time to discuss options with the

LUMBAR LAMINECTOMY

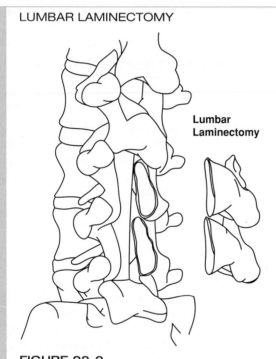

Lumbar Laminectomy

FIGURE 22-2
A lumbar laminectomy with a section of lumbar spine being removed

The patient is positioned prone, and the area of the back is prepped. An incision over the area to be decompressed is made, and dissection through the erector spinae muscles eventually reveals the spinal column. The muscles are dissected on both sides and the laminae are removed, being careful to preserve the facet joints, leaving the dural sheath exposed. Careful trimming of the facet joints may be performed to allow a wider decompression. The dura is inspected for inadvertent injury and, if present, repaired to avoid a cerebrospinal fluid leak. The skin is closed.

patient, but they all still warrant surgical decompression. The only true surgical emergency is cauda equina syndrome or acute foot drop.

Cauda Equina Syndrome

This syndrome is caused by severe compression of the cauda equina at or distal to the conus medularis. The patients present typically with severe **bilateral leg pain** and weakness and usually complain of **fecal incontinence** and **urinary retention** or incontinence. It can occur gradually, such as in cases of severe spinal stenosis and extra- or intradural tumors. Acute causes include large extruded HNP, trauma, and epidural hematomas. Acute cases are true **surgical emergencies** and should be decompressed immediately (within 6 hours if possible), since the literature suggests that rapid decompression provides the best chance or recovery, although many patients are left with some residual neurologic deficits. Chronic cases also warrant urgent decompression, although recovery is very variable.

Acute weakness in specific myotomes such as foot drop or arm weakness is somewhat controversial, but most authors would agree that urgent decompression is warranted. These conditions are typically caused by a large HNP. Acute cervical myelopathy like cauda equina syndrome is a surgical emergency. It is typically caused by a large central HNP that fills the central canal. Patients present with similar symptoms as cauda equina syndrome but also with upper extremity involvement, loss of coordination, and upper extremity hyperreflexia.

Spinal Canal Stenosis

Spinal stenosis results from narrowing of the spinal canal, nerve root canals, or intervertebral foramina owing to spondylosis (arthritis) and degenerative disk disease. The spine responds to physiological stresses by growing osteophytes, to increase the surface and thereby decreasing the contact stresses, and the ligamentum flavum hypertrophies and ossifies. Posterior osteophytes narrow the spinal canal diameter and also cause lateral recess stenosis. This results in spinal cord or nerve root compression. Furthermore, degeneration causes facet joint hypertrophy and synovial cysts, which further narrows the canal and the neural foramina.

In the **cervical spine**, this typically presents as a progressive myelopathy or radiculopathy in a specific dermatome. In the **lumbar spine**, it can manifest itself as lower back pain, unilateral or bilateral radiculopathy, and possibly bladder and bowel difficulties. The classic presentation commonly known as **neurogenic claudication** consists of radiating leg pain associated with walking, which is relieved by rest, and buttock or thigh pain. When patients bend forward (to sit or go up stairs), the pain diminishes (**shopping cart sign**). Rarely, patients with lumbar stenosis present with cauda equina syndrome.

Make the diagnosis on **plain radiographs** and **MRI**. CT myelogram may be ordered if MRI is contraindicated or severe scoliosis coexists. Nonsurgical treatments include **physical therapy, anti-inflammatory** medications, and epidural **steroid injections**. These are aimed at treating the symptoms but do not address the actual stenosis. In the patient who has mild symptoms or is not a surgical candidate, these can be very effective. Surgical treatment includes laminectomy and posterior foraminotomy, with or without a fusion, at the stenotic levels in the lumbar spine (Figure 22-2). For cervical stenosis, either an anterior or a posterior approach can be used to decompress the spinal canal and or the neural foramen (Figure 22-3).

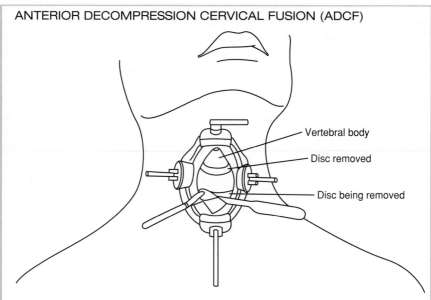

ANTERIOR DECOMPRESSION CERVICAL FUSION (ADCF)

Vertebral body

Disc removed

Disc being removed

FIGURE 22-3

The anterior approach to the cervical spine to perform a decompression and fusion.

In the supine position, a horizontal incision is made along the medial border of the sternocleidomastoid muscle. The structures of the neck are mobilized with the trachea and esophagus retracted medially and the carotid sheath retracted laterally. The anterior spine is then exposed. The level of vertebrae is determined by fluoroscopy or plain radiograph by placing a probe into the wound and noting the position on the radiograph. The involved discs and hypertrophied intravertebral joints are removed, relieving the compression. Removal of the vertebral body along with the disc, a corpectomy, may be needed to fully decompress the spinal space. Care is taken to remove all tissues that are causing pressure on the spinal cord and nerve roots.

After removal of the disc and possibly the vertebral bodies, the spine must be stabilized by reconstructing the support previously provided by the structures. Options for stabilization include inserting a bone graft (from the iliac crest or cadaveric) between the remaining vertebrae or spanning the area with an implantable strut that is anchored to the existing vertebrae. A plate and screw construct is usually added for increased stability. A completion radiograph confirms proper spinal alignment, and the wound is closed over a Jackson–Pratt drain.

Fractures

Fractures occur from trauma, from nontraumatic causes, and secondary to infections.

Osteoporotic Fracture

This is often seen in elderly or younger patients who have predisposing factors such as a metabolic bone disease, chronic steroid use, and chronic seizure medications. Spine fractures are the most common osteoporosis-induced fracture and can be quite debilitating. Order plain X-rays and MRI to asses the acuteness of the fracture. If indicated, include tumor markers in the laboratory workup.

The treatment of these types of fracture is currently undergoing a paradigm shift. It was initially thought that nonoperative treatment is the preferred treatment modality and that all of these heal without consequence. However, recent literature suggests that osteoporotic compression fractures are a major cause of long-term morbidity in the form of chronic back pain, decreased mobility, and health care expenditure. For these reasons, consider one of the following procedures in these patients. **Vertebroplasty** involves the injection of cement directly into the trabeculae of the vertebrae, whereas **kyphoplasty** uses an inflatable balloon to first create a cavity, in which cement is injected. Both procedures have theoretical advantages and disadvantages. No significant clinical difference has been found between the two procedures.

Nonosteoporotic Fracture

This is a consequence of high-energy trauma. It can be associated with significant neurologic injury, and thus a careful neurologic examination is always performed. Order **plain radiographs** or a **CT scan** of any section of the spine where there is a complaint of pain. The cervical spine is also imaged, since many thoracic and lumbar fractures are associated with cervical injury.

The vertebra is divided into three columns. The anterior half is defined as the **anterior column**; the posterior half, including the posterior wall, of the body is defined as the middle column; and everything posterior (pedicles, lamina, and ligaments) is defined as the **posterior column**. If the posterior column is thought to be involved or if there are any neurologic findings, then obtain a MRI to better evaluate the ligamentous structures and the neural elements. Treatment is once again controversial. In patients who are neurologically intact, nonoperative treatment has been shown to be equally effective as operative treatment in stable fractures. If the fracture is unstable (all three columns are involved), then most practitioners would recommend surgical stabilization in the form of an instrumented fusion. If the patient has a progressive neurologic deficit then urgent surgical decompression and fusion is performed.

Infections

Typically spread to the spine by hematogenous means. Batson's plexus (a venous plexus that drains the spinal cord and vertebrae) is a conduit for bacteria to seed the spine. Spinal infection frequently manifests in the disc first (septic discitis) and then spreads to the vertebral bodies, in contradistinction to tumors that typically involve the vertebrae first. Patients usually present with increasing pain and, in the later stages, deformity. Typically, they will have a history of intravenous drug abuse, a recent interventional procedure, or a remote infection that caused bacteremia.

Have a high suspicion for this in a high-risk patient who complains of back pain. Plain radiographs can be "normal" for several weeks, since the infection is in the disc. Only when the vertebrae are involved will the X-ray be beneficial. It is important to obtain laboratory studies (CBC, ESR, and C-reactive protein), and if the infection can be localized then an MRI should be ordered and if not then a bone scan will help identify the location.

Treatment depends on the amount of destruction of the disc/vertebrae. If no significant deformity or instability exists then bracing and long-term intravenous antibiotics are appropriate. If possible the bacteria should be identified, by either blood culture or direct biopsy, so that the appropriate antibiotic can be chosen. Typically, an infectious disease specialist is involved. If instability or deformity has ensued then operative debridement and stabilization should be performed.

Tumors

Primary tumors in the vertebrae or spinal cord are rare but should be treated aggressively, depending on the type and the location. Metastatic tumors are much more common, and once again the treatment is dependent on the location, type, and whether a deformity and/or instability exist. The workup is typically the same as in infection, but identifying the primary tumor is paramount. Some can be treated with radiation and or chemotherapy, while others require surgical intervention.

23

Hematuria

Courtney C. Morton, MPA, PA-C ■ *C. William Schwab II, MD*

Key Points

- Hematuria can originate anywhere along the patient's genitourinary tract from multiple possible etiologies. The appropriate workup must evaluate the kidneys, ureters, bladder, urethra, and prostate.

- It is important to characterize the type of hematuria present—gross (macroscopic) or microscopic—as well as whether or not pain is involved.

- The initial assessment of new-onset hematuria should include a urinalysis, urine culture, urine cytology, and upper tract imaging.

- Gross hematuria is the presenting symptom in up to 85% of patients with bladder cancer and 40% of patients with renal cell carcinoma (RCC) (kidney cancer). Thus, in the urologist's view, hematuria in a patient older than 40 years suggests a malignancy until proven otherwise.

■ HISTORY

Gross or macroscopic hematuria exists when blood is visible in the urine to the naked eye. **Microscopic hematuria** exists when more than three red blood cells (RBCs) per high-power field is detected in the urine by microscopy. Patients generally present to the emergency department with **gross hematuria**, noticed either in the toilet after voiding or as a small drop of blood in his or her underwear (Table 23-1).

TABLE 23-1.
Causes of Isolated Microscopic Hematuria*

Origin	<50 Yr of Age	≥50 Yr of Age
Glomerular	IgA nephropathy (increased incidence in Asians)	IgA nephropathy
	Thin basement membrane disease (begin familial hematuria)	Hereditary nephritis (Alport's syndrome)
	Hereditary nephritis (Alport's syndrome)	Mild focal glomerulonephritis of other causes
	Mild focal glomerulonephritis of other causes	
Nonglomerular		
Upper urinary tract causes	Nephrolithasis	Nephrolithasis
	Pyelonephritis	Renal-cell cencer
	Polysystic kidney disease	Polysystic kidney disease
	Medullary sponge kidney	Pyelonephritis
	Hypercalciuria, hyperuricosuria, or both, without documented stone	Renal-pelvis or ureteral transitional-cell cencer
	Renal trauma	Papillary necrosis
	Papillary necrosis	Renal infraction
	Ureteral stricture and hydronephrosis	Ureteral stricture and hydronephrosis
	Sickle cell trait or disease in blacks	Renal tuberculosis
	Renal tuberculosis in endemic areas or in patients with HIV infection	
Lower urinary tract causes	Cystitis, prostatitis, and urethritis	Cystitis, prostatitis, and urethritis
	Benign bladder and ureteral polyps and tumors	Bladder cencer
	Bladder cencer	Prostate cencer
	Prostate cencer	Benign bladder and ureteral polyps and tumors
	Ureteral and meatal strictures	
	Schistosoma haematobium in North Africans	
Uncertain	Exercise hematuria	Exercise hematuria
	"Benign hematuria" (unexplained microscopic hematuria)	Over-anticoagulation (usually with warfarin)
	Over-anticoagulation (usually with warfarin)	
	Factitious hematuria (usually present with gross hematuria)	

Disorders causing microhematuria are presented roughly in order of descending frequency of presentation, according to avialable data.

Document in what setting the patient noticed his/her hematuria, since spotting in the underwear may represent gastrointestinal bleeding, vaginal bleeding in females, or bloody semen in males.

Further categorize gross hematuria in terms of when it occurs. **Initial hematuria** suggests a urethral source. **Terminal hematuria** in males suggests a prostatic source as the prostate constricts at the end of micturition, forcing small amounts of urine from the prostatic urethra. **Total hematuria** occurs throughout the entire stream and indicates a source at the level of the bladder or higher (i.e., ureters or kidneys).

The presence or absence of **lower urinary tract symptoms** (LUTS) is valuable in determining the etiology of the patient's hematuria. The most frequent LUTS that accompany hematuria are dysuria, frequency, urgency, and incontinence, indicating a possible urinary tract infection, as well as hesitancy or decreased caliber of stream, suggesting bladder outlet obstruction or prostatic etiology.

Elicit prior history of hematuria as well as any prior history of genitourinary diseases, malignancies, surgeries, and/or interventions. Also, determine if the patient ever had pelvic radiation.

Review risk factors that may suggest significant underlying disease: **Cigarette smoking** is a known risk factor for transitional cell carcinoma (TCC) of the bladder. Smoking increases the risk of bladder cancer three- to fivefold; **occupational exposure** to aromatic amides and amines (often occurring in leather, rubber, and dye manufacturing) also increases a person's risk for developing bladder cancer. **Medications** can alter the appearance of urine, giving the appearance of blood, whereas others may induce hematuria. The most notable hematuria-inducing medications are the chemotherapeutic agents cyclophosphamide (Cytoxan®) and mitotane. Chronic NSAID ingestion can result in papillary necrosis and resultant hematuria. Penicillins and cephalosporins have been associated with an allergic interstitial nephritis. Lastly, anticoagulants such as warfarin place a person at increased risk of hematuria.

A patient with hematuria on one or more of the abovementioned medications **must still undergo a complete evaluation** to rule out other etiologies. Research shows that 75% of patients presenting with gross hematuria while on anticoagulation will have urologic findings.

■ PHYSICAL EXAMINATION

Review the **vital signs** for fever higher than 101°F, chills, or rigors that may suggest infection and warrant further workup for a urinary tract infection or pyelonephritis.

Inspect the **abdomen** for a flank mass, bruit, or a pulsatile aortic aneurysm. A bruit could indicate a vascular process relating to the bleeding (i.e., aneurysm or arteriovenous malformation). A lower, midline abdominal (suprapubic) mass that is dull to percussion suggests a distended bladder. Small pencil-tip tattoo markings on the skin may suggest prior external beam radiotherapy.

Examine the **back** by inspection, palpation, and percussion to reveal ecchymosis, suggesting a retroperitoneal bleed or recent trauma. Differentiation of

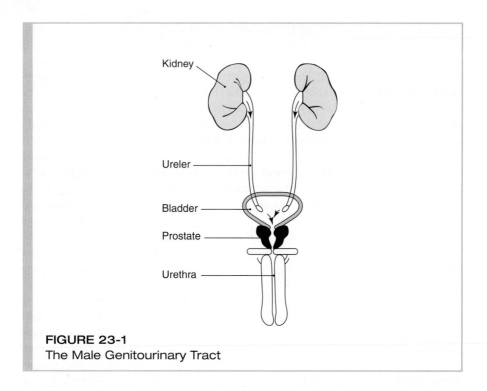

FIGURE 23-1
The Male Genitourinary Tract

tenderness over one or both flanks (costovertebral angle tenderness) could suggest presence of a stone (nephrolithiasis), infection (pyelonephritis), obstruction of a kidney (hydronephrosis), or inflammation.

Perform a complete **genital** and **rectal** examination. A male's genital examination should include retraction of the foreskin in uncircumcised patients and gentle spreading of the urethral meatus to look for polyps, condyloma, or meatal stenosis (Figure 23-1). Palpate the penis and urethra and examine the testicles for masses, hernias, swelling, tenderness, varicoceles, or other pathology. Additionally, examination of the prostate must be performed via a digital rectal examination (DRE) with a well-lubricated, gloved finger, in an effort to detect evidence of prostatitis or prostate cancer. Tenderness, warmth, and bogginess of the prostate can correlate with acute prostatitis, whereas a hard, irregular prostate could reveal prostate cancer. In women, urethral and vaginal examinations can exclude local causes of hematuria such as lacerations or menstruation. Furthermore, inspection of the urethra might reveal a caruncle, prolapse, or tumor.

■ LABORATORY STUDIES

Order a **CBC**, **chemistry** panel, and a **PT/PTT** to evaluate for the presence of an infection, severity of anemia, degree of renal insufficiency, and possible coagulopathy.

Initial testing of urine is usually performed using a chemical reagent strip known as a dipstick **urinalysis**. A comprehensive dipstick includes a test of urine pH, glucose, ketones, blood, leukocyte esterase (indicating presence of white blood cells), nitrates (indicating presence of uropathogenic bacteria), bilirubin and/or urobilinogen, and specific gravity. The presence of hemoglobin is detected by a color change on the testing strip, signifying the presence of blood. False positives may be observed in the presence of myoglobin, free hemoglobin, and antiseptic solutions such as povidone-iodine. Emphasis must be placed on proper specimen collection, especially in uncircumcised males, obese females, or menstruating females.

Consider **urine microscopy**. A urine specimen is centrifuged and the sediment resuspended and then observed under a high-power microscope to observe for the presence and number of RBCs. Microscopic hematuria is defined as the presence of more than three RBCs per high-power field. Additional information reported includes the number of white blood cells, an estimate on the amount of bacteria (none, few, moderate, and many), numbers of epithelial cells, presence and appearance of casts, and presence and type of crystals. The presence of red cell casts, dysmorphic cells, and proteinuria suggest a glomerular source of hematuria, whereas RBCs with normal morphology are nonspecific. An important additional piece of information obtained in the urinalysis is the presence of bacteria, leukocyte esterase, and/or nitrates, suggesting an **infectious source** of bleeding. Patients with hematuria and evidence of a UTI should be rechecked several weeks after antibiotic therapy to determine if the hematuria persists.

Obtain a **urine culture** and sensitivity (C&S). Although it takes time for this test to return, it provides definitive evidence as to whether or not there is an infectious etiology of the patient's complaints. A urine specimen should be sent for C&S prior to administration of any antibiotics.

Cytologic examination of exfoliated cells within the urine is a useful way to noninvasively test for urothelial malignancy. Cytology results are usually reported in one of three categories: (1) negative for malignant cells, (2) atypical cells where you cannot rule out TCC, and (3) positive for cells consistent with TCC. It is important to understand that while urine cytology is highly specific, overall it is poorly sensitive, especially in the presence of low-grade TCC. Additionally, false positives can occur, most commonly in the presence of bladder inflammation or urinary infection. **Fluorescent in situ hybridization** (FISH) is a newer specialized urine cytology analysis for chromosomal alterations, which is usually performed in those patients whose results are unclear. It has a specificity and sensitivity in the 85%–90% range. Studies have indicated that a positive FISH, even in the presence of a normal cystoscopy, strongly implies that the patient will develop clinically evident transitional cell cancer within 1 year of the positive test.

■ **RADIOGRAPHIC STUDIES**

In the emergent setting for hematuria, a **computed tomography** (CT) scan of the abdomen and pelvis will often provide the maximum information and will be most readily available. If urolithiasis or renal colic is suspected, a "stone protocol CT" should be requested. This finer-cut CT of the abdomen and pelvis without contrast provides greater sensitivity for the evaluation of stones. The administration of intravenous contrast (if the serum creatinine level is not elevated and the patient is not allergic to IV dye) provides improved evaluation of the renal blood flow and parenchyma. Delayed CT imaging following contrast excretion can suggest the presence of urinary obstruction or lesions within the ureters.

Newer technology allows reconstruction of these images into views similar to those previously obtained with flat-plate intravenous pyelography (IVP), with the advantage of providing simultaneous cross-sectional imaging. This modality, termed **CT urography**, has largely replaced IVP as the imaging study of choice in the evaluation of hematuria.

The selection of initial imaging studies should be tailored to the individual patient, based on history and physical examination findings. For example, in those patients who are at low risk of malignancy, or with a presentation consistent with renal colic, a noncontrast (or stone protocol) CT scan is usually sufficient. However, in patients without evidence of stones or at a higher risk of malignancy, subsequent imaging with IV contrast is necessary.

Contrast nephropathy is a potentially serious reaction some individuals experience after being subjected to IV contrast. Risk factors include patients with preexisting renal disease, who are dehydrated, and with diabetes mellitus. For this reason, a serum creatinine level should be obtained in all patients to identify renal insufficiency before any contrast study. Also, those patients taking metformin for management of diabetes should avoid taking this medication for 48 hours before or after IV contrast administration, if possible, to avoid potential lactic acidosis.

Renal ultrasonography is a popular form of imaging in a patient who cannot tolerate radiation, such as in a pregnant female, or IV contrast, such as those with contrast allergies or elevated creatinine. It is especially useful in determining the presence of **hydronephrosis** and in differentiating a solid renal mass from a cyst with clearly defined walls. Ultrasound, however, cannot clearly delineate the lining of the collecting system or the ureters and therefore does not adequately evaluate for the presence of some urothelial malignancies. Furthermore, a renal sonogram poorly defines small renal calculi (<4 mm), and it is not a useful study for a nondilated ureter. Lastly, complex cystic lesions in the kidney frequently require additional cross-sectional imaging with the use of IV contrast to be fully characterized.

Plain radiographs such as the "kidneys, ureters, and bladder" (KUB) are often useful if a kidney or ureteral calculus is suspected, as up to 85% of symptomatic urinary calculi will be seen. Otherwise, it generally provides very little detailed urologic-specific soft-tissue anatomy.

IVP had traditionally been the study of choice for evaluating the upper urinary tract prior to the refinement of the CT scan. An IVP involves a series of X-rays, usually consisting of a plain film prior to IV contrast administration, to detect any calcifications and bony structures; 1-minute delay to visualize the renal parenchyma; 5-minute delay to visualize the upper collecting system to the level of the upper ureter; and a 15–20-minute delay to evaluate the lower ureters and bladder. In general, an IVP is unable to differentiate a cyst from a solid mass or tumor. An IVP is also of little diagnostic value in a patient with a serum creatinine greater than 2.0 because there is poor renal function and the kidneys and upper ureters will be inadequately visualized. For these reasons, the CT scan has largely replaced the IVP in initial imaging for hematuria.

Retrograde pyelography is an imaging study performed during cystoscopy, by injecting radiographic contrast into a ureter through the ureteral orifice in the bladder. Using fluoroscopy, the entire course of the ureter is observed from the bladder up to the kidney and then into its collecting system. Filling defects observed may be due to a calculus, blood clot, or tumor. This study is generally performed by a urologist in the operating suite, as most patients require a regional or a general anesthetic.

Although **magnetic resonance imaging** (MRI) provides excellent resolution of soft tissue and bone, it rarely offers additional information in the initial assessment of the kidneys, ureters, or bladder. Additionally, most stones in the urinary tract are not visible on MRI. Moreover, the higher cost of MRI studies and less availability compared to CT make it less favorable as the initial imaging study in the workup of hematuria.

■ DIAGNOSTIC PLAN

After the patient has been deemed hemodynamically stable, the most important aspect in initial care of a patient with urologic abnormalities is to ensure adequate bladder emptying. If a patient presents with **gross hematuria** with the presence of clots, he or she is at increased risk of developing clot retention, as some clots may be too large to pass through the urethra. A postvoid residual via portable bladder ultrasound, stationary ultrasound, or straight catheter can reveal if the patient is failing to empty appropriately (or reveals a large amount of clot in the bladder). In the event of an elevated bladder residual, or clots, placement of a **urinary catheter** is indicated (Figure 23-1). There are many different catheters available for urinary drainage, and, depending on the patient's presenting history and complaints, special catheters may need to be inserted. Consider a urologist consult if severe hematuria with clots is noted or if initial attempts at placing a catheter are unsuccessful. In these cases, further intervention may cause damage to the urethra or bladder.

If infection is suspected, send a urine culture and start **empiric antibiotics** as soon as possible. The goal in treatment is to eradicate the infection by selecting the appropriate antibiotics that would target specific bacterial susceptibility. Therefore, the general principles for selecting the proper antibiotics include consideration of the possible infecting pathogen, the patient, and the site of infection.

Patients presenting with urologic abnormalities frequently suffer from dehydration, especially if there is accompanying nausea and vomiting. For these patients, **fluid resuscitation** is generally warranted.

Although some etiologies of hematuria are painless, there are several that may cause extreme discomfort for the patient in the acute setting (i.e., urolithiasis, pyelonephritis, or prostatitis). In these patients, order oral or **parenteral analgesics** (and frequently antiemetics) throughout further workup and treatment.

A patient with recurrent or persistent gross hematuria can easily become **anemic**, just as in the case of a patient with chronic gastrointestinal bleeding. For this reason, such patients may require treatment for this condition (i.e., transfusions) as part of their overall management. Additionally, if the patient is coagulopathic, correction of the coagulopathy is indicated.

Despite the usefulness of radiographic imaging in evaluating upper urinary tract abnormalities, its use is limited in identifying abnormalities distal to the ureters. **Cystoscopy** provides direct visualization and evaluation of the urethra and bladder mucosa. It is prudent to perform upper tract imaging prior to cystoscopy so that any upper tract abnormalities can be addressed concurrently. Depending on the indications, cystoscopy can be performed in the office setting under local anesthesia, using a flexible cystoscope or, in the operating room suite, using a rigid cystoscope that has a larger working channel, which allows for the passage of various urologic instruments. Common findings identified by cystoscopy are prostatic enlargement, urethral trauma, bladder stones, and bladder tumors.

■ DIFFERENTIAL DIAGNOSIS AND TREATMENTS

Cystitis

Acute, recurrent, or radiation cystitis refers to a urinary infection of the lower urinary tract, most commonly the bladder. Literally meaning "inflammation of the bladder," cystitis is associated with the hallmark symptoms of frequency, urgency, nocturia, and dysuria. **Urinalysis** typically shows hematuria as well as pyuria and bacteriuria, in the case of bacterial cystitis. The primary mode of infection is ascent of the periurethral/vaginal and fecal flora. For this reason, *Escherichia coli* is the most common pathogen in acute cystitis.

The diagnosis is usually made clinically and does not normally require extensive radiologic imaging. Uncomplicated lower urinary tract infections can usually be treated with a 3–5-day course of **oral antibiotic**. Severe infections or infections in individuals with diabetes, a solitary kidney, or multiple medical comorbidities may require **IV antibiotics** for a short time before starting PO antibiotics. Trimethoprim–sulfamethoxazole (TMP–SMX) was once recommended as first-line treatment for symptomatic UTIs, but increased bacterial resistance in certain geographic regions has limited its usefulness. Therefore, in areas where resistance to TMP–SMX is between 10% and 20%, **fluoroquinolones** are now recommended as first-line therapy for uncomplicated UTIs. The two most commonly used fluoroquinolones in the treatment of genitourinary tract infections are ciprofloxacin and levofloxacin.

Recurrent cystitis/UTI is caused either by bacterial persistence or by reinfection with another organism. Identification of the cause of the recurrent infection is important because the management of bacterial persistence and reinfection are distinct. Preventative therapy (in the form of either low-dose continuous prophylactic antibiotic or intermittent self-start antibiotic therapy) is often effective in treating reinfection. In the latter of these two options, patients self-identify episodes of infection on the basis of their symptoms and treat themselves with a single dose of antibiotics, such as TMP–SMX. Patients with frequent reinfections or infections caused by unusual bacteria should be evaluated for potential sources of bacterial persistence, including asymptomatic stones, bladder diverticulum, and urethral diverticulum.

Radiation cystitis can occur months to years after receiving external beam radiation therapy for various pelvic cancers (i.e., cervical, prostate, etc.). This condition is not caused by bacterial invasion, but rather a change in the physical characteristics of the bladder itself, as a result of radiation injury. Bladder capacity is usually appreciably reduced, and cystoscopic evaluation reveals pale bladder mucosa with multiple areas of fragile telangiectatic blood vessels. The initial treatment in such patients includes management of gross hematuria and evaluation of concurrent pathology (urinary tract infection, tumor recurrence, etc.). Patients with recurrent episodes of gross hematuria secondary to radiation cystitis may benefit from hyperbaric therapy. Intractable cases may ultimately require cystectomy and urinary diversion.

Benign Prostatic Hyperplasia

As men age, the prostate gland enlarges. Fifty percent of men older than 50 years have evidence of an enlarged prostate. The symptoms caused by an enlarged prostate are directly related to the obstruction that the prostate creates on the bladder opening/proximal urethra. The spectrum of LUTS associated with benign prostatic hyperplasia (BPH) includes decreased force and caliber of stream, hesitancy and straining to void, interruption of stream, postvoid dribbling, sensation of incomplete emptying, frequency and nocturia, and/or urinary retention. To adequately diagnose BPH, a thorough history is needed. Also, a DRE is important to assess the size, shape, and consistency of the prostate.

If BPH is suspected, order a **prostate-specific antigen** (PSA) for the possibility of prostate cancer. It should be noted that the presence of symptoms consistent with BPH and an enlarged prostate on DRE does not permit one to attribute hematuria to a prostatic origin. A full workup including imaging studies should still be undertaken. Treatment of BPH is most effectively managed by an urologist, as there are many medical and surgical therapies that may be recommended, based on the patient's severity of symptoms. Medical management often includes an α_1-**adrenergic blocking** agent (i.e., tamsulosin, terazosin, or doxazosin) to relax prostatic smooth muscle fibers and decrease bladder outlet resistance, thereby relieving the symptoms associated with BPH. There are also several **5-α-reductase inhibitors** that can shrink hyperplastic glands and reduce further progression of BPH over the course of several months. Surgical intervention can range from office procedures using transurethral microwave thermotherapy (**TUMT**) to hospital-based procedures such as transurethral resection of the prostate (**TURP**) or the newer and less invasive photovaporization of the prostate (**PVP**).

Urolithiasis

Stone disease can further be characterized by location of the stone in the kidney (nephrolithiasis), ureter, or bladder. A **noncontrast CT** of the abdomen and pelvis combined with the patient's physical examination and laboratory findings provide the clinician with enough information to determine whether acute intervention needs to occur. In patients with a high-grade obstruction, infection, or any complicating medical problem (i.e., diabetes or solitary kidney), early intervention in the form of **cystoscopy** with retrograde pyelography and ureteral stent placement is indicated to allow drainage of the affected side. An alternative to stent placement is **percutaneous nephrostomy** tube placement performed by an interventional radiologist. This external form of drainage through the patient's back is considered when stent placement is unsuccessful or cannot be performed. While each of these techniques can provide urinary drainage, neither definitively treats the stone.

Initial stone management in the inpatient setting involves vigorous fluid resuscitation, **analgesics** (usually in the form of narcotics), **antibiotics** as indicated, and the straining of urine for stones. For the otherwise healthy individual with an acute stone of less than 5 mm in diameter, outpatient management is appropriate. Patients are encouraged to drink plenty of **fluids**, strain their urine to catch the stone, and save the stone for analysis. Order an adequate supply of oral analgesics. Follow-up includes interval imaging to monitor progress of the stone passage. Patients with stones larger than 5 mm are less likely to pass their stone spontaneously and should therefore be considered for elective intervention.

Definitive stone management usually occurs in the outpatient setting and is overseen by a urologist. Intervention may involve **extracorporeal shockwave lithotripsy** (ESWL) or ureteroscopy with laser lithotripsy. Pregnant patients with renal colic and microscopic hematuria present with a diagnostic challenge due to concerns of fetal radiation with diagnostic testing. Additionally, such patients often have some degree of physiologic right-sided hydronephrosis caused by partial compression by the gravid uterus. A **plain abdominal film** and renal **ultrasonography** are the initial imaging studies of choice. In the second and third trimesters, a tailored IVP (scout, 30-second film, and 20-minute film) provides excellent imaging with minimal fetal risk. Approximately 65%–80% of pregnant women will pass stones spontaneously. Should conservative measures fail, **ureteral stent** placement under fluoroscopic guidance is a safe option. Because of the increased risk of encrustation, stents must be replaced every 6–8 weeks until definitive treatment of the stone can be undertaken. Patients may continue to have symptoms, and, if intolerable, **percutaneous nephrostomy** placement should be entertained.

Transitional Cell Carcinoma

Cancer of the bladder is the second most common cancer of the genitourinary tract. Nearly all tumors arising from the bladder urothelium are transitional cells in origin. In general, smokers have approximately a three to fivefold increased risk of bladder cancer than nonsmokers, and the association seems to be dose related. Hematuria (gross or microscopic) is the presenting symptom in 85%–90% of patients with bladder cancer. Cytology should be ordered in any patient suspicious for having bladder cancer.

Initial management of bladder tumors involves **cystoscopy** with transurethral resection of the tumor under anesthesia. Random bladder **biopsies** are generally performed to evaluate for the presence of microscopic disease. **Treatment** of TCC is dependent on the stage of the tumor. Tumors not invading the bladder detrusor muscle are effectively treated with transurethral resection and surveillance. Patients with residual papillary tumors, carcinoma in situ, tumors invading the lamina propria, or those who experience superficial tumor recurrence should be considered for intravesicle therapy. **Bacille Calmette–Guerin** (BCG) (immunotherapy) or **mitomycin C** (chemotherapy) are the most commonly employed agents. These are instilled intravesically via Foley catheter in the office setting as an outpatient. Both have been shown to decrease rates of recurrence. Following initial treatment, patients are placed on strict surveillance regimens including cystoscopy and cytology every 3 months for 1–2 years, every 6 months for an additional 2 years, and annually thereafter. Muscle-invasive bladder tumors are initially treated with **transurethral resection**. Most patients with muscle-invasive tumors will be treated with cystectomy and urinary diversion. **Partial cystectomy** may be considered for solitary invasive tumors in a location such as the dome of the bladder where adequate margins can be obtained. Metastatic disease usually is treated with a chemotherapy combination, such as methotrexate, vinblastin, doxorubicin, and cisplatin (MVAC). Radiation is also used, both on a palliative basis and occasionally as a definitive therapy with salvage cystectomy. Five-year survival rates following cystectomy are approximately 50%.

Adenocarcinoma of the Prostate (Prostate Cancer)

Prostate cancer is a common problem among elderly men; rarely does it cause hematuria in its initial presentation. Usually, the diagnosis of prostate cancer is made by a high **PSA level** during routine screening or an abnormal prostate on **DRE**. As with BPH, clinical evidence of prostate cancer warrants a serum PSA level and follow-up with a urologist. Additional tests (including a prostate biopsy and advanced imaging studies) are often performed by the urologist to definitively diagnosis the patient and formulate a treatment plan. Treatment of prostate cancer is beyond the scope of this book and, therefore, will not be discussed here. However, it is important to remember the prostate as a potential cause for hematuria, especially in elderly males.

Acute Pyelonephritis

Pyelonephritis is a clinical syndrome of chills, fever, and flank pain because of a bacterial infection of the renal parenchyma and pelvis. The most common causative organisms are **E. coli** and **enterococci**. Infection usually results from bacteria ascending from the lower urinary tract. Cultures (both urine and blood) are paramount in the diagnosis as well as treatment assessment. For patients requiring hospitalization, **intravenous antibiotics** should be started immediately after cultures have been sent. A common choice for empiric treatment is a quinolone or ampicillin with gentamicin for adequate coverage of both Gram-negative and Gram -positive organisms. Antibiotic adjustments can then be made once the sensitivities return.

Another crucial aspect in the management of a patient with pyelonephritis is a form of **upper tract imaging** (either renal ultrasound or CT scan of the abdomen and pelvis) to rule out possibility of obstruction. If **hydronephrosis** is found, the obstruction must be relieved (either by retrograde placement of a **ureteral stent** by an urologist or a **percutaneous nephrostomy** tube placed by an interventional radiologist). The decision to proceed with a specific form of drainage depends on the cause of obstruction, available resources, patient preference, and anesthesia risk. Patients treated for **pyelonephritis** will often have persistent fevers for several days, despite appropriate antibiotic therapy and sterile urine. Clinically, patients experience a continued "saw-tooth" pattern of temperature spikes; however, the frequency and severity should decrease. If symptoms have not resolved or the urine remains infected, reimaging may be warranted to rule out possibility of an abscess or obstruction. If the patient remains afebrile for 24–48 hours, he or she may be switched to PO antibiotics for an additional 2–3 weeks, depending on the severity of infection and coexisting conditions. A follow-up urinalysis and culture should be obtained to ensure adequate treatment.

Prostatitis

Classify prostate infection as acute or chronic and bacterial or nonbacterial. Of these, hematuria is associated with **acute bacterial prostatitis**, an inflammation of the prostate associated with a UTI. It is the most common urologic diagnosis in men younger than 50 years of age. Signs and symptoms are consistent with inflammation and/or infection of the prostate gland and include fever, dysuria, perineal pain, urinary frequency, and positive urine cultures. Clinically, the prostate is **tender** and **boggy**. Treatment with antibiotics is essential in the management of acute prostatitis. Empiric therapy directed against gram-negative bacteria and enterococci should be instituted immediately, while awaiting the culture results. Either trimethoprim or fluoroquinolones have high drug penetration into prostatic tissue and are recommended for 4–6 weeks. The long duration of antibiotic treatment is to allow the complete sterilization of the prostatic tissue to prevent complications such as chronic prostatitis and abscess formation.

Patients who have sepsis are immunocompromised and are in acute urinary retention, or who have significant medical comorbidities often benefit from hospitalization and treatment with IV antibiotics. Ampicillin and an aminoglycoside provide effective therapy against both gram-negative bacteria and enterococci. Transurethral catheterization is contraindicated in such patients with urinary retention; suprapubic catheter placement should be performed instead.

Renal Cell Carcinoma

RCC accounts for roughly 3% of adult malignancies but 90% of primary malignancies of the kidney. Commonly, individuals with RCC are diagnosed between 40 and 60 years of age. RCC is typically **unilateral**. Pain, hematuria, and **flank mass** comprise the classic triad of presenting symptoms of RCC. However, this constellation is rarely seen today and, if present, usually indicates advanced disease.

Hematuria is the most common presenting sign, occurring in 60% of patients with a renal tumor. With the variety of complaints these days, most renal masses are discovered incidentally. The diagnosis of RCC is usually based on radiographic findings. CT scanning with and without intravenous contrast is the method of choice for detecting and staging RCC. CT assessment of the renal vein and inferior vena cava, adrenal glands, and regional lymph nodes, as well as evaluation of the liver and lungs for distant metastases, is necessary for staging. **Surgical removal** of the early-stage lesion remains the only potentially curative therapy available for RCC patients. Following treatment, the disease-specific cancer survival rates are tightly linked to the tumor stage. Tumors less than 4 cm are associated with a disease-free survival approaching 100% at 5 years.

Partial nephrectomy and **wedge resection** with an adequate margin of normal parenchyma are now largely employed as a nephron-sparing option for tumors <4 cm. Larger and more invasive tumors are associated with lower rates of cancer-free survival. **Radical nephrectomy** is the gold standard for treatment of clinically localized RCC. Radical nephrectomy entails the removal of the kidney and its enveloping fascia (Gerota's fascia), including the ipsilateral adrenal, proximal ureter, and lymph nodes to the area of transection of the renal vessels. Renal artery embolization has been used both as a surgical adjunct for radical nephrectomy in the preoperative setting and as a palliative treatment in patients with nonresectable tumors and significant symptoms. In select patients with metastatic disease, **palliative nephrectomy** can be undertaken to minimize severe hemorrhage, pain, or paraneoplastic syndromes. Immunotherapy has shown promise in cases of advanced disease, but, unfortunately, radiation therapy, chemotherapy, and hormonal therapy have not been shown to influence overall survival in patients with advanced disease. Metastatic RCC has a natural history that is typically aggressive and rapidly progressive, with 5-year survival rates typically less than 10%.

FIGURE 23-2
Insertion of a Bladder Catheter

Urethral catheterization may be performed for diagnostic or therapeutic indications. Familiarity with the anatomy of the urethra (both males and females) and with the catheters that are available will increase the ease and success of bladder catheterization. Catheter size is noted in French. As the number increases, the size increases. A commonly used adult catheter size is 16 French.

With the patient in the supine position, cleanse the urethral meatus and the surrounding area with an antiseptic solution and isolate the genitalia with sterile drapes or towels. Wearing sterile gloves, instill 10 cc water-soluble lubricant (or 2% lidocaine jelly, if available) into the urethra. For female patients, insert the Foley catheter into the urethra and allow the catheter to follow the normal course of the urethra.s Watch for urine return and pass the catheter an additional 2–3 inches into the urethra to ensure adequate placement in the bladder. Then, inflate the balloon with 10 cc of sterile water per the balloon port. The catheter may then be pulled outward until the balloon is resting against the bladder neck.

For males, the catheter should be passed the full length of the tubing until the junction of the catheter and inflation port for the balloon is resting against the patient's urethral meatus. This is done to ensure that the balloon will be inflated in the patient's bladder and not in his urethra. Urine return should be noted prior to balloon inflation. If the balloon does not inflate easily or if the patient experiences discomfort as the balloon is being inflated, you should stop and reposition the catheter. Once the balloon has successfully been inflated, pull it gently down against the bladder neck.

For male patients older than 50 years, a Coudé tip catheter may be needed. These catheters are similar to standard straight Foley catheters, except that the terminal 2 inches are curved upward. The curve of the catheter should be directed at the 12 o'clock position, which allows the catheter to glide over an enlarged median lobe of the prostate or an elevated bladder neck. If the catheter does not pass easily, it should be removed and the process repeated. *Do not, however, force the catheter, as creation of a false passage can occur.* If you cannot pass a 16 French Foley or Coudé catheter into the male urethra, there is usually a urethral stricture, bladder neck stenosis, or very large median lobe of the prostate. In such a case, you may consider using a 12 French catheter. If however, this proves unsuccessful, a urology consultation is advised.

Once the catheter is in place and the balloon is inflated, drainage tubing and a drainage bag should be connected to the catheter's drainage port. Remember to secure the patient's catheter in a tension-free manner to his or her upper thigh with a catheter-securing device or tape. Monitor and record the initial amount and character of urine obtained with catheter placement.

Genitourinary Injury

In the 1% of these additional possible causes for hematuria, genitourinary trauma is by far the most serious. **Trauma to the kidney** in hemodynamically stable patients presenting with a history of blunt or penetrating injury to the torso and hematuria should undergo immediate imaging, usually in the form of a CT scan with intravenous contrast. Management strategies depend on the extent of parenchymal and/or vascular injury; however, there has been an increasing trend toward conservative management of most blunt renal trauma. Penetrating trauma involving the kidney generally requires **surgical exploration**. When appropriate, renal unit salvage with **debridement** and reconstruction should be considered.

Ureteral injury usually occurs as a result of surgical misadventure. However, occasionally penetrating trauma will involve the ureter. Hematuria is variably present, and therefore a high suspicion is key to making the diagnosis. Contusions or incomplete tears can often be managed with ureteral stenting. More extensive injuries will require debridement and **ureteral reanastomosis** or **reimplantation** into the bladder.

Bladder or urethral injury is suggested by evidence of a pelvic fracture, blood at the urethral meatus, or displacement of the prostate on DRE. Hematuria is present in almost 100% of lower urinary tract injuries, with gross hematuria occurring >90% of the time. Diagnosis requires a cystogram, obtained by filling the bladder with 300–400 cc of dilute contrast via Foley catheter under fluoroscopic evaluation. Intraperitoneal bladder ruptures require surgical exploration, repair, and urinary diversion. Extraperitoneal bladder injuries can usually be managed conservatively with Foley catheter drainage for 7–10 days and a follow-up cystogram prior to Foley removal (Figure 23-2).

Urethral injuries are relatively rare and are usually only associated with straddle-type injuries. **Blood at the meatus** is often present. Any suspicion of a urethral injury should prompt retrograde urethrography prior to any attempts at Foley catheter placement. If there is any evidence of contrast extravasation, a urology consult should be obtained. Successful placement of a urethral catheter with urinary drainage for 2–3 weeks is often sufficient to allow healing of the urethral injury. Complete disruptions may require **suprapubic tube** placement and delayed repair of the primary injury. Subsequent urethral stricture formation is a common long-term complication.

Selected Readings

James RE, Palleschi JR. Bladder catheterization. In: Pfenninger JL, Fowler GC, eds. *Procedures for Primary Care Physicians*. Philadelphia: Mosby; 1994:495–499.

Macfarlane MT. *House Officer Series: Urology*. 3rd ed. Louisville, KY: Lippincott, Williams, and Wilkins; 1998.

Resnick MI, Schaeffer AJ. In: Sahn SA, Heffner JE, eds. *Urology Pearls*. Philadelphia: Hanley & Belfus; 2000.

Rosenstein D, McAninch JW. Urologic emergencies. In: Resnick MI, ed. *Medical Clinics of North America*. Vol 88. No 2. Philadelphia: Saunders; 2004:495–518.

Tanagho EA, McAninch JW, eds. *Smith's General Urology*. 16th ed. New York: McGraw-Hill; 2004.

Yun EJ, Meng MV, Carroll PR. Evaluation of the patient with hematuria. In: Resnick MI, ed. *Medical Clinics of North America*. Vol 88. No 2. Philadelphia: Saunders; 2004:329–334.

24

Scrotal Pain

Courtney C. Morton, MPA, PA-C ■ *C. William Schwab II, MD*

Key Points

■ Acute scrotal pain, also termed as the "acute scrotum," represents a true urologic emergency. Indecisive action or delay in care may result in substantial morbidity or mortality.

■ The importance of the initial evaluation remains the most powerful tool in correctly diagnosing and treating the acute scrotum. The primary distinction that needs to be made in any case of acute scrotal pain is testicular torsion versus nontorsion.

■ The most important differential diagnoses in acute scrotal pain are testicular torsion, epididymitis/orchitis, torsion of the appendix testis, and necrotizing fasciitis/Fournier's gangrene.

■ If testicular torsion or Fournier's gangrene is suspected, an immediate urologic consultation should be obtained to expedite surgical intervention.

■ HISTORY

Use **age** is a useful indicator of potential etiologies for a patient's acute scrotal pain. Torsion of the appendix testis is the most common cause of scrotal pain in children aged 2–10 years. Testicular torsion, a much more serious condition, tends to occur in early childhood and preadolescence (ages 12–18 years). Acute epididymitis, on the other hand, occurs more frequently in postadolescent males, correlating with increased sexual activity.

Elicit from the patient the **onset** and **duration** of symptoms and a history of **similar symptoms**. Testicular torsion usually begins suddenly, whereas torsion of the appendix testis and epididymitis present with a more gradual onset of pain. One-third of boys with testicular torsion report previous episodes of scrotal pain. This is thought to be secondary to intermittent torsion and spontaneous detorsion.

Enquire as to whether or not there was a **precipitating event** to the onset of pain. A history of forceful trauma should raise suspicion for testicular rupture. Assess for **associated symptoms** (dysuria, urgency, frequency, etc.) that may point to an infectious or inflammatory cause such as epididymitis. Nausea and vomiting seem to be more specific for torsion than epididymitis.

■ PHYSICAL EXAMINATION

The **scrotum** and its contents should first be inspected to determine the presence of any scrotal edema, erythema, or ecchymosis. Inguinal fullness, suggesting the presence of an inguinal hernia, should also be noted. Documentation of the position, axis, and lie of the testicle can provide important clues to the underlying cause. A torsed testis tends to lie high in the scrotum and may have a more horizontal orientation of its superior–inferior axis. Conversely, in acute epididymitis, the testicle has a normal lie and axis. Presence of urethral discharge or any scrotal rashes should also be noted. Before palpating the testicles, evaluate the **cremasteric reflex** by lightly stroking the superomedial aspect of the patient's thigh. An intact cremasteric reflex results in brisk retraction of the testicle on that side. Absence of this reflex is highly sensitive for testicular torsion. **Palpate** the testis, noting size, uniformity, and location of tenderness. A torsed testis is usually enlarged because of venous congestion and, as a result, diffusely tender to palpation.

In contrast, epididymitis tends to produce more localized pain in the superior pole of the testis or at the head of the epididymis. A torsed appendix testis typically produces focal point tenderness at the head of the epididymis. Traditional teaching describes the **"Phren's sign"** as a way to differentiate between epididymitis and testicular torsion. Historically thought to be indicative of epididymitis, patients with a "positive" Phren's sign experience temporary relief of scrotal pain with elevation of the scrotum. Research has shown that this finding is **not reliable** and must **not** be considered a definitive way to diagnose a patient with either torsion or epididymitis. Another physical examination finding related to scrotal pain is the **"blue dot sign."** This infrequent finding is actually the torsed and necrotic **appendix testis** and is pathognomonic for torsion of the appendix testis. If present, this tiny blue spot can be seen through the patient's skin on the upper pole of the testicle.

■ LABORATORY STUDIES

Order routine laboratory examinations such as a **urinalysis** and a **urine culture**. If an infectious etiology is suspected, a **CBC** may be helpful. Presence of pyuria or bacteriuria on urinalysis suggests epididymitis. In the case of torsion, the urinalysis is often normal. Sexually active men should have **urethral cultures** sent for evaluation of gonococcal and nongonococcal urethritis, especially if urethral discharge is noted.

■ RADIOGRAPHIC STUDIES

The dominant form of imaging for cases of acute scrotal pain is **duplex scrotal ultrasonography**. Although dependent on the operator's level of experience, color doppler ultrasound is close to 90% sensitive in detecting scrotal pathology. Findings can identify blood flow to the affected testis, enlargement or increased flow suggesting inflammation, enlargement of the epididymitis, collections of blood within the testicle or scrotum, and the integrity of the testicular capsule. Of note, if the testicle is torsed less than 360 degrees, a color Doppler ultrasound can be normal.

■ DIAGNOSTIC PLAN

Patients with acute scrotal pain are assessed as quickly as possible to minimize serious consequences to the patient. Three etiologies of acute scrotal pain that require immediate surgical intervention are testicular torsion, Fournier's gangrene, and testicular rupture. If one of these diagnoses is suspected based on patients' history or physical examination, a urologic consultation should be called immediately. Accordingly, the patients should be prepped for surgery by restricting their PO intake and initiating a broad-spectrum antibiotic.

In the case of acute scrotal pain, it is critical to point out that ultrasonography should in no way take the place of or obviate the clinical examination. Moreover, radiologic imaging is *not* indicated in cases where obtaining the images would cause a delay in treatment. Thus, if the clinical diagnosis strongly suggests testicular torsion, urologic consultation and expeditious surgical exploration are the most appropriate next steps.

Involve the general surgeon in addition to the urologist if the patients exhibit signs or symptoms to suggest perirectal involvement of their scrotal pain.

■ DIFFERENTIAL DIAGNOSIS AND TREATMENT

Epididymitis and Orchitis

Acute epididymitis is an infection of the epididymis acquired by retrograde spread of organisms down the vas from the urethra or bladder. It is the most frequent cause of acute scrotal pain in postadolescents. Patients normally present with heaviness and a dull, aching discomfort in the affected hemiscrotum, which can radiate up to the flank. The epididymis is usually **tender** and **indurated** in the early stages of the infection. Later, orchitis may make the testicle more tender or produce a reactive hydrocele. Fever and chills may be present in severe cases. A scrotal ultrasound with Doppler reveals normal to increased blood flow to the testis and epididymis. The most common causes of epididymitis or orchitis in sexually active patients younger than 35 years are **gonorrhea** and **Chlamydia**. Conversely, in children and in males older than 35 years, *Escherichia coli* is the most common cause. Antibiotic selection is based on the most likely causative organism: intramuscular ceftriaxone plus a course of doxycycline for suspected sexually transmitted infection or a 3-week course of an oral fluoroquinolone for a presumed *E. coli* infection. A urine culture, and if appropriate, a urethral culture should be sent and antibiotics adjusted as appropriate. Patients should also be encouraged to utilize bedrest and scrotal elevation. Analgesics are usually necessary in the acute phase. NSAIDs can be very effective. It is important to educate patients that complete resolution of pain and swelling may take several weeks to months. Abscess formation can complicate a prolonged, untreated episode of epididymitis. This is clinically suggested by scrotal fluctuance or fixation of the testicle to the scrotal wall.

Trauma

Injury to the testes and scrotum may result from either blunt or penetrating insults. Direct blows to the testicle (as in the case of assault or certain sports-related injuries) can cause rupture of the fibrous tunica albuginea, which surrounds the testicle causing what is known as "testicular fracture." Clinical findings are usually nonspecific and include scrotal pain and a swollen, ecchymotic scrotum. Because of rapid expansion of the scrotal hematoma, it is often difficult to appreciate the testicular contour on physical examination. Although scrotal imaging may serve as a useful adjunct to the physical examination in cases of suspected testis trauma, the definitive diagnosis is made surgically. Early scrotal exploration and repair of testicular rupture result in the highest testis salvage rates. Scrotal contusions, which do not rupture the tunica, can be treated conservatively.

Testicular Torsion

This refers to a twisting of the testis and spermatic cord around its vertical axis, causing venous obstruction, progressive swelling, arterial compromise, and eventual testicular infarction (Figure 24-1). Although testicular torsion is not the most common cause of the acute scrotum, it should be highest in the differential diagnosis because testicular viability is inversely related to the amount of time it is ischemic. Salvage of testicular parenchyma and function is highest in patients whose testicles are detorsed within **6 hours** of the onset of pain. However, beyond 12 hours, the salvage rates drop below 20%. A thorough but efficient physical examination is crucial in this condition. Certain details in the history, such as adolescent age, acute onset, nausea, vomiting, and a history of prior episodes, are particularly suggestive of torsion. Additionally, the episode is typically preceded by a history of trauma, exercise, or sexual activity.

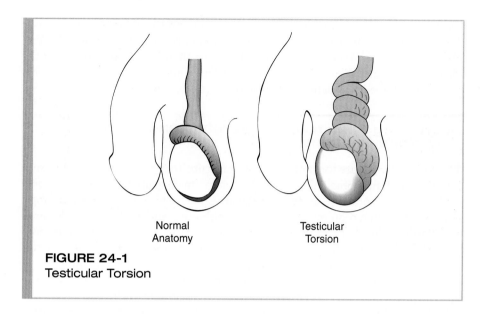

Normal
Anatomy

Testicular
Torsion

FIGURE 24-1
Testicular Torsion

If testicular torsion is suspected by evidence of an abnormally high, horizontal lying testicle, a urologic consultation should immediately be obtained, so as to expedite the time to surgical intervention. **Manual detorsion** can be attempted while awaiting surgical intervention. This is performed by externally rotating the testicle from medial to lateral on its vertical axis. Classically, this maneuver is described as "opening a book." If detorsion is successful, patients will experience relief of their pain. Beware, not all testicles will torse laterally and some torse more than 360 degrees. Such testicles will not have blood flow reestablished by manual detorsion. Regardless, all patients with torsion should proceed with surgical intervention to secure the testicles to the scrotal wall, in an effort to prevent future recurrent torsion. Some studies have shown that cooling the torsed testis with an ice pack while awaiting surgery can decrease the degree of ischemia. **Surgical exploration** involves a scrotal incision through which the affected testicle is visualized and then detorsed. Its viability is assessed after the contralateral testicle is anchored to the scrotal wall, thus preventing future episodes of torsion on that side. If the affected testicle is deemed viable, it too undergoes an orchiopexy to the scrotal wall. Testicles deemed unviable are removed (orchiectomy).

Torsion of Appendix Testis

It is an embryologic remnant of the mullerian duct and sits on the upper pole of the testis. It, like the testis itself, has the ability to twist and infarct. Although the blue dot sign may be visible early in the process, it is eventually obscured by edema and erythema. There are rarely any voiding complaints or fevers associated with this condition. Doppler ultrasound usually shows normal testicular blood flow with a small hyperechoic area adjacent to the testis. Once the diagnosis is definitively made, management of a torsed appendix testis is nonoperative with use of analgesics and scrotal support. If, however, there is any question about the diagnosis, an immediate urologic consultation should be obtained for possible surgical exploration to definitively rule out testicular torsion.

Necrotizing Fasciitis of the Scrotum and Perineum (Fournier's Gangrene)

This is a relatively rare form of necrotizing fasciitis that presents as a progressive, fulminant polymicrobial infection involving the male genitalia, most commonly arising in the skin of the urethral or rectal regions. This condition is a **urologic emergency**, which requires resuscitation, antibiotics, and aggressive, wide surgical debridement of the involved skin and subcutaneous tissue. Mortality rates average 30%, with higher mortalities in those patients with predisposing factors such as diabetes mellitus, immunosuppression, or chronic alcohol abuse.

On physical examination, patients usually present with early systemic toxicity. The genital examination may be limited to induration of the penis or scrotal skin early in the course of the infection; however, with progression, erythema and crepitus may extend over the perineum and abdominal wall. Often, a foul, feculent odor may be present. A plain film of the abdomen or CT may demonstrate air within the soft tissues. Initial treatment includes rapid **fluid resuscitation** and broad-spectrum **antibiotic coverage** (usually ampicillin, gentamicin, and metronidazole), followed by immediate, aggressive **surgical debridement** of all involved tissues. At the time of surgical debridement, **fecal diversion** (via a diverting colostomy) or **urinary diversion** (by means of a suprapubic tube) may be necessitated, depending on colonic or urethral involvement. The wound is usually packed open, with a second surgical look and debridement occurring within 24–48 hours. Strict local wound care is necessary on a BID or TID basis. **Hyperbaric oxygen** therapy may be of benefit, if available. Strict control of diabetes and adequate nutrition are essential to wound healing.

Other Etiologies of Scrotal Pain

An **incarcerated inguinal hernia** is evidenced by a scrotal mass, which is often accompanied by signs or symptoms of intestinal obstruction. A **testicular tumor** is only acutely painful, if there has been hemorrhage into the tumor. A **varicocele** rarely presents with acute pain unless there is acute thrombus. **Henoch–Schonlein purpura** is a systemic vasculitis seen in young children, which sometimes can cause scrotal pain.

Selected Readings

James RE, Palleschi JR. Bladder catheterization. In Pfenninger JL, Fowler GC, eds. *Procedures for Primary Care Physicians*. Philadelphia: Mosby; 1994:495–499.

Macfarlane MT. *House Officer Series: Urology*. 3rd ed. Louisville, KY: Lippincott, Williams, and Wilkins; 1998.

Resnick MI, Schaeffer AJ. In: Sahn SA, Heffner JE, eds. *Urology Pearls*. Philadelphia: Hanley & Belfus. 2000.

Rosenstein D, McAninch JW. Urologic emergencies. In: Resnick MI, ed. *Medical Clinics of North America*. Vol 88. No 2. Philadelphia: Saunders; 2004:495–518.

Tanagho EA, McAninch JW, eds. *Smith's General Urology*. 16th ed. New York: McGraw-Hill; 2004.

Yun EJ, Meng MV, Carroll PR. Evaluation of the patient with hematuria. In: Resnick MI, ed. *Medical Clinics of North America*. Vol 88. No 2. Philadelphia: Saunders; 2004:329–343.

25

Obesity

Mary E. Haskell, APN, TNS ■ *J. Stephen Marshall, MD, FACS*

Key Points

- The problem of morbid obesity and the diseases caused by morbid obesity has increased markedly across the world. The lack of significant long-term weight loss by dietary therapy has led to the development of bariatric surgery, the surgery to cause loss of weight.

- Surgery should be considered an adjunct to weight loss, not a replacement for good eating habits.

- Today, in the United States, there are three common options for surgically induced weight loss. These include the Roux-en-Y gastric bypass, the laparoscopic adjustable gastric band, and the biliopancreatic diversion (BPD) with or without duodenal switch (DS).

- Surgical weight-loss methods can be classified as restrictive, malabsorptive, or a combination of these methods.

- Restrictive methods, such as the laparoscopic adjustable gastric band, promote early satiety, with the resulting intake of fewer calories.

- Malabsorptive procedures do not restrict the intake of food as drastically as restrictive procedures, but because of the rearrangement of the normal intestinal anatomy do not allow for absorption of the calories into the system. The BPD with or without DS is an example of a primarily malabsorptive procedure, and the Roux-en-Y gastric bypass is a combination of the two procedures.

- Because of the significant life style changes required and the risk that may occur as a result of the surgery, the process of preparing the bariatric patient is important.

- Morbidly obese patients have an increased risk of developing deep venous thrombosis (DVT) with subsequent pulmonary embolus (PE).

- There are complications in the perioperative phase that may include leaks and bleeding. In the late phases of recovery, complications include hernia and inadequate weight loss.

- Obese patients provide a challenge for the nursing staff. Extra staffing is required, as well as assistive devices and equipment designed for obese patients, to ensure proper care.

■ PREOPERATIVE CARE

Candidates for bariatric surgery are those who are considered **morbidly obese**. Patients are considered for surgery if their body mass index (BMI) is greater than 40 or greater than 35 with other comorbid conditions caused by obesity, such as type II diabetes, hypertension, or obstructive sleep apnea (OSA). **BMI is** calculated by dividing the weight in kilograms by the height in meters squared $(BMI = Wt \ (kg)/Ht^2 \ (m^2))$

Patients are introduced to an educational program that helps them understand their disease and the **goal of surgery**, which is the creation of tools to help modify their life and improve their health. This program introduces them to the **dietary changes** that will be required for successful weight loss, as well as exercise education. Patients are also required to attend **support group** meetings where they can meet people who have had bariatric surgery.

Elicit a thorough **medical history** to identify and characterize all preexisting conditions. Especially important is respiratory function including reactive airway disease or sleep apnea, exercise tolerance, previously diagnosed heart disease, and previous venous thrombosis.

Perform a **physical examination** in conjunction with a surgeon and an advanced practice nurse. Identify possible challenges to successful surgery such as previous abdominal surgery scars, potential airway problems, venous stasis disease of the legs, and existing decubitus lesions.

Consider radiographic studies such as an **upper GI series** to define existing anatomy or a gallbladder **ultrasound** to determine if cholelithiasis needs to be addressed at the time of surgery. A preoperative **CXR** will identify pleural lesions and set a baseline for postoperative care.

Order standard preoperative laboratory studies including a **CBC** to document the initial hemoglobin and to rule out platelet disorders. The **PT** and **PTT** are checked and corrected if needed. All patients should have a **thyroid** profile and a *Helicobacter pylori* screen to guide preoperative treatment if required.

If symptoms indicate, **consult** with a cardiologist, pulmonologist, or sleep specialist for sleep apnea symptoms. Arrange for a **psychological screening** to detect behavior patterns that may impede success of bariatric surgery. Some examples of this are schizophrenia, untreated depression, addictive behavior, or an educational handicap.

In the immediate preoperative period, administer a prophylactic dose of a broad-spectrum **antibiotic**. Begin prophylaxis for DVT with pneumatic antiembolic devices, low-molecular-weight **heparin (LMWH)**, and inferior vena cava (IVC) filters when indicated.

DVT Prophylaxis

The morbidly obese patient has several factors that contribute to the development of DVT. Virchow described the triad of venous injury, hypercoagulability, and venous stasis as leading to the development of venous thrombosis. The morbidly obese patient often has several of these factors as a result of the obese state. It has been shown that obese patients may have an associated chronic inflammatory condition. This condition along with elevated levels of estrogen can contribute to a **hypercoagulable state**. The veins of the lower extremity often suffer intimal damage from chronic venous insufficiency. Venous stasis can be caused in some patients simply because their obesity decreases their mobility.

The best treatment of DVT and PE is prevention. Consider one of several regimens that are available. These include the administration of LMWH preoperatively, the use of **sequential compression devices**, and the early institution (within 12 hours postoperatively) of ambulation.

The **dosing** of LMWH is not standardized. Most surgeons feel that some form of LMWH is indicated and the minor risk of bleeding complications is less than the consequence of DVT/PE.

The recent introduction of temporary **IVC filters** has made it possible to offer certain patients who are at high risk of PE, another level of PE prophylaxis. Placement of IVC filters should be predicated on history. A history of **previous PE or DVT** is an indication for IVC filter placement, as is a prior history or **family history** of coagulation disorders. Patients with **pulmonary hypertension** or hypoxia who cannot tolerate a small decrease in oxygenation should be considered candidates for IVC filter placement. **Venous stasis**, as evidenced by brawny indurations or history of venous-stasis ulcers, may indicate damaged veins that are more susceptible to thrombosis, which should prompt consideration of placement of IVC filters. None of these indications is absolute but should prompt concern about the increased risk of a PE.

The obese patient who is in a postoperative condition may experience a prolonged period of immobility. It is a matter of debate whether anticoagulation for several weeks postoperatively would benefit these patients. To date, no conclusive evidence mandates this practice.

■ OPERATIVE PLAN

There are three bariatric procedures in wide use. The **laparoscopic adjustable gastric band** (Figure 25-1) is a silastic ring with an inner balloon that is placed around the top of the stomach just distal to the gastroesophageal junction. The balloon is connected to a subcutaneously placed port by a catheter, which will allow filling of the balloon. This becomes necessary as the postoperative edema dissipates and the patient begins to lose fat from around the stomach. The band system is a purely restrictive procedure, which should be used to help the patient achieve early satiety, thereby making it easier for the patient to make healthy food choices.

The Biliopancreatic Diversion (BPD) with or without Duodenal Switch (DS) is, as mentioned above, primarily a malabsorptive procedure. While the stomach

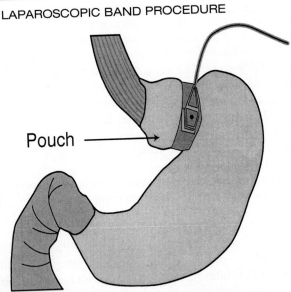

LAPAROSCOPIC BAND PROCEDURE

Pouch

FIGURE 25-1
A Band Placed Around the Proximal Stomach to Produce Early Satiety

By way of a laparoscopic or laparotomy approach, a silastic band is placed around the proximal stomach, creating a very small area of the stomach that is stretched as food is eaten. This results in early satiety. The band is connected to a subcutaneously placed port (not shown) by the catheter shown in the diagram. Thus, the band can be inflated and deflated to allow the right amount of restriction, without causing complete obstruction.

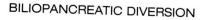

BILIOPANCREATIC DIVERSION

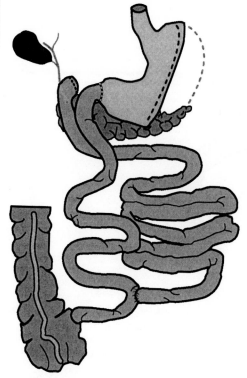

FIGURE 25-2
Anatomic Reconstruction after the Biliopancreatic Diversion

The BPD consists of a sleeve gastrectomy, which creates early satiety. The duodenum is then transected with an anastomosis of the stomach to the small bowel limb. The divided small bowel is then anastomosed to the ileum, resulting in a short common channel and a short alimentary channel. This results in malabsorption of food.

size is altered to decrease the intake of food, the resulting size of the stomach is not as small as that with restrictive procedures (Figure 25-2). The BPD/DS incorporates a very short length of common channel small bowel. The common channel is that part of the intestine that has both food and biliary pancreatic fluid and enzymes. This then results in less time for exposure of food to the digestion process and a resultant decrease in absorption of nutrients.

The Roux-en-Y **gastric bypass** has been described as a combination procedure (Figure 25-3). It is probably more restrictive than malabsorptive. The small pouch created in the operation creates early satiety. The roux limb is created to bypass the stomach and results in some phenomena that contribute to weight loss. If a patient eats food with a high osmotic load (typically a food high in simple sugars and not recommended for the diet), the small gastric pouch cannot dilute

GASTRIC BYPASS

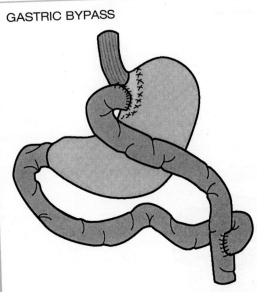

FIGURE 25-3
Reconstruction after a Roux-en-Y Gastric Bypass

The procedure can be accomplished laparoscopically or by way of an exploratory laparotomy. The stomach is stapled or divided near the esophagus, resulting in a very small pouch (15–30 cc). The small bowel is then divided, and the roux limb is anastomosed to the stomach pouch. The proximal limb of the divided small bowel is then connected to the roux limb to restore bowel continuity.

this to the usual iso-osmotic load that is delivered to the jejunum. The exposure of the jejunum to this osmotic load results in acute distention of the jejunum, as it secretes fluid to dilute the food. This then causes cramping abdominal pain, hypovolemia, and diarrhea, which characterize the **dumping syndrome**. A decrease in appetite has also been noted in gastric bypass patients. It has also been shown that the hormone **ghrelin**, which contributes to hunger, is markedly decreased in gastric bypass patients. The exact mechanism of this is not well known.

■ POSTOPERATIVE CARE

Pulmonary

Immediately postoperatively, assess the **respiratory function** for a phenomenon called **obesity hypoventilation syndrome** (OSA). The patient's decreased lung and chest wall expansion secondary to increased weight result in decreased functional reserve capacity, decreased expiratory reserve volume, and retained CO_2. Take measures to promote ventilation including **head elevation** 30–45 degrees to improve their tidal volumes and promote adequate oxygenation. This position also reduces abdominal pressure on the lungs and promotes ventilation.

Careful attention should be paid to symptoms of **OSA**. OSA involves the partial or complete obstruction of the upper airway, which is associated with decreased oxygen saturations and awakening from sleep. These symptoms include daytime sleepiness, snoring, and symptoms of gastroesophageal reflux disease. Offer continuous positive pressure mask ventilation (**CPAP or BiPAP**) to improve ventilation and comfort. Many patients have this technology at home and are encouraged to bring in their machines for use in the postoperative period. Be prepared for **airway compromise**, including acute obstruction.

The obese patient's neck is often short and wide with excessive oropharyngeal tissue, which provides an extra challenge for intubation. Be prepared for the use of **fiberoptic intubation**, if the need for intubation occurs. In addition, tracheostomy kits are available in case of emergency. Postoperatively, aggressive **pulmonary toilet** is encouraged. Consider hourly use of **incentive spirometry**, continuous oxygen saturation monitoring, and frequent **arterial blood gas** analysis to assess respiratory status.

Cardiovascular

Obese patients have an **increase in circulating blood volume** because of increased blood flow requirements of adipose tissue. This increase in blood volume leads to increased preload, stroke volume, and cardiac output, which, in turn, cause increased myocardial demand. The demand on the heart leads to ventricular dilation and hypertrophy and reduced effectiveness of contractions. The increased myocardial demand puts obese patients at risk of myocardial infarction, congestive heart failure, arrhythmias, and sudden cardiac death. Assess patients postoperatively, with special attention to **vital signs**. Order at least hourly vital signs, which include heart rate, blood pressure, cardiac rhythm, and urine output. Blood pressure should be done with an appropriate-sized cuff, and consideration should be given to placement of the blood pressure cuff, such as considering placing the cuff on the forearm.

More than half of obese patients experience **hypertension** as one of their comorbid conditions. When auscultating heart sounds, it may be necessary to position the patient supine or leaning forward in order to clearly auscultate heart tones. **Hypovolemia**, a serious side effect of bariatric surgery, is evidenced by tachycardia, decreased urine output, and hypotension. Many patients are placed on a clear liquid diet 3 days prior to surgery; this may also contribute to the hypovolemia postoperatively. Electrolytes should also be monitored, since some preoperative bowel preparations may lead to disturbances in the sodium, potassium, and calcium.

Medications

Use special consideration when **dosing medications** in obese patients. Special attention should be given to absorption, distribution, and elimination of medicines.

Many obese patients are malnourished and have low protein stores. **Low protein stores** limit the ability of drug binding and leads to an increased amount of the circulating drug in the body. Obese patients have a greater **percentage of adipose tissue**, a decreased percentage of water in the body and lean body mass. Lipophilic drugs should be calculated on the actual body weight of the patient and may require increased dosing to penetrate the adipose tissue. The increased amount of lipophilic drugs that remain in the adipose tissue will also lead to a **longer half-life** of the drug and a delayed onset of the action of the drug because of decreased blood supply to the adipose tissue. Nonlipophilic drugs should be dosed based on ideal body weight. Use caution when administering medications via the intramuscular route, owing to the increased risk for actually administering the drug into the adipose tissue. If an intramuscular injection is needed, special consideration is given to the length of the needle by using at least a 1½-inch needle.

Postoperative pain control is managed with **patient-controlled analgesia** (PCA). Frequent monitoring for respiratory depression as a side effect of the pain medication should be implemented on all postoperative bariatric patients. All medications administered after bariatric surgery will need to be in **liquid or crushed** form. Conversion of medications to liquid or crushed form should ideally take place before surgery to prevent confusion postoperatively.

Integument

Since obese patients are at an increased risk of **skin breakdown** secondary to decreased vascularity of adipose tissue, frequently assess skin folds of the breasts, back, abdomen, groin, and perineum. Frequently reposition to remove pressure from bony prominences. Use of **powders is discouraged** in obese patients, since the abrasive nature of the powder coupled with the weight of the skin folds can lead to skin breakdown. Skin should be kept as dry as possible, and, if a powder is used, an **antifungal powder** should be used to prevent the accumulation of yeast. It is important to pay special attention to lines and tubing to make sure that they are not trapped in skin folds while repositioning obese patients. Because of the large size of the abdomen, obese patients are more prone to urine and **fecal incontinence**. The abdomen impinging on the bowel and bladder, coupled with the inability to cleanse the perineum owing to size, can lead to skin breakdown. A moisture barrier can be used to prevent further skin breakdown. **Delayed wound healing** is another risk of bariatric surgery. The adipose tissue is poorly vascularized and may affect wound healing. Wound assessment involves detailed documentation of wound edges, color of drainage, odor, and color of tissue. An abdominal binder may be a useful tool to relieve pressure along the wound edges and promote healing.

Nutrition

It is important to appreciate that many obese patients are **malnourished** despite their weight. Fat stores are not readily mobilized as an energy source, which leads to the consumption of protein as the patient's primary energy source. Obese patients are also prone to a syndrome known as a **metabolic syndrome**, which is characterized by insulin resistance, hyperinsulinemia, hyperglycemia, coronary artery disease, hypertension, and hyperlipidemia. Institute a strict diet regimen postoperatively. On day 1, the patient will begin a clear liquid diet of 2 ounces, six times daily. Drinking from a medicine cup may be encouraged to aid the bariatric patient in understanding the capacity of the new stomach. The diet will be advanced to full liquids after 3 days and after 1 week; a pureed diet will be initiated for 4–6 weeks. The bariatric diet consists of a high-protein, low-fat, and low cholesterol diet, with avoidance of simple sugar and carbonated beverages.

Bariatric patients are at risk of **dumping syndrome** (rapid gastric emptying), which is characterized by nausea, weakness, sweating, faintness, cramps, and diarrhea. This dumping syndrome can occur 90 minutes after eating and is caused by food entering the small bowel rapidly without the partial digestion of the food by gastric enzymes. Instruct patients to **eat slowly**, at least 30 minutes for meals three times a day; not to drink during the meal, but rather before or after; and to sit in an upright position after meals. The diet is also supplemented with protein shakes for the first 3 months postoperatively to maintain a diet with 70 g of protein daily. Assess the patient's risk for **vitamin deficiency**. This occurs because the nutrients bypass the duodenum when they are ingested, and the duodenum is the primary source for absorption of these nutrients. Patients are instructed to take a multivitamin with iron and B complex and B12, as well as calcium supplements.

The staff should be educated on proper body technique as well as the use of assistive devices when **repositioning** the obese patients. **Assistive devices** can include larger beds, air-assist transfer devices, mechanical patient lifts, and trapezes. Patients are encouraged to participate as much as possible in their own transfers. Adequate staff are utilized when repositioning the obese patient—at least five people are recommended. Tests should be scheduled during the daytime, so that there is a maximum number of staff available to assist the obese patient in transfers. Postoperatively, bariatric patients are **mobilized** early to prevent complications such as pneumonia and PE. Nursing should expect that the bariatric patient could ambulate as soon as 2 hours postoperatively and frequently thereafter.

Behavioral

Patients often have **low self-esteem** and decreased socialization secondary to disability from their weight, inability to work, and isolation. These issues may lead to **manipulative behaviors** such as refusing to walk and not following the dietary restrictions. Patients may also report feelings of **shame and embarrassment**, which makes it essential for nursing care to be consistent, emotionally supportive, and professional. Obese patients have faced a lifetime of discrimination and bias and may need behavioral therapy to develop skills to identify and modify eating behaviors. **Family participation** is encouraged to enhance compliance with treatment regimens of the postoperative patient. Creation of a **therapeutic partnership** between the nurse and the patient will promote success with the strict treatment regimen of the bariatric patient. Obese patients know that they are difficult to care for, and the therapeutic relationship will alleviate concerns by the patient.

Care of bariatric patients provides many challenges for the hospital as a whole. The hospital must provide **operating room tables** that can accommodate up to 800 pounds. Extra large beds, wheelchairs, commodes, and patient gowns need to be available for these patients. The structure of the facility should include **wall-mounted toilets**, as well as widened door frames and ceiling lifts. Private rooms will provide for privacy and dignity of this population. Many family members of bariatric patients may also be obese, so **extra large furniture** is made available for the visitors. Staff in-service training on the benefits of bariatric surgery and a routine orientation regarding the care of obese patients should be included for all new employees.

■ COMPLICATIONS

Anastomotic Leak

The development of a leak can be a life-threatening event if left untreated. Leaks develop in approximately 2%–5% of gastric bypass patients, with a slightly lower risk in BPD/DS patients and a low risk in band patients. The presence of a new onset of tachycardia must be considered a leak until proven otherwise. Other signs that indicate a leak include tachypnea; decrease in urine output, abdominal or back pain, and acidosis; and a change in mental status or sense of impending doom. Order a **gastrograffin swallow** study or **CT scan** to aid in the diagnosis of a leak. Neither of these tests is 100% accurate, and suspicion of a leak, even in the face of normal radiographic examinations, should prompt surgical exploration. If a leak is discovered at surgery, revision of the anastomosis is ill advised, as this will probably also leak. Options include an attempt to control the leak. The area should be generously drained.

Pulmonary Embolism

PE is a dramatic and potentially life-threatening complication. The signs of a PE often mimic those of a leak. A **spiral CT** is sensitive and specific for making the diagnosis, as is a **ventilation/perfusion scan** (see Chapter 5). Occasionally, a bariatric patient will exceed the limits of the CT equipment. The clinical situation would then dictate whether exploration for a leak or empiric therapy with heparin for a PE is performed.

Postoperative **bleeding** may occur after bariatric surgery. This may present as tachycardia and hypotension, which should prompt surgical exploration. The bariatric patient, particularly the gastric bypass patient, may develop hematemesis. Hematemesis that develops in the immediate postoperative period is typically suture-line hemorrhage that needs **reexploration** (Chapter 13). If this happens at a time distant from surgery, correction of coagulopathies and observation may often be sufficient. In the early postoperative period, **endoscopic** approaches to the upper gastrointestinal bleed should be approached with extreme caution, as should **angiographic embolization**.

Wound Infection

The obese patient has a propensity to **wound infection**. There is no clear understanding of this, but the large space of poorly perfused tissue in the wound, combined with the immunologic changes of obesity and major surgery, certainly plays a role. The rate of wound complications including seromas approaches 40% in some reports. The incidence of serious wound infection is much less, in the range of 5%. The development of laparoscopic surgery has lessened this problem considerably. Seromas should be drained if possible. Should a wound become infected, **simple drainage** is usually adequate, with **antibiotic therapy** to be reserved for those who are systemically symptomatic.

Stricture and Fistula

The rate of **stricture formation** at the gastrojejunal anastomosis of a gastric bypass has been reported to be as high as 20%. Symptoms of stricture formation are the gradual development of **food intolerance**, with severe strictures limiting the ability of the patient to drink fluids, leading to dehydration. Most strictures form from 4 to 8 weeks postoperatively. Strictures can usually be treated by endoscopy and balloon dilation, although several dilations may be necessary. If a stricture forms at a point beyond 1 year after a gastric bypass, biopsy is recommended, as this may indicate the development of a malignancy.

A **gastrogastric fistula** may occur. If the gastric pouch is created by applying multiple rows of staples to the stomach without dividing the stomach (a partitioned stomach), the rate of this can be as high as 9%. If the stomach is physically divided, as in most laparoscopic cases, this incidence decreases but may still occur at a rate of approximately 1%, probably as a result of a local infection or an unrecognized leak. Chronic overeating will allow the small pouch to distend and will allow the gastrojejunal anastomosis to dilate, resulting in a loss of early satiety, with **weight regain**. Therefore, it is important to remember that the pouch is not a tool to simply limit how much food the patient can eat, but rather a tool to allow the patient to reach satiety with a small amount of food.

Because of the decreased intake of food and the anatomic rearrangement from a gastric bypass and BPD/DS, the absorption of vitamins and minerals may be decreased. In particular, iron and B_{12} deficiency may be noted with a resulting **iron deficiency anemia**. Chronic nausea and vomiting can also lead to **thiamine deficiency**. Rapid weight loss can contribute to B_6 and folate deficiency. Reports of deficiencies include potassium, calcium, magnesium, phosphorus, copper, zinc, iodine, and vitamins A, C, D, E, K, B_1, B_2, and B_6. Vitamin supplements are a part of a standard protocol, but close monitoring of the patient for a lifetime is required, as reports have noted occasional deficiencies in those patients following accepted replacement protocols. The malabsorptive procedures can result in protein calorie malnutrition, thus mandating careful lifelong monitoring.

Hernia and Mechanical Complications

The gastric bypass and the BPD/DS patients may develop **internal hernias**. Several potential hernia defects are created suturing the operative procedure, and these are closed as part of the procedure. In spite of this, 5%–10% of patients may develop hernias over the course of their lifetime. These may present as pain out of proportion to physical examination, which should warrant urgent exploration to free strangulated, ischemic bowel. The patient may present with vomiting and pain of an acute-onset, or an insidious, nagging pain that may occur after meals, mimicking the pain of biliary colic. Three hernias are of note.

Herniation through the **transverse mesocolic defect** will usually cause an acute onset of vomiting with abdominal pain. A hernia through the **jejunojejunostomy defect** will often present similarly. These hernias may present as obstruction on a plain abdominal radiograph. CT scan may show the obstruction, but clinical suspicion coupled with the knowledge that some of these obstructions will not be present on radiographic studies would support exploration. Laparoscopic repair of these hernias may be possible if treated early. **Peterson's defect**, the space created by passing the small bowel in front of or behind the colon to the stomach, often presents with more subtle symptoms. This can be very hard to diagnose on radiographs, and laparoscopic investigation is often the only way to diagnose this hernia. This hernia presents with cramping postprandial pain and is much more frequent in the laparoscopic population than the open cases.

Ventral incisional hernias occur in open bariatric procedures at an increased rate over the nonobese population. The increased rate of wound infection and the weight of the abdominal pannus pulling on the abdominal wall contribute to this. Consider repair if the hernia is significantly symptomatic, but, if asymptomatic, consider elective repair when maximum weight loss has been achieved. The advent of laparoscopic surgical approaches to the bariatric patient has lessened the rate of hernias markedly, but hernias at **trochar sites** occur in approximately 1% of patients.

The laparoscopy-adjustable gastric band is a soft band that is placed around the top of the stomach. **Dysphagia** immediately postoperative is usually caused by acute outlet obstruction, often caused by a large perigastric fat pad. This can often be treated by laparoscopic revision. The risk of injury to the stomach or distal esophagus is present during the placement of the band, although this risk is exceedingly small. However, the clinical suspicion of this would warrant a workup, possibly even exploration. The band has several unique late complications. The first of these is **band erosion**. This is seen in approximately 2%–3% of cases. The band can be seen endoscopically to have eroded into the stomach.

This presents as bleeding or pain. This can usually be treated by band removal, with weight regain unless the band is converted into a gastric bypass. The distal stomach can **herniate** through the band, causing an acute onset of dysphagia and vomiting consistent with obstruction. The stomach is secured over the band during band placement, in an attempt to avoid both herniation and rotation of the band, which may cause erosion. The herniated stomach may be reduced laparoscopically and secured, or removal of the band may be necessary. The band requires **adjustment** to maintain the sensation of early satiety. This requires an access site to the band, which is a port placed on the anterior abdominal wall. This port can leak or become infected, necessitating repair. If the band is adjusted too tightly, the patient will experience dysphagia, owing to obstruction. If, however, the band is a little less tight and the patient chronically overeats, the distal esophagus may dilate. This is treated by deflation of the band to allow this to resolve, with careful reinflation of the band and patient education at a later date.

Occasionally, gastric bypass patients will develop epigastric pain, and a **marginal ulcer** will be found. This is at the gastrojejunal anastomosis, usually on the side of the jejunum. These may also cause bleeding. Treatment is with proton pump inhibitors. If symptoms persist, surgical revision of the anastomosis and creation of a small pouch with repair of any fistulas will be required.

Selected Readings

Buchwald H. Overview of bariatric surgery. *J Am Coll Surg.* 2002;194(3):367–375.

Buchwald H, Avidor Y, Braunwald E, et al. Bariatric surgery: A systematic review and meta-analysis. *JAMA.* 2004;292(14):1724–1737.

Brolin RE. Bariatric surgery and long-term control of morbid obesity. *JAMA.* 2002;288(22):2793–2796.

Martin L.*Obesity Surgery.* New York: McGraw-Hill; 2004.

Hydock CM. A brief overview of bariatric surgical procedures currently being used to treat the obese patients. *Crit Care Nurse* Q. 2005;28(3):217–226.

26

Soft-Tissue Lesions

Joanna C. Ellis, MSN, CRNP-BC ■ *Mary Kate FitzPatrick, RN, MSN, CRNP* ■ *Benjamin Braslow, MD*

Key Points

■ As the largest organ in the body, the skin is responsible for several very important functions, including temperature regulation, fluid balance, and soft-tissue protection.

■ Rash is a generic term used to describe any skin lesion that affects color or texture in the skin, typically acute in nature.

■ Cellulitis is an acute bacterial infection to the skin, subcutaneous tissue, and, in some cases, superficial fascia.

■ Have a high degree of suspicion for masses on the extremities that grow quickly, are greater than 5 cm, or appear fixed to surrounding tissue.

■ Always consider the possible need for a wide resection of a soft-tissue mass and plan the biopsy incision accordingly.

■ HISTORY

Most skin lesions are able to be visualized by the patient or clinician. Since skin lesions can often be a manifestation of systemic disease, a complete medical history is sought on all patients. A **history of the present illness** is elicited by using the mnemonic OLD CART—onset, location, duration, characteristics, associated symptoms, relieving agents, and treatments already tried. Probe the **past medical history** for evidence of systemic diseases that have cutaneous involvement. **Diabetes** can put patients at risk of various skin infections. Several **immune disorders** such as allergies and autoimmune disease can cause certain rashes. **Cellulitis** typically occurs when the protective barrier of the skin is compromised, allowing bacteria to enter, usually from an operative or traumatic wound and burns. Review current and recent **medications** that could be responsible for drug reactions involving the skin, such as antibiotics. Explore the use of **illicit drugs** that could be responsible for skin infections from needle sticks of cutaneous manifestations of endocarditis. Review recent **exposure** and **travel** history. Both of these situations can introduce new allergens to the patient, causing immune and infectious skin problems.

■ PHYSICAL EXAMINATION

Evaluation should begin with a thorough inspection of all skin surfaces. Identify and characterize the **primary skin lesions** using the appropriate terminology. Flat lesions are identified by a skin color change. A **macule** is a nonpalpable color change in the skin. This should be differentiated from a **wheal**, which is a slightly raised area of tense edema in the dermis. Raised lesions are distinguished by their character. A **papule** is solid with distinct borders, no more than 1 cm in diameter, whereas a **nodule** connotes a larger lesion more like a mass. **Vesicles** and **pustules** are similar in that they are small (<1 cm). However, the former is filled with clear fluid, the latter with pus. A **plaque** is a solid flat lesion with distinct borders and epidermal changes greater than 1 cm in diameter. Larger mass lesions include a **cyst,** which is a palpable sac filled with liquid or solid material. A **bulla** is similar to a vesicle but is larger that 1 cm. Any solid, unidentified growth greater than 1 cm is often referred to as a "mass" until the diagnosis is made.

Identify **secondary skin** changes that can accompany the primary lesion. Progressive loss of epidermis causes characteristic changes in the skin. **Scaling** is a partial separation of the superficial layer of skin, resulting in the presence of thin white plates on the skin surface. **Erosions** are depressed lesion from loss of epidermis that results from rupture of vesicles or bullae. **Excoriation** is often self-induced by scratching with resulting redness and irritation at the site of inflammation or injury. Finally, an **ulcer** is a deep depression from loss of epidermis and part of the dermis.

Abnormal dryness or ongoing inflammation can cause **lichenification** or thickening of the skin with increased skin markings. **Crusting** occurs with healing and consists of dried exudates from skin surface. A **fissure** is the presence of linear wedge-shaped cracks, and **atrophy** is thinning of the skin with associated decrease in skin markings. Note the **appearance** of skin color in the lesion. Determine if the discoloration is blanchable. Note the **arrangement of the lesions as** discrete such as abscesses, linear such as in shingles, or annular like the target lesion in Lyme disease or grouped such as in furnuculosis. Note the **distribution** as generalized, acral (limited to hands), or localized.

If infection is suspected, such as cellulitis, visualize and palpate the affected area. Mark the affected area to assess the progression and severity of the infection. Skin over the area is typically warm, erythematous, edematous, and exquisitely tender to palpation. This is usually seen in the area immediately surrounding the assumed entry site for the bacteria. Borders are vague and ill defined. When palpating the area, assess for any **fluctuance** or bogginess that may indicate an associated abscess. The presence of lymphangitis or lymphadenitis, although rare, can be indicative of a more serious infection, and further workup is indicated.

■ LABORATORY STUDIES

Order a **CBC** to evaluate the white blood cell count. Eosinophilia is sometimes associated with allergic reactions and certain parasitic diseases. Consider a calcium and **parathyroid hormone** level only in patients suspected of having calciphylaxis. Consider a **coagulation** workup (PT, PTT, DIC panel, and a bleeding time) if the lesions are suspected to be related to bleeding, such as purpura with thrombocytopenia or ecchymosis associated with a high prothrombin time. Obtain **wound cultures** in patients presenting with severe infection. Order **blood cultures** if an underlying bacteremia is suspected.

Selectively obtain a **skin biopsy** to diagnose a persistent dermatitis, palpable purpura, skin tumor, or blister that was not already diagnosed by clinical appearance and presentation. Also, consider **fungal scraping** to diagnose a dermatophyte or fungal infection.

■ RADIOGRAPHIC STUDIES

In patients with an infectious process, obtain **plain films** of the affected area to identify possible gas in the soft tissue or a retained foreign body as the causative agent. In soft-tissue infections, consider **CT scan** or **MRI** to determine the presence of a fluid collection and/or abscess and degree of tissue involvement. It can also help to identify the presence of metastatic disease from cutaneous cancer. Occasionally, **ultrasound** may also help to determine the presence of an underlying fluid collection.

■ DIFFERENTIAL DIAGNOSIS AND TREATMENTS

Traumatic Wounds

The skin can be broken by different mechanisms, and the way the skin is torn affects the type of repair. An **incision wound** is made by a cutting object like a knife. The edges are often clean and straight, making repair fairly easy with simple suture techniques. A **laceration** is a tear in the skin caused by a blunt force that makes the skin seperate in a jagged pattern. Repair often requires debridement of the edges and complex repair (Figure 26-1). Other types of

SUTURING TECHNIQUES

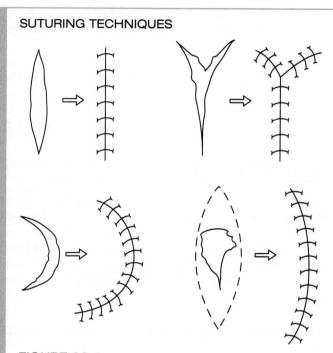

FIGURE 26-1
Suture Repair for Different Types of Wounds

Many institutions stock prepackaged laceration trays, which contain the necessary equipment for laceration repair. Often, however, the appropriate suture material must be selected from a separate suture cart.

One percent lidocaine is an appropriate local anesthetic for most lacerations repairs. The addition of epinephrine to the anesthetic causes localized vasoconstriction, which prevents systemic absorption of the anesthetic agent, which extends the duration of action, reduces the bleeding, and increases the amount of anesthetic that can be used. However, solutions containing epinephrine should be avoided in areas with only a single blood supply: nose, pinna of the ear, penis, fingers, and toes. Bupivacaine (0.25%) can be added in situations requiring extended postprocedure analgesia (up to 6 hours). Its longer time to onset and lower maximum dose lend it more to a supplemental role.

For percutaneous stitches, nonabsorbable monofilament nylon or polypropylene suture material is the standard. Sizes 3-0, 4-0, or 5-0 should be used on the torso and extremities (including hands and feet), choosing the larger suture size (3-0) for wounds subject to higher static or dynamic skin tension. Size 6-0 is often utilized for facial lacerations to minimize scaring. In hair-bearing areas, choose a suture of different color than the hair to facilitate suture removal at the appropriate time. Absorbable sutures (i.e., vicryl) are intended for subcutaneous placement in deep lacerations, which often require multiple layer repairs to obliterate dead space and disperse tension. Reverse-cutting needles are preferred, and the needle should be large enough to pass through the required depth and width of the tissue without difficulty.

Prep the skin around the laceration with a skin-cleansing agent. Anesthetize the tissues adjacent to the laceration using the preferred local anesthetic and a 25-gauge needle. Once the anesthetic has taken effect, the wound should be copiously irrigated with normal saline solution. Irrigate the wound until it is visibly clean. Sharply debride devitalized tissue before beginning laceration repair.

The wound should be kept covered and dry for the first 24 hours as re-epithelialization proceeds. Subsequently, the patient should be encouraged to wash the wound gently with soap and water. Showering is OK after 24 hours, but bathing should be discouraged for several days, as prolonged immersion in water should be minimized. Prophylactic antibiotics are not needed for simple clean lacerations; however, they should be considered for patients with grossly contaminated wounds, crush injuries, tendon injuries, and bite wounds or for immuno-compromised patients.

Assess the patient's tetanus-immunization status. Administer tetanus prophylaxis if the last dose was given more than 10 years earlier, more than 5 years for heavily contaminated or extensive tissue damage. Tetanus immune globulin should be given to patients with grossly contaminated or extensive wounds, if no previous tetanus prophylaxis has been given.

The timing of suture removal depends largely on the location of the wound. Facial sutures should be removed within 5 days to prevent scarring. Sutures placed in the scalp, torso, or extremities should stay in for 7–10 days. Sutures exposed to significant intermittent tension, such as those overlying joints, should be removed in 10–14 days.

wounds include penetrating and perforating, with the latter defined as a penetrating wound that exists out a separate side leaving a through and through wound. Typically these wounds are left open and not repaired as they are classified as contaminated.

Cellulitis

Acute bacterial infection of the skin, subcutaneous tissue, and, in some cases, superficial fascia are associated with pain, erythema, and edema in the involved skin with nonspecific borders. The most commonly isolated **organisms** to cause cellulitis are group A β-hemolytic streptococci, and *Staphylococcus aureus*. Cellulitis caused by gram negatives is typically seen in patients who are immunosuppressed or are granulocytopenic. Other atypical organisms include those found in fresh or salt water (*Aeromonas hydrophila/Vibrio vulnificus*). They can cause severe cellulitis, which can lead to rapid decompensation and death. Typically, classic cellulitis is associated with **pain**, **erythema**, and **edema** in the involved skin with nonspecific borders. Depending on its severity and progression, systemic symptoms may also be present, including fever, malaise, and rigors. In extreme cases, such as a cellulitis that has been left untreated or a rapidly progressive cellulitis, sepsis and septic shock can occur, requiring intensive-care management.

Treatment includes **antibiotic therapy** with penicillins and first-generation cephalosporins. The emergence of community-acquired methicillin-resistant *S. aureus* (ca-MRSA) often necessitates alternative therapy. Bactrim, doxycycline, clindamycin, linezolid, and vancomycin have all proven effective against ca-MRSA. Consider **hospital admission** and the use of parenteral antibiotics in patients who present with systemic symptoms, are hemodynamically unstable, or have already failed an appropriate oral regimen. Special consideration should also be given to those who have comorbid conditions that may place them at increased risk or those who are already immunocompromised. **Blood** and **wound** cultures and sensitivities are obtained upon admission to the hospital, to help with the choice of antibiotic.

Adverse Cutaneous Drug Reaction

Hypersensitivity reaction to any topical or systemically administered drug can mimic any dermatologic manifestation and, therefore, should be considered as a differential diagnosis for any spontaneous skin eruption. Assessment of adverse cutaneous drug reaction (ACDR) includes physical examination and ruling out all other possible causes. Note the **time interval** between drug administration and onset of symptoms. Look for clinical improvement after withdrawal of medication. **Reaction** can vary in severity from minor to life threatening. Most reactions are mild with pruritis and will resolve once the offending drug is discontinued. However, severe life-threatening reactions can occur and be unpredictable, requiring critical care management. The most common form is an **exanthematous** reaction typically presenting <14 days after administration of drug. A **fixed drug reaction** is an ACDR that occurs after ingestion of a drug. It presents as a solitary (or multiple) erythematous patch, plaque, bulla, or erosion. If rechallenged, the patient will present with the same lesion in the same location within hours of reingestion.

Uticaria and **angioedema** will occur within 36 hours of initial administration and within minutes after rechallenge. Typically present with transient **wheals** and large areas of edema, which involve both the dermis and the subcutaneous tissue. **Anaphylaxis** is the most serious of the ACDRs and can occur within minutes to hours of administration of the drug. It manifests as a respiratory distress, vascular collapse, and/or shock. Serum sickness occurs within 5–21 days after initial administration and is classified as minor or major (complete). The **minor form** presents with fever, uticaria, and arthralgia. The **major form** (complete) presents with fever, uticaria, angioedema, arthralgia, arthritis, lymphadenopathy, eosinophilia, nephritis, and/or endocarditis. Treatment of choice for any drug reaction is the **discontinuation** of the offending agent, use of **antihistamines,** and symptom management. Again, in extreme cases, intensive care management may be necessary.

Dermatitis and Eczema

These represent inflammatory responses to a stimulus in the superficial dermis and epidermis, with resulting skin surface disruption. Typically, the primary lesions include papules, erythematous macules, and vesicles, which can coalesce to form patches and plaques. **Atopic dermatitis** is a chronic superficial inflammation of the skin. The diagnostic criteria are based on clinical findings of pruritic, exudative, or lichenified eruption on face, neck, trunk, wrists, and hands and in the antecubital and popliteal folds. It is characterized by chronic recurrences and is often associated with a family history of allergic manifestations. Fifty percent of individuals with this diagnosis will have respiratory manifestations such as asthma or allergic rhinitis. Treatment is largely directed toward prevention, reducing inflammatory response and symptom management. Short-term use of topical steroids and oral antibiotics for acute flare-ups can be used. Other management includes avoidance of aggravating factors, keeping the skin well hydrated, avoiding overheating, and the use of drying agents.

Contact dermatitis is an acute inflammatory response in the skin caused by a direct contact from substances that may directly or indirectly injure the skin. It is further distinguished between primary **irritant contact dermatitis (ICD)** and **allergic contact dermatitis (ACD)**. The response seen in ICD is due to the characteristics of the substance that is in contact with the skin, whereas ACD is due to an antigen-specific immune response to the agent. Presentation for both ICD and ACD can be acute or chronic, depending on the length and intensity of exposure. ICD lesions are strictly demarcated to exposed areas and to areas that were occluded with the irritant. This usually affects areas with very thin skin.

Lesions in ICD and ACD can range from minimal erythema to edema, vesicles, and ulceration with oozing and crusting. Treatment is directed toward **prevention** and symptom management. Patients should eliminate, avoid, or protect them from causative agents. In severe dermatitis, short course of topical steroids will aid to clear up the dermatitis and provide some relief.

Necrotizing Fasciitis

A true surgical emergency, necrotizing fasciitis, is an aggressive, fast-spreading, infection within deep fascia. It causes secondary necrosis of subcutaneous tissue and is often characterized by a presence of gas-forming organisms within subcutaneous tissue. It most commonly occurs after trauma or recent surgical procedures because of localized tissue injury and the invasion of bacteria. Patients who have multiple comorbid disease or those who are immunosuppressed have a greater risk of developing necrotizing infections.

Physical examination findings include pain that may be present in the general area but not necessarily at the site of injury and may be disproportionate to injury. Symptoms such as diarrhea, nausea, fever, confusion, dizziness, weakness, and general malaise are typically seen. The hallmark finding is an area of **erythema** that **rapidly spreads** over a course of hours to days. Advanced symptoms occur within hours to days. The affected area begins to swell, and a dusky, purplish rash may be exhibited. In the critical stage, the patient begins to exhibit signs of shock secondary to the toxins the bacteria emit. Hypotension occurs, and unconsciousness may result as the body becomes too weak to fight infection without treatment. Have a **high index of suspicion** for this disease, since physical examination findings can be unimpressive.

The gold standard in confirming the presence of necrotizing fasciitis is **operative exploration**. Radiographic studies should not delay surgical diagnosis and debridement but may be helpful in determining the extent of the disease. Consider a plain film of the affected area to determine the presence of foreign bodies and reveal gas in the subcutaneous fascia. Consider **CR scan** or **MRI** to identify the anatomic site of involvement by demonstrating necrosis with asymmetric fascial thickening and gas formation.

Early **surgical consultation** and rapid surgical **debridement** is the key to survival. General anesthesia is needed to facilitate complete exploration and debridement. The patient should return to the OR frequently until all necrotic tissue is removed. Appropriate **antibiotic coverage** is essential. The drug of choice in treating streptococci infections is penicillin G, with clindamycin to prevent toxin formation. Adequate treatment must include coverage for aerobic and anaerobic bacteria, as these are typically polymicrobial infections. An infectious disease specialist may be useful in determining initial empiric antibiotic therapy. Hyperbaric oxygen therapy (HBO) can be considered as an adjunct to surgical debridement and antibiotic therapy (Figure 15-1).

Soft-Tissue Mass

Basal Cell Carcinoma

It is the most common malignant cutaneous neoplasm. Commonly it is found on the face (Figure 26-2). It occurs in several clinical forms: nodular, pigmented, cystic, sclerosing, and superficial. Most common appearance of basal cell cancer is small, dome-shaped bump that has a pearly white color. It does not normally metastasize or travel in the blood stream.

Normal evaluation includes a physical examination, and, if suspicious, a biopsy is performed. This involves local anesthesia followed by a "punch" (cookie cutter type) biopsy. If biopsy reveals basal cell carcinoma, the dermatologist may utilize one of several techniques. **Electrodessication and curettage** involves removing the bulk of the mass with cautery of the base skin. Alternatively, a simple **surgical excision** is performed by a surgeon or dermatologist.

Squamous Cell Carcinoma

It is a malignant tumor that arises in the epithelium. It is most commonly found in sun-exposed areas like the back of the hands, scalp, lower lip, and ears (Figure 26-2). The lesions are soft, mobile, and elevated masses with a surface scale. The base of the lesion may be inflamed, and these cancers are generally locally destructive. If left untreated, squamous cell carcinoma can destroy much of the tissue surrounding the tumor. Make the diagnosis by skin biopsy. Most treatments are office-based procedures utilizing local anesthesia. Surgical excision to remove the entire cancer is the most commonly utilized option. "Mohs," micrographic surgery, can be used to remove the whole tumor, while sparing as much normal skin as possible. Larger masses will require more extensive surgery in the operating room with general anesthesia.

Malignant Melanoma

It is a skin cancer that develops from melanocytes (Figure 26-2). These cells migrate into the skin, eye, central nervous systems, and mucous membranes. The characteristics are best remembered by utilizing the mnemonic ABCD: asymmetry of the lesion, borders are irregular, color is blue/black or variegated, and the diameter >6 mm. Suspicious lesions are removed by performing an **excisional biopsy** (Chapter 18). There is no role for shave or incisional biopsies, since these will fail to make the diagnosis histologically and have the potential to seed cancer away from the primary lesion.

COMMON SKIN CANCERS

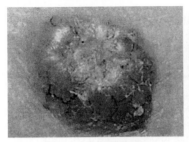

Basal cell carcinoma

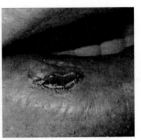

Squamous cell carcinoma

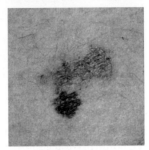

Melanoma

FIGURE 26-2
Images of Common Skin Cancers

Soft-Tissue Sarcoma

These are rare tumors most often found on the extremities. Any palpable mass that is new, enlarging, or larger than 5 cm should be considered a soft-tissue malignancy, until proven otherwise. Biopsy is performed with a **Tru-Cut** needle or by an **open excision**. There is no role for fine needle aspiration, since the histological diagnosis requires examination of the cellular ultrastructure, which is lost on FNA. Take care to perform the incisional biopsy, with consideration for the need of possible wide excisional surgery if the biopsy is positive (Figure 26-3). The most common **tumor types** are liposarcoma, malignant fibrous histiocytoma, and leisomyosarcoma. Offer limb-sparing, wide resection with postoperative radiation as the treatment of choice for most extremity sarcomas. Chemotherapy has not been shown to be effective. The most common form of treatment failure is local recurrence, which often is amendable to re-resection.

Fungal Infection

Dermatophytes are fungi that invade the outer layer of the epidermis, hair, and nails. Toxins released by the dermatophytes initiate the inflammatory response. It is known by various names, depending on the part of body affected, such

THE SOFT TISSUE BIOPSY

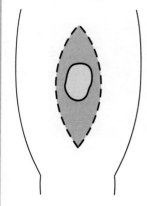

FIGURE 26-3
The Proper Orientation of a Planned Biopsy of a Lesion on the Thigh

Care must be taken when planning a soft-tissue biopsy of a mass. In most cases, an excisional biopsy is warranted, where the entire lesion is removed with an amount of normal tissue around the edges (margin). When there is concern that the lesion may be a sarcoma or melanoma, attempt to get at least a 5 cm margin in all directions, including deep into the soft tissue. Use an incision that is in the proper position if a larger resection is needed in the future. For example on the thigh, orient the elliptical incision vertically so that a second wide excision is possible.

as "jock itch," athlete's foot, or "diaper rash." These infections typically present as circular erythematous patches with a clear center. Specific characteristics of the patches will vary, based on the responsible dermatophyte. Diagnosis is often made by inspection; however, confirmation can be made by a positive potassium hydroxide (KOH) examination of the scaly border of the lesion. Cultures are reserved for a persistent infection that has not responded to conventional therapy. Treatment includes topical antifungal creams, which are the treatment of choice. Treatment should extend 2 weeks beyond clinical resolution to ensure complete eradication of the causative fungus. Use of oral or systemic antifungals are reserved for extensive or resistant infections.

Selected Readings

Stevens DL. Infections of the skin, muscle and soft tissues. In: *Harrison's Principles of Internal Medicine*. 16th ed. McGraw-Hill; 2005.

Folstad SG. Soft tissue infections. In: *Tintinalli's Emergency Medicine*. 6th ed. McGraw-Hill; 2004.

A

List of Procedures

Chapter 3

Spinal and epidural analgesia

Chapter 4

Thoracostomy
Thoracostomy removal
Nasoenteric Intubation
Surgical drain removal

Chapter 5

Interpretation of the arterial blood gas
Interpretation of the chest radiograph
Needle thoracostomy and thoracentesis
Rapid sequence intubation (RSI)

Chapter 6

Central venous access
Pulmonary artery catheterization
Interpretation of the pulmonary artery catheter waveform

Chapter 7

Continuous renal replacement therapy (CRRT)

Chapter 9

The surviving sepsis campaign

Chapter 10

Appendectomy
Laparoscopic cholecystectomy

Chapter 17

Craniotomy with clipping of intracranial aneurysm
Cerebral angiogram and endovascular embolization
Carotid endarterectomy

Chapter 18

Thyroid resection
Radical neck dissection
Modified radical mastectomy
Whipple procedure
Liver resections

Chapter 19

Perirectal abscess drainage
Surgery for hemorrhoid disease
Lateral internal sphincterotomy

Chapter 20

Total abdominal hysterectomy

Chapter 21

Diagnostic laparoscopy

Chapter 22

Lumbar laminectomy
Anterior decompression cervical fusion (ADCF)

Chapter 23

Insertion of a bladder catheter

Chapter 25

Gastric band
Gastric bypass
The biliary diversion procedure

Chapter 26

Common techniques for laceration repair
Soft tissue biopsy

Index

Page numbers followed by "t" denote tables; those followed by "f" denote figures.